FOURTH EDITION

Guide to Evidence-Based Physical Therapist Practice

Dianne V. Jewell, PT, DPT, PhD, FAACVPR
The Rehab Intel Network
Ruther Glen, Virginia

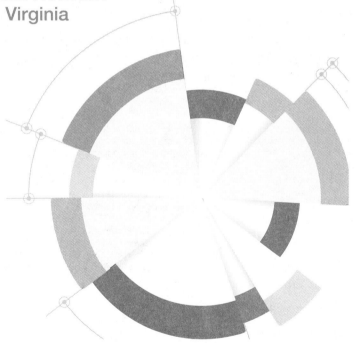

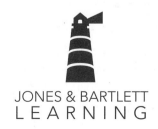

JONES & BARTLETT
LEARNING

World Headquarters
Jones & Bartlett Learning
5 Wall Street
Burlington, MA 01803
978-443-5000
info@jblearning.com
www.jblearning.com

Jones & Bartlett Learning books and products are available through most bookstores and online booksellers. To contact Jones & Bartlett Learning directly, call 800-832-0034, fax 978-443-8000, or visit our website, www.jblearning.com.

Production Credits
VP, Executive Publisher: David D. Cella
Publisher: Cathy L. Esperti
Acquisitions Editor: Sean Fabery
Associate Editor: Taylor Maurice
Senior Vendor Manager: Sara Kelly
VP, Manufacturing and Inventory Control: Therese Connell
Product Fulfillment Manager: Wendy Kilborn

Composition and Project Management: S4Carlisle Publishing Services
Cover Design: Kristin E. Parker
Rights & Media Specialist: Merideth Tumasz
Media Development Editor: Troy Liston
Cover Image: © LFor/Shutterstock
Printing and Binding: Edwards Brothers Malloy
Cover Printing: Edwards Brothers Malloy

To order this product, use ISBN: 9781284104325

Library of Congress Cataloging-in-Publication Data
Names: Jewell, Dianne V., author.
  Title: Guide to evidence-based physical therapist practice / Dianne V. Jewell.
  Description: Fourth edition. | Burlington, MA : Jones & Bartlett Learning,
    [2018] | Includes bibliographical references and index.
  Identifiers: LCCN 2017013147 | ISBN 9781284130836 (pbk.)
  Subjects: | MESH: Physical Therapy Modalities | Evidence-Based
    Practice—methods
  Classification: LCC RM700 | NLM WB 460 | DDC 615.8/2—dc23 LC record available at https://lccn.loc.gov/2017013147

6048
Printed in the United States of America
21 20 19 18 17   10 9 8 7 6 5 4 3 2 1

To my physical therapist colleagues at
Sheltering Arms Physical Rehabilitation Centers,
Richmond, VA. Your quest for excellence in the art
and science of what we do and your dedication to
our mission inspire me to do better every day.

CONTENTS

PREFACE

Guide to Evidence-Based Physical Therapist Practice, Fourth Edition provides foundational groundwork in research methods and teaches physical therapist students and clinicians alike how to integrate evidence in clinical practice. Its goal is to make the evidence-based physical therapist practice (EBPT) process accessible and relevant to nonresearchers who need to *apply* research as well as conduct it.

Consistent with prior versions, the patient/client management model described in the American Physical Therapy Association's *Guide to Physical Therapist Practice 3.0* remains the framework for discussion. The definitions and labels used to describe the evidence-based practice approach to patient care are consistent with the World Health Organization's *International Classification of Functioning, Disability and Health*. A new clinical scenario introducing each chapter provides the context for use of evidence in practice in conjunction with the physical therapist's clinical judgment and the patient's or client's preferences, values, and goals. Updated citations provide current examples throughout the book of the various forms of evidence available to students and practitioners.

Organization of the *Fourth Edition*

The organization and goals of the sections are described here. Every effort has been made to have a structure that promotes ease-of-use for the physical therapist student and practicing clinician.

Part I: Principles of Evidence-Based Physical Therapist Practice

Part I comprises three chapters that set the stage for the use of evidence in patient/client management. Tools and resources from organizations and individual authors recognized as leaders in the evidence-based practice movement are adapted or referenced in the context of physical therapist practice.

Part II: Elements of Evidence

The first five chapters of Part II describe the different components of a research article with an emphasis on the features that enhance or diminish a study's quality. The goal of these chapters is unchanged. They are intended to increase readers' understanding of and confidence with the evidence they review, not to train new researchers. The remaining chapters review statistical methods relevant to physical therapist practice and their application in different research designs.

Part III: Appraising the Evidence

The underlying principle remains; evidence-based physical therapist practice requires students and clinicians to work with the best available evidence that, often times, is weakly designed. The chapters in this section assist readers in determining for themselves whether the evidence they locate is useful *despite* its limitations.

Part IV: Evidence in Practice

Part IV continues its focus on the application of evidence in the context of patient/client management. A fundamental tenet of this book is that evidence must be considered with respect to the individual patient or client.

Updates to the *Fourth Edition*

As previously mentioned, a new Clinical Scenario feature has been included at the beginning of each chapter which provides context for the use of evidence in practice. Additionally, key updates to select chapters are listed below. My hope is that these updates serve readers in their quest to engage effectively in evidence-based physical therapist practice.

- *Chapter 1 Evidence-Based Physical Therapist Practice.* The physical therapist patient/client management model and related terminology have been updated to reflect the changes included in the American Physical Therapy Association's *Guide to Physical Therapist Practice 3.0.*
- *Chapter 2 What is Evidence?* Hierarchies of evidence have been expanded to include application of a model for pre-appraised evidence as well as a proposed model for use with qualitative research designs.
- *Chapter 3 The Quest for Evidence: Getting Started.* An adaptation of the "Problem, Intervention, Comparison, Outcome" (PICO) method for developing answerable clinical questions has been added. Updated features and functionality of the most commonly used electronic search engines have been included. The American Physical Therapy Association's PTNow web portal has been added in place of the discontinued Hooked on Evidence portal. New to this edition are descriptions of the Turning Research into Practice (TRIP) database and the National Guideline Clearinghouse database.
- *Chapter 17 Appraising Collections of Evidence: Systematic Reviews* and *Chapter 18 Appraising Collections of Evidence: Clinical Practice Guidelines.* This content, originally combined into one chapter, has been split into separate chapters to facilitate better understanding of the material and to allow for expansion of content regarding clinical practice guidelines.
- *Chapter 19 Appraising Qualitative Research Studies.* This is a new chapter that provides guidance regarding the quality assessment of evidence that is developed from the words that subjects and researchers use to describe experiences, perceptions, perspectives, and observations.
- *Chapter 20 Patient or Client Preferences and Values.* This chapter has been renumbered to reflect the changes in Chapters 17, 18, and 19.
- *Chapter 21 Putting It All Together.* This chapter has also been renumbered. A new scenario illustrating the search for, appraisal, and application of a qualitative research study has been added.

Resources for the Instructor

In addition to the updates described, *Guide to Evidence-Based Physical Therapist Practice, Fourth Edition* includes a comprehensive suite of instructor resources. These resources are provided so instructors can effectively map and incorporate the book into their course.

- Test Bank
- Slides in PowerPoint format
- Instructor Manual (*New to this edition!*)
- Sample Syllabus
- Image Bank

Resources for the Student

In the hopes of supplying students with all the tools they need to practice and apply the material in the book, each new copy of the *Fourth Edition* comes with access to the Navigate Student Companion Website. Resources on the Companion Website include:

- Practice Quizzes
- Flashcards
- Interactive Glossary
- Web Links
- Crossword Puzzles

ACKNOWLEDGMENTS

Special thanks for this *Fourth Edition* go to Jones & Bartlett Learning team members Sean Fabery for clearing the path whenever creative boulders appeared to block the way forward, and Taylor Maurice for her persistence in taking on the unenviable role of keeping me on task and on time! Thanks also to Escaline Charlette Aarthi for wrangling the overwhelming number of minute editorial details into submission.

REVIEWERS

Mary Ann Holbein-Jenny, PT, PhD, DPT
Professor
Graduate School of Physical Therapy
College of Health, Environment, and Science
Slippery Rock University
Slippery Rock, PA

John J. Jeziorowski, PT, PhD
Associate Professor
School of Health Sciences
Cleveland State University
Cleveland, OH

Neeraj Kumar, PT, PhD
Regional Dean and Assistant Program Director
School of Allied Health Sciences
Texas Tech University Health Sciences Center
Odessa, TX

Genevieve Pinto Zipp, PT, EdD
Professor
Department of Interprofessional Health Sciences & Health Administration
Director
Center for Interprofessional Education in Health Sciences
Seton Hall University
South Orange, NJ

PRINCIPLES OF EVIDENCE-BASED PHYSICAL THERAPIST PRACTICE

CHAPTER 1

EVIDENCE-BASED PHYSICAL THERAPIST PRACTICE

OBJECTIVES

Upon completion of this chapter, the student/practitioner will be able to do the following:

1. Discuss the circumstances that have resulted in an emphasis on the use of evidence in practice.
2. Distinguish among definitions of evidence-based medicine, evidence-based practice, and evidence-based physical therapist (EBPT) practice.
3. Discuss the use of evidence in physical therapist decision making in the context of the American Physical Therapy Association's *Guide to Physical Therapist Practice 3.0*.[1]
4. Describe focus areas of EBPT practice.
5. Describe the general steps involved in EBPT practice.
6. Discuss the barriers to EBPT practice and possible strategies for reducing them.

TERMS IN THIS CHAPTER

Activity limitations (ICF model): "Difficulties an individual may have in executing activities."[2]

Biologic plausibility: The reasonable expectation that the human body could behave in the manner predicted.

Clinical expertise: Proficiency of clinical skills and abilities, informed by continually expanding knowledge, that individual clinicians develop through experience, learning, and reflection about their practice.[3,4]

Diagnosis: A process of "integrating and evaluating the data that are obtained during the examination to describe the individual condition in terms that will guide the physical therapist in determining the prognosis and developing a plan of care."[1]

Evaluation: The "process by which physical therapists
- interpret the individual's response to tests and measures;
- integrate the test and measure data with other information collected in the history;
- determine a diagnosis or diagnoses amenable to physical therapist management;
- determine a prognosis, including goals for physical therapist management; and,
- develop a plan of care."[1]

Evidence: "A broad definition of evidence is any empirical observation, whether systematically collected or not. Clinical research evidence refers to the systematic observation of clinical events. . . ."[5]

Examination: "Physical therapists conduct a history, perform a systems review, and use tests and measures in order to describe and/or quantify an individual's need for services."[1]

Impairment (ICF model): "Problems in body functions or structure such as a significant deviation or loss."[2]

Intervention: "Physical therapists purposefully interact with the individual and, when appropriate, with other people involved in his or her care, using various" procedures or techniques "to produce changes in the condition."[1]

Outcome: "The actual results of implementing the plan of care that indicate the impact on functioning;" may be measured by the physical therapist or determined by self-report from the patient or client.[1]

Participation restrictions (ICF model): "Problems an individual may experience in involvement in life situations."[2]

Patient-centered care: Health care that "customizes treatment recommendations and decision making in response to patients' preferences and beliefs. . . . This partnership also is characterized by informed, shared decision making, development of patient knowledge, skills needed for self-management of illness, and preventive behaviors."[6(p.3)]

Prevention: "The avoidance, minimization, or delay of the onset of impairment, activity limitations, and/or participation restrictions."[1]

Prognosis: "The determination of the predicted optimal level of improvement in function and the amount of time needed to reach that level and also may include a prediction of levels of improvement that may be reached at various intervals during the course of therapy."[1]

Introduction

Use of systematically developed *evidence* in clinical decision making is promoted extensively across health care professions and practice settings. Gordon Guyatt, MD, David L. Sackett, MD, and their respective colleagues published the original, definitive works that instruct physicians in the use of clinical research evidence in medical practice.[5,7] In addition, federal agencies, including the Agency for Healthcare Research and Quality and the Centers for Medicare and Medicaid Services, evaluate the strength of published evidence during the development of clinical guidelines and health care policies.[8,9] Professional associations such as the American Medical Association, the American Heart Association, and the American Occupational Therapy Association also have developed resources to help their members and consumers access evidence regarding a wide variety of diseases, treatments, and outcomes.[10-12]

The physical therapy profession also has expressed a commitment to the development and use of published evidence. The American Physical Therapy Association envisioned that by 2020 physical therapists would be autonomous practitioners who, among other things, used evidence in practice.[13] Numerous articles regarding the methods for, benefits of, and barriers to evidence-based practice have been published in the journal *Physical Therapy*.[14-17] For several years, the journal also included a recurring feature, "Evidence in Practice," in which a patient case was described and the subsequent search for, evaluation, and application of evidence was illustrated.[18] The journal also added features such as "The Bottom Line" and podcasts in 2006 and 2008, respectively, to facilitate the translation of evidence into practice. Finally, the American Physical Therapy Association has created PTNow, a web-based portal designed to facilitate efficient access to the latest evidence related to physical therapist practice.[19]

The historical ground swell of interest in the use of evidence in health care resulted from the convergence of multiple issues, including (1) extensive documentation of apparently unexplained practice variation in the management of a variety of conditions, (2) the continued increase in health care costs disproportionate to inflation, (3) publicity surrounding medical errors, (4) identification of potential or actual harm resulting from previously approved medications, and (5) trends in technology assessment and outcomes research.[20-23] In addition, the rapid evolution of Internet technology increased both the dissemination of and access to health care research.

Related issues stimulated the drive for EBPT practice, the most dramatic of which was the use of evidence by commercial and government payers as a basis for their coverage decisions. For example, the Centers for Medicare and Medicaid Services ruled that insufficient scientific evidence existed to support the use of transcutaneous electrical stimulation for chronic low back pain and stated that patients must be enrolled in a clinical trial as a condition of coverage for this modality under the Part B benefit.[24] In light of these important developments, physical therapists needed an understanding of what evidence-based practice is, how it works, and how it may improve their clinical practice.

CLINICAL SCENARIO

Meet Your Patient

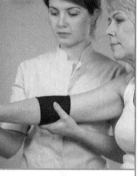

© Photographee.eu/Shutterstock

Anne is a 41-year-old, right-handed, high school chemistry teacher, and married mother of two boys aged 9 and 11. She presents to your outpatient physical therapy clinic with a 4-week history of progressively increasing pain that extends from her right elbow to midway down her lateral forearm. She denies previous injury to this upper extremity but notes that she spent several hours shoveling heavy wet snow from her front walk prior to the onset of her symptoms. Her pain makes it difficult for her to use a keyboard and mouse, grasp and manipulate pens and utensils, and maintain a grip on a full coffee mug or glass beaker. She also has discontinued her upper extremity strength training regimen and switched from an elliptical aerobic device to a recumbent cycle ergometer due to her symptoms.

She states that ice packs temporarily relieve her pain. She sought physical therapy because her primary care physician recommended anti-inflammatory medication and an orthopedic surgeon recommended a corticosteroid injection. She does not want to take medication in any form. She is anxious to resolve this problem as it interferes with her work and daily exercise program. Anne also has many questions about her options and any research available to prove or disprove their usefulness in her case.

How will you describe the role of evidence in your clinical decision making?

Evidence-Based What?

The use of evidence in health care is referred to by a variety of labels with essentially similar meanings. *Evidence-based medicine*, a term relevant to physicians, is defined as "the conscientious, explicit, and judicious use of current best evidence in making decisions about the care of individual patients. The practice of evidence-based medicine means integrating individual *clinical expertise* with the best available clinical evidence from systematic research."[3(p.71)]

"Evidence-based practice" and "evidence-based health care" are labels that have been created to link the behavior described by evidence-based medicine to other health care professionals. Hicks provided this expanded definition: "care that 'takes place when decisions that affect the care of patients are taken with due weight accorded to all valid, relevant information.'"[25(p.8)] In all cases, evidence does not replace clinical expertise; rather, evidence is used to inform more fully a decision-making process in which expertise provides one perspective to the clinical problem.

Regardless of the label, the implicit message is that the use of evidence in clinical decision making is a movement away from unquestioning reliance on knowledge gained from authority or tradition. Authority may be attributed to established experts in the field, as well as to revered teachers in professional training programs. Tradition may be thought of as practice habits expressed by the phrase "this is what I have always done for patients like this one." Habits may be instilled by eminent authority figures, but they also may be based on local or regional practice norms reinforced by their use in payment formulas ("usual and customary") and in legal proceedings ("local standard of care"). Practice habits also may be reinforced by errors in clinical reasoning related to various biases and the inadequacies of experience-based problem solving, such as those described in **Table 1-1**.[26]

TABLE 1-1	Examples of Biases and Heuristic Failures in Clinical Reasoning	
Type of Reasoning Error	**Nature of the Problem**	**Clinical Management Consequences**
Ascertainment Bias	Occurs when a clinician draws a conclusion based on previously held expectations of a particular outcome (e.g., a physical therapist determines that a woman is catastrophizing her back pain experience because she has expressed job dissatisfaction).	The physical therapist forgoes clinical examination procedures that would have identified joint restrictions in the woman's lumbar spine.
Confirmation Bias	Occurs when a clinician selectively focuses on information that confirms a hypothesis (e.g., a physical therapist remembers only those people with adhesive capsulitis of the shoulder who improved following application of ultrasound and forgets those people who did not improve with the same technique).	The physical therapist applies ultrasound to all people with adhesive capsulitis of the shoulder regardless of their response to the modality.

TABLE 1-1	Examples of Biases and Heuristic Failures in Clinical Reasoning (*Continued*)	
Type of Reasoning Error	**Nature of the Problem**	**Clinical Management Consequences**
Recency Effect	Occurs when a clinician believes that a particular patient presentation or response is a common phenomenon because it is easily remembered (e.g., a physical therapist believes that fibromyalgia is more common in men than in women because her last two patients with this diagnostic label were male).	The physical therapist classifies all men with generalized pain in the upper back as having fibromyalgia.
	OR	
	Occurs when a clinician believes that a particular patient presentation or response is an uncommon phenomenon because it is not easily remembered (e.g., a new graduate physical therapist does not remember how to differentiate among various sources of painful conditions that express themselves in dermatomal patterns).	The physical therapist mistakes pain due to herpes zoster for radicular pain due to vertebral joint restriction in a person with an idiopathic acute onset of symptoms.
Representativeness Exclusivity	Occurs when a clinician draws conclusions about patient presentation or response based only upon those people who return for scheduled treatment sessions (e.g., a physical therapist believes all people with Parkinson's disease benefit from a particular balance program based on experience with people who have completed an episode of treatment versus those who have not).	The physical therapist applies the balance program exactly the same way for all people with Parkinson's disease who are referred to him for management.
Value Bias	Occurs when the importance of an outcome in the eyes of the clinician distorts the likelihood of the outcome occurring (e.g., a physical therapist's concern about undiagnosed fractures in acute painful conditions outweighs the data about prevalence of fractures under specific situations).	The physical therapist forgoes application of validated clinical prediction rules and refers all people with acute painful conditions for radiographic testing.

Modified with permission from John Wiley and Sons. Croskerry P. Achieving quality in clinical decision making: Cognitive strategies and detection of bias. *Acad Emerg Med*. 2002;9(11):1184–1204.

Knowledge derived from authority and tradition often reflects an initial understanding of clinical phenomena from which diagnostic and treatment approaches are developed based on *biologic plausibility* and anecdotal experience. As such, this form of knowledge will continue to have a role as new clinical problems are encountered that require new solutions. The fundamental weakness in a clinician's dependence on this type of knowledge, however, is the potential for selection of ineffective, or even harmful, tests, measures, or interventions as a result of the lack of inquiry into their "true" effects. These cognitive and heuristic failures can lead to incomplete or incorrect conclusions about what is wrong with an individual patient and what is the most effective means for treating the problem.

Straus et al. offer as an example the use of hormone replacement therapy in women without a uterus or those who are postmenopausal.[27] Women in these situations were observed to have an increased risk of heart disease that, from a biologic perspective, appeared connected to the loss of estrogen and progestin. Replacing the lost hormones in an effort to reduce the risk of heart disease in these women made sense. The success of this treatment was confirmed further by observational studies and small randomized controlled trials.[28] However, the early termination in 2002 of a large hormone replacement therapy trial sponsored by the National Institutes of Health challenged the concept of protective effects from this intervention. The study's initial results indicated, among other things, that estrogen replacement did not protect postmenopausal women against cardiovascular disease as had been hypothesized. Moreover, long-term estrogen plus progestin therapy increased a woman's risk for the development of heart attacks, strokes, blood clots, and breast cancer.[22] In effect, years of clinical behavior based on a biologically plausible theory supported by lower quality evidence were invalidated by a well-designed piece of evidence. This example is extreme, but it makes the point that health care providers should willingly and knowingly reevaluate the assumptions that underlie a practice that is based on authority and tradition supported by limited evidence.

Evidence-Based Physical Therapist Practice

With that background in mind, this text has adopted the term *evidence-based physical therapist (EBPT) practice* to narrow the professional and clinical frame of reference. The definition of EBPT should be consistent with previously established concepts regarding the use of evidence, but it also should reflect the specific nature of physical therapist practice.

The American Physical Therapy Association's *Guide to Physical Therapist Practice 3.0* describes physical therapy as a profession informed by the World Health Organization's International Classification of Functioning, Disability, and Health (ICF).[1,2] This framework is an expansion of the biopsychosocial model of health that provides "a means not only to describe the states of illness and disability, but also to classify the components and magnitude of the level of health."[1] The model illustrated in **Figure 1-1** depicts the clinical aspects of a patient or client's situation, as well as the social context that shapes perceptions of health, wellness, illness, and disability for each individual. Within this framework, physical therapists examine, evaluate, diagnose, prognosticate, and intervene with individuals with identified *impairments*, *activity limitations, and participation restrictions*, as well as with persons with health, *prevention*, and wellness needs. These professional behaviors are summarized in the term "patient/client management." Finally, the management process incorporates the individual patient or client as a participant whose knowledge, understanding, goals, preferences, and appraisal of his or her situation are integral to the development and implementation of a physical therapist's plan of care.

Structure of the International Classification of Functioning, Disability and Health (ICF) model of functioning and disability.[5]

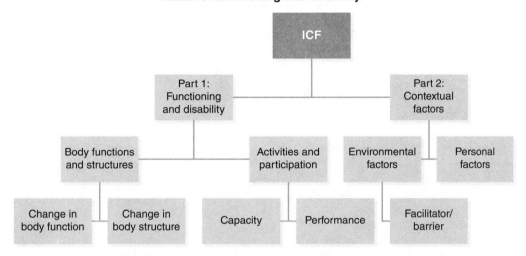

Reprinted from Guide to Physical Therapist Practice 3.0 (http://guidetoptpractice.apta.org), with permission of the American Physical Therapy Association. Copyright © 2006 American Physical Therapy Association. All rights reserved.

A definition of EBPT practice that reflects the intent of evidence-based medicine as well as the nature of physical therapist practice is offered here:[1,29]

> Evidence-based physical therapist practice is "open and thoughtful clinical decision making" about physical therapist management of a patient or client that integrates the "best available evidence with clinical judgment" and the patient or client's preferences and values, and that further considers the larger social context in which physical therapy services are provided, to optimize patient or client outcomes and quality of life.

The term "open" implies a process in which the physical therapist is able to articulate in understandable terms the details of his or her recommendations, including (1) the steps taken to arrive at this conclusion, (2) the underlying rationale, and (3) the potential impact of taking and of refusing action. "Thoughtful clinical decision making" refers to the physical therapist's appraisal of the risks and benefits of various options within a professional context that includes ethics, standards of care, and legal or regulatory considerations.[30] "Best available evidence" refers to timely, well-designed research studies relevant to the question a physical therapist has about a patient or client's management. "Preferences and values" are the patient or client's "unique preferences, concerns, and expectations"[7] against which each option should be weighed and which ultimately must be reflected in a collaborative decision-making process between the therapist and the patient or client. This point is consistent with the emphasis on *patient-centered care* as articulated by the Institute of Medicine.[6]

FIGURE 1-2   Evidence-based physical therapist practice in a societal context.

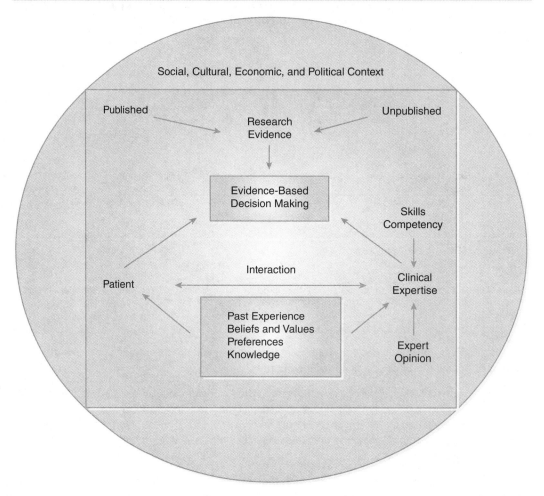

Finally, "larger social context" refers to the social, cultural, economic, and political influences that shape health policy, including rules governing the delivery of and payment for health care services.[31] **Figure 1-2** provides an illustration of EBPT.

Evidence-Based Physical Therapist Practice Focus Areas

A clinician interested in EBPT practice rightly might ask, "Evidence for what?" The process of patient/client management provides the answer to this question when one considers its individual elements

FIGURE 1-3   The process of physical therapist patient/client management.

The process of physical therapist patient and client management.

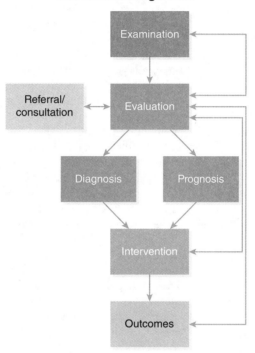

(**Figure 1-3**).[1] To conduct an *examination* and *evaluation*, physical therapists must choose, apply, and interpret findings from a wide variety of tests and measures, such as ligament stress techniques and quantifications of strength and range of motion. Similarly, accurate *diagnosis* of conditions resulting in pain depends on a properly constructed and tested classification scheme. Well-designed research may assist the physical therapist in selecting the best techniques to correctly identify, quantify, and classify an individual's problem, a result that will enhance the efficiency and effectiveness of service delivery.

Prognosis refers to a prediction of the future status of the patient or client that may reflect the natural course of a condition or result following physical therapy treatments or prevention activities. Predictive ability depends on the physical therapist's understanding of the phenomenon in question (i.e., accurate diagnosis), as well as the identification of indicators or risk factors that signal a particular direction. In all cases, the therapist must determine which of the numerous characteristics of the individual's physical, psychological, behavioral, and environmental situation will be most predictive of the outcome of interest. Evidence may identify the most salient factors that will produce the most accurate prediction.

The choice of *interventions* is the step in the patient or client management process that carries particular weight because of the dual responsibilities of the provider to "do good" (beneficence) and to "do no harm" (nonmaleficence). The stakes in this balancing act increase when the intervention in question has a risk of serious consequences, such as permanent disability or mortality. Most treatment options physical therapists implement are not "high risk" in this sense; however, the application of low-risk interventions that produce no positive effect does not meet the test of beneficence. A common clinical scenario is one in which a patient presents with a painful condition and the therapist must decide which manual techniques, exercise, or some combination of both, will be most effective for this individual. Relevant studies may assist the therapist and the patient in a risk–benefit analysis by providing information about effectiveness and harm.

The products of the patient or client management process are referred to as the *outcomes*, which should be distinguished from treatment effects.[31] The former focus on results that occurred at the conclusion of the episode of care from the individual's point of view. For example, return-to-work represents a common outcome following outpatient orthopedic physical therapy management. In contrast, treatment effects represent the change, if any, in the underlying problems that prevented the individual from working. Outcomes usually are stated in functional terms such as "The patient will work 6 hours without pain." Such statements reflect the individual's goals for the physical therapy episode of care. Use of measures of standardized outcomes, however, permits an analysis of progress over the course of an episode for a single individual, as well as a comparison across patients or clients with similar issues. As with the selection of tests and measures used to quantify impairments and aid in diagnosis, a physical therapist must decide which instrument of standardized outcomes will provide the most discriminating information with respect to changes in impairment of body functions and structures, activity limitations, participation restrictions, or health-related quality of life. A review of available evidence may assist the therapist to determine what outcomes are possible and which measurement tool is able to detect change in a consistent and meaningful fashion.

Evidence also may inform a physical therapist's understanding of patients' or clients' perspectives, beliefs, attitudes, or opinions as they experience health, disease, and/or disability and navigate health care services. The impact of these experiences on their relationships with others, their ability to engage in their environment, and their sense of self and relatedness to a larger community also may be relevant to physical therapists' clinical decision making and anticipated outcomes. A review of studies that capture these experiences through the individual's own words may facilitate the therapist's effort to deliver patient-centered care (or "person-centered" services for clients).

The Process of Evidence-Based Physical Therapist Practice

Evidence-based physical therapist practice as a process starts with a question in response to a patient or client's problem or concern. A search for relevant studies to answer the question is then followed by a critical appraisal of their merits and conclusions, as well as a determination of their applicability to the individual. At the conclusion of the appraisal, the therapist will consider the evidence in the context of his or her clinical expertise and the individual's values and preferences during an explicit discussion with that individual.[4] Finally, the therapist and that individual will collaborate to identify and implement the next steps in the management process.

Evidence-based physical therapist practice depends on a variety of factors. First, physical therapists require sufficient knowledge about their patient or client's condition to recognize the unknown. In other words, physical therapists must be willing to suspend the assumption that they have complete information about an individual's situation. In addition, they must have, or have access to, knowledge of the evidence appraisal process—that is, which features characterize stronger versus weaker study designs. Second, physical therapists need access to the evidence, a situation that has improved considerably with the advent of online databases and electronic publication of journals. Availability of these resources, however, does not ensure their efficient use, particularly when it comes to developing effective search strategies. Third, physical therapists need the time to search for, appraise, and integrate the evidence into their practice. In busy clinical settings, time is a limited commodity that usually is dedicated to administrative tasks, such as documentation of services and discussions with referral sources and payers. Unless the entire clinic or department adopts the EBPT philosophy, it may be difficult for a single physical therapist to incorporate the behavior into his or her patient or client management routine.

Results from a survey conducted by Jette et al. in 2003 suggested that some of the requirements of EBPT practice are obstacles to its implementation.[16] Although most respondents (*n* = 488) believed evidence was necessary for practice and improved quality of care, 67% of the subjects listed "lack of time" as one of the top three barriers to implementation of EBPT practice. Nearly all respondents (96%) indicated they had access to evidence; however, 65% reported performing searches for clinical studies less than twice in a typical month. In addition, notable proportions of the sample indicated lower confidence levels in their abilities to search effectively (34%), appraise the study designs (44%), and interpret results using terms such as "odds ratio" (47%) and "confidence interval" (37%). Finally, older therapists with more years since licensure were less likely to have the necessary training, familiarity with, and confidence in the skills necessary for effective EBPT practice.

Subsequent studies have suggested an overall improvement in physical therapists' knowledge of and self-efficacy with evidence-based practice skills. However, changes in clinical decision making in response to available evidence continue to lag.[32-34] This disparity between EBPT knowledge and actual practice fuels the current interest in knowledge translation methods.[34-38] Jones et al. published a systematic review of the evidence regarding knowledge translation interventions in rehabilitation.[35] Thirteen of the articles included in the review were specific to physical therapist practice. All of these studies included some form of professional education regarding EBPT practice. Only two included audit and feedback mechanisms to study participants. Results were mixed, a finding Jones and colleagues attributed to the low methodological quality of most of the studies. Clearly, more work is needed to close the gap between the EBPT knowledge and skills acquired in professional physical therapist education and their application in clinical practice.

So, what can be done to reduce the barriers to effective EBPT practice? Perhaps most importantly, a philosophical shift is required to develop consistent behavior during a busy day of patient or client care. Physical therapists must value the contribution trustworthy evidence can make when integrated with clinical judgment and a patient or client's values and preferences. Management support also is necessary in terms of EBPT education, access to evidence, time allotted in a therapist's schedule, and ongoing feedback about the impact evidence has on patient or client outcomes. Use of services that locate, summarize, and appraise the evidence for easy review by practitioners may also help the time issue. However, physical therapists must determine whether the methodology used by these services is sufficiently stringent to provide an appropriate assessment of evidence quality. Databases dedicated to physical therapy evidence also may enhance the efficiency of the search process.

Ultimately, the ability to engage in EBPT practice consistently requires practice, just like any other skill. The process starts with the individual patient or client and the questions generated from the initial encounter, such as the following:

- Which tests will provide accurate classification of this person's problem?
- What activity limitations can be anticipated if this problem is not addressed?
- What is the most effective intervention that can be offered for documented impairments in body functions and structure?
- How will we know if we have been successful?
- How can changes in this person's quality of life that result from this episode of care be captured?
- Can the perspectives of other people who have similar issues or concerns inform my decision making for this individual?

A physical therapist's willingness to consider these questions *consciously* is the first step in EBPT practice. The word "consciously" is emphasized because it takes practice to develop the habit of openly challenging one's assumptions and current state of knowledge. Until this behavior becomes a routine part of one's practice, EBPT practice will be difficult to implement in a consistent and time-efficient manner.

Summary

The use of systematically developed evidence in clinical decision making is promoted among many health professions in response to documented practice variation and increasing health care costs, as well as in response to a desire for improved quality of care. Evidence-based practice in any profession promotes less dependence on knowledge derived from authority or tradition through the use of evidence to evaluate previously unquestioned information. EBPT practice is open, thoughtful decision making about the physical therapist management of a patient or client that integrates the best available evidence, clinical expertise, and the patient or client's preferences and values, within the larger social context of the individual and the therapist. Well-designed research studies may inform decision making regarding measurement, diagnosis, prognosis, interventions, and outcomes, as well as the perspectives and experiences of individuals seeking physical therapist services. Requirements for EBPT practice include a willingness to challenge one's assumptions, the ability to develop relevant clinical questions about a patient or client, access to evidence, knowledge regarding evidence appraisal, and the time to make it all happen, as well as a willingness to acquire, practice, and evaluate the impact of the necessary skills described in this text.

Exercises

1. Describe two factors that have prompted the emphasis on evidence-based practice in health care. How might evidence address these issues or concerns?
2. Discuss the strengths and weaknesses of clinical knowledge derived from the following:
   a. Authority
   b. Evidence
   c. Tradition
3. Describe a specific example in current physical therapist practice of each type of knowledge listed in question #2.
4. Use Anne's case history and provide examples for each of the potential errors in clinical reasoning described in Table 1-1.
5. Discuss the potential contribution of evidence to each step of the patient or client management process. Provide clinical examples relevant to physical therapist practice to support your points.
6. Discuss the role of the patient or client in EBPT practice. Provide a clinical example relevant to physical therapist practice to support your points.
7. Think about your experiences in the clinical setting and complete the survey in **Figure 1-4** modified from Jette et al.[16] What do your answers tell you about your willingness and readiness to participate in EBPT practice?
8. Based on your results from the previous question, identify two changes you would need to make to enhance your ability to participate in EBPT practice. For each change, identify one strategy you could implement to move you in the right direction.

FIGURE 1-4 **Survey of beliefs and attitudes regarding evidence-based physical therapist practice.**

Appendix.
Evidence-Based Practice (EBP) Questionnaire

This section of the questionnaire inquires about personal attitudes toward, use of, and perceived benefits and limitations of EBP.

For the following items, place a mark ☒ in the appropriate box that indicates your response.

1. Application of EBP is necessary in the practice of physical therapy.
   ☐ Strongly disagree   ☐ Disagree   ☐ Neutral   ☐ Agree   ☐ Strongly Agree

2. Literature and research findings are useful in my day-to-day practice.
   ☐ Strongly disagree   ☐ Disagree   ☐ Neutral   ☐ Agree   ☐ Strongly Agree

3. I need to increase the use of evidence in my daily practice.
   ☐ Strongly disagree   ☐ Disagree   ☐ Neutral   ☐ Agree   ☐ Strongly Agree

4. The adoption of EBP places an unreasonable demand on physical therapists.
   ☐ Strongly disagree   ☐ Disagree   ☐ Neutral   ☐ Agree   ☐ Strongly Agree

5. I am interested in learning or improving the skills necessary to incorporate EBP into my practice.
   ☐ Strongly disagree   ☐ Disagree   ☐ Neutral   ☐ Agree   ☐ Strongly Agree

6. EBP improves the quality of patient care.
   ☐ Strongly disagree   ☐ Disagree   ☐ Neutral   ☐ Agree   ☐ Strongly Agree

7. EBP does not take into account the limitations of my clinical practice setting.
   ☐ Strongly disagree   ☐ Disagree   ☐ Neutral   ☐ Agree   ☐ Strongly Agree

8. My reimbursement rate will increase if I incorporate EBP into my practice.
   ☐ Strongly disagree   ☐ Disagree   ☐ Neutral   ☐ Agree   ☐ Strongly Agree

9. Strong evidence is lacking to support most of the interventions I use with my patients.
   ☐ Strongly disagree   ☐ Disagree   ☐ Neutral   ☐ Agree   ☐ Strongly Agree

10. EBP helps me make decisions about patient care.
    ☐ Strongly disagree   ☐ Disagree   ☐ Neutral   ☐ Agree   ☐ Strongly Agree

11. EBP does not take into account patient preferences.
    ☐ Strongly disagree   ☐ Disagree   ☐ Neutral   ☐ Agree   ☐ Strongly Agree

For the following items, place a mark ☒ in the appropriate box that indicates your response for a typical month.

12. Read/review research/literature related to my clinical practice.
    ☐ ≤ 1 article   ☐ 2-5 articles   ☐ 6-10 articles   ☐ 11-15 articles   ☐ 16+ articles

13. Use professional literature and research findings in the process of clinical decision making.
    ☐ ≤ 1 time   ☐ 2-5 times   ☐ 6-10 times   ☐ 11-15 times   ☐ 16+ times

14. Use MEDLINE or other databases to search for practice-relevant literature/research.
    ☐ ≤ 1 time   ☐ 2-5 times   ☐ 6-10 times   ☐ 11-15 times   ☐ 16+ times

The following section inquires about personal use and understanding of clinical practice guidelines. Practice guidelines provide a description of standard specifications for care of patients with specific diseases and are developed through a formal, consensus-building process that incorporates the best scientific evidence of effectiveness and expert opinion available.

For the following items, place a mark ☒ in the appropriate box that indicates your response.

15. Practice guidelines are available for topics related to my practice.
    ☐ Yes   ☐ No   ☐ Do Not Know

16. I actively seek practice guidelines pertaining to areas of my practice.
    ☐ Strongly disagree   ☐ Disagree   ☐ Neutral   ☐ Agree   ☐ Strongly Agree

17. I use practice guidelines in my practice.
    ☐ Strongly disagree   ☐ Disagree   ☐ Neutral   ☐ Agree   ☐ Strongly Agree

18. I am aware that practice guidelines are available online.
    ☐ Yes   ☐ No

19. I am able to access practice guidelines online.
    ☐ Yes   ☐ No

20. I am able to incorporate patient preferences with practice guidelines.
    ☐ Strongly disagree   ☐ Disagree   ☐ Neutral   ☐ Agree   ☐ Strongly Agree

The following section inquires about availability of resources to access information and personal skills in using those resources.

For the following items, place a mark ☒ in the appropriate box that indicates your response. In items referring to your "facility," consider the practice setting in which you do the majority of your clinical care.

21. I have access to current research through professional journals in their paper form.
    ☐ Yes   ☐ No

22. I have the ability to access relevant databases and the Internet at my facility.
    ☐ Yes   ☐ No   ☐ Do Not Know

(continues)

FIGURE 1-4 **Survey of beliefs and attitudes regarding evidence-based physical therapist practice. (*Continued*)**

---

23. I have the ability to access relevant databases and the Internet at home or locations other than my facility.
☐ Yes   ☐ No   ☐ Do Not Know   ☐ Agree   ☐ Strongly Agree

24. My facility supports the use of current research in practice.
☐ Strongly disagree   ☐ Disagree   ☐ Neutral   ☐ Agree   ☐ Strongly Agree

25. I learned the foundations for EBP as part of my academic preparation.
☐ Strongly disagree   ☐ Disagree   ☐ Neutral   ☐ Agree   ☐ Strongly Agree

26. I have received formal training in search strategies for finding research relevant to my practice.
☐ Strongly disagree   ☐ Disagree   ☐ Neutral   ☐ Agree   ☐ Strongly Agree

27. I am familiar with the medical search engines (e.g., MEDLINE, CINAHL).
☐ Strongly disagree   ☐ Disagree   ☐ Neutral   ☐ Agree   ☐ Strongly Agree

28. I received formal training in critical appraisal of research literature as part of my academic preparation.
☐ Strongly disagree   ☐ Disagree   ☐ Neutral   ☐ Agree   ☐ Strongly Agree

29. I am confident in my ability to critically review professional literature.
☐ Strongly disagree   ☐ Disagree   ☐ Neutral   ☐ Agree   ☐ Strongly Agree

30. I am confident in my ability to find relevant research to answer my clinical questions.
☐ Strongly disagree   ☐ Disagree   ☐ Neutral   ☐ Agree   ☐ Strongly Agree

For the following item, place a mark ☒ in one box in the row for each term.
31. My understanding of the following terms is:

Term	Understand Completely	Understand Somewhat	Do Not Understand
a) Relative risk	☐	☐	☐
b) Absolute risk	☐	☐	☐
c) Systematic review	☐	☐	☐
d) Odds ratio	☐	☐	☐
e) Meta-analysis	☐	☐	☐
f) Confidence interval	☐	☐	☐
g) Heterogeneity	☐	☐	☐
h) Publication bias	☐	☐	☐

For the following items, rank your top 3 choices by placing number in the appropriate boxes (1 = most important).
32. Rank your 3 greatest barriers to the use of EBP in your clinical practice.
☐ Insufficient time
☐ Lack of information resources
☐ Lack of research skills
☐ Poor ability to critically appraise the literature
☐ Lack of generalizability of the literature findings to my patient population
☐ Inability to apply research findings to individual patients with unique characteristics
☐ Lack of understanding of statistical analysis
☐ Lack of collective support among my colleagues in my facility
☐ Lack of interest

References

1. American Physical Therapy Association. *Guide to Physical Therapist Practice 3.0.* Available at: http://guide toptpractice.apta.org. Accessed July 16, 2016.

2. World Health Organization. *Towards a Common Language of Functioning, Disability and Health. ICF.* Geneva, Switzerland: World Health Organization; 2002. Available at: http://www.who.int/classifications/icf/icfbeginners guide.pdf. Accessed July 16, 2016.

3. Sackett DL, Rosenberg WM, Gray JA, Haynes RB, Richardson WS. Evidence-based medicine: what it is and what it isn't. *BMJ.* 1996;312(7023):71–72.

4. Higgs J, Jones M, Loftus S, Christensen N, eds. *Clinical Reasoning in the Health Professions.* 3rd ed. Oxford, England: Butterworth-Heinemann; 2008.

5. Guyatt G, Rennie D. *Users' Guides to the Medical Literature: A Manual for Evidence-Based Clinical Practice.* 3rd ed. Chicago, IL: AMA Press; 2014.

6. Greiner AC, Knebel E, eds. *Health Professions Education: A Bridge to Quality.* Institute of Medicine Website. Available at: https://www.nap.edu/read/10681/chapter/1. Accessed July 16, 2016.

7. Sackett DL, Straus SE, Richardson WS, et al. *Evidence-Based Medicine: How to Practice and Teach EBM.* 2nd ed. Edinburgh, Scotland: Churchill Livingstone; 2000.

8. EPC Evidence-based Reports. Agency for Healthcare Research and Quality Website. Available at: http://www .ahrq.gov/research/findings/evidence-based-reports/index.html. Accessed July 16, 2016.

9. Medicare Evidence Development and Coverage Advisory Committee. Centers for Medicare and Medicaid Services Website. Available at: www.cms.gov/Regulations-and-Guidance/Guidance/FACA/MEDCAC.html. Accessed July 16, 2016.

10. JAMA evidence. American Medical Association Website. Available at: http://jamaevidence.mhmedical.com. Accessed July 16, 2016.

11. Process for Evidence Evaluation. American Heart Association Website. Available at: http://cpr.heart .org/AHAECC/CPRAndECC/ResuscitationScience/InternationalLiaisonCommitteeonResuscitationILCOR /UCM_476509_Process-for-Evidence-Evaluation.jsp. Accessed July 16, 2016.

12. Evidence-based Practice & Research. American Occupational Therapy Association Website. Available at: http://www.aota.org/Practice/Researchers.aspx. Accessed July 16, 2016.

13. Vision 2020. American Physical Therapy Association Website. Available at: www.apta.org/Vision2020/. Accessed July 16, 2016.

14. Schreiber J, Stern P, Marchetti G, Providence I. Strategies to promote evidence-based practice in pediatric physical therapy: a formative evaluation project. *Phys Ther.* 2009;89(9):918–933.

15. Stevans JM, Bise CG, McGee JC, et al. Evidence-based practice implementation: case report of the evolution of a quality improvement program in a multicenter physical therapy organization. *Phys Ther.* 2015;95(4):588–599.

16. Jette DU, Bacon K, Batty C, et al. Evidence-based practice: beliefs, attitudes, knowledge, and behaviors of physical therapists. *Phys Ther.* 2003;83(9):786–805.

17. Salbach NM, Jaglal SB, Korner-Bitensky N, et al. Practitioner and organizational barriers to evidence-based practice of physical therapists for people with stroke. *Phys Ther.* 2007;87(10):1284–1303.

18. Rothstein JM. Editors Notes. *Phys Ther.* 2002;82. Physical Therapy Journal Website. Available at: http://ptjournal. apta.org/content/82/1/6.full. Accessed July 16, 2016.

19. PTNow. American Physical Therapy Association Website. Available at: www.ptnow.org/Default.aspx. Accessed July 16, 2016.

20. Eddy DM. Evidence-based medicine: a unified approach. *Health Affairs.* 2005;24(1):9–17.

21. Steinberg EP, Luce BR. Evidence based? Caveat emptor! *Health Affairs.* 2005;24(1):80–92.

22. Women's Health Initiative Participant Information. Women's Health Initiative Website. Available at: https:// www.nhlbi.nih.gov/whi/. Accessed July 16, 2016.

23. The National Academies of Sciences, Engineering, Medicine Website. Available at: https://www.national academies.org/hmd/. Accessed July 16, 2016.

24. CMS Retains Clinical Study Requirement in Final TENS Decision Memo. American Physical Therapy Association Website. Available at: www.apta.org/PTinMotion/NewsNow/2012/6/12/FinalTENSMemo/. Accessed July 16, 2016.

25. Hicks N. Evidence-based healthcare. *Bandolier.* 1997;4(39):8.

26. Croskerry P. Achieving quality in clinical decision making: cognitive strategies and detection of bias. *Acad Emerg Med.* 2002;9(11):1184–1204.

27. Straus SE, Richardson WS, Glaziou P, Haynes RB. *Evidence-Based Medicine: How to Practice and Teach EBM.* 3rd ed. Edinburgh, Scotland: Elsevier Churchill Livingstone; 2005.

28. Mobasseri S, Liebson PR, Klein LW. Hormone therapy and selective receptor modulators for prevention of coronary heart disease in postmenopausal women: estrogen replacement from the cardiologist's perspective. *Cardiol Rev.* 2004;12(6):287–298.

29. American Physical Therapy Association. *Normative Model of Physical Therapist Education: Version 2004.* Alexandria, VA; 2004.

30. Guyatt GH, Haynes RB, Jaeschke RZ, et al. Users' Guides to the Medical Literature: XXV. Evidence-based medicine: principles for applying the Users' Guides to patient care. Evidence-Based Medicine Working Group. *JAMA.* 2000;284(10):1290–1296.

31. Herbert R, Jamtvedt G, Hagen KB, Mead J. *Practical Evidence-Based Physiotherapy.* 2nd ed. Edinburgh, Scotland: Elsevier Butterworth-Heinemann; 2011.

32. Manns PJ, Norton AV, Darrah J. Cross-sectional study to examine evidence-based practice skills and behaviors of physical therapy graduates: is there a knowledge-to-practice gap? *Phys Ther.* 2015;95(4):568–578.

33. Olsen NR, Bradley P, Lomborg K, Nortvedt NW. Evidence-based practice in clinical physiotherapy education: a qualitative interpretive discussion. *BMC Med Educ.* 2013;13:52.

34. Tilson JK, Mickan S, Howard R et al. Promoting physical therapists' use of research evidence to inform clinical practice: part 3 – long term feasibility assessment of the PEAK program. *BMC Med Educ.* 2016;16(1):144.

35. Jones CA, Roop SC, Pohar SL, Albrecht L, Scott SD. Translating knowledge in rehabilitation: a systematic review. *Phys Ther.* 2015;95(4):663–677.

36. Deutsch JE, Romney W, Reynolds J, Manal TJ. Validity and usability of a professional association's web-based knowledge translation portal: American Physical Therapy Association's PTNow.org. *BMC Med Inform Decis Mak.* 2015;15:79.

37. Hudon A, Gervais M-J, Hunt M. The contribution of conceptual frameworks to knowledge translation interventions in physical therapy. *Phys Ther.* 2015;95(4):630–639.

38. Schreiber J, Marchetti GF, Racicot B, Kaminski E. The use of a knowledge translation program to increase the use of standardized outcome measures in an outpatient pediatric physical therapy clinic: administrative case report. *Phys Ther.* 2015;95(4):613–629.

CHAPTER 2

WHAT IS EVIDENCE?

OBJECTIVES

Upon completion of this chapter, the student/practitioner will be able to do the following:
1. Discuss the concept of "best available clinical evidence."
2. Describe the general content and procedural characteristics of desirable evidence and their implications for the selection of studies to evaluate.
3. Describe different forms of evidence and their uses for answering clinical questions in physical therapist practice.
4. Discuss and apply the principles and purposes of evidence hierarchies for each type of clinical question.
5. Discuss the limitations of evidence hierarchies and their implications for the use of evidence in practice.

TERMS IN THIS CHAPTER

Bias: Results or inferences that systematically deviate from the truth "or the processes leading to such deviation."[1](p.251)

Biologic plausibility: The reasonable expectation that the human body could behave in the manner predicted.

Case report: A detailed description of the management of a patient or client that may serve as a basis for future research,[2] and describes the overall management of an unusual case or a condition that is infrequently encountered in practice or poorly described in the literature.[3]

Clinical practice guidelines: ". . . statements that include recommendations intended to optimize patient care. They are informed by a systematic review of evidence and an assessment of the benefits and harm of alternative care options."[4] also referred to as "summaries."[5]

Cross-sectional study: A study that collects data about a phenomenon during a single point in time or once within a single defined time interval.[6]

Effectiveness: The extent to which an intervention or service produces a desired outcome under usual clinical conditions.[1]

Efficacy: The extent to which an intervention or service produces a desired outcome under ideal conditions.[1]

Evidence: "A broad definition of evidence is any empirical observation, whether systematically collected or not. Clinical research evidence refers to the systematic observation of clinical events. . . ."[7]

Experimental design: A research design in which the behavior of randomly assigned groups of subjects is measured following the purposeful manipulation of an independent variable(s) in at least one of the groups; used to examine cause and effect relationships between an independent variable(s) and an outcome(s).[8,9]

Longitudinal study: A study that looks at a phenomenon occurring over an extended period of time.[1]

Narrative review (also referred to as a *literature review*): A description of prior research without a systematic search and selection strategy or critical appraisal of the studies' merits.[10]

Nonexperimental design (also referred to as an *observational study*): A study in which controlled manipulation of the subjects is lacking[8]; in addition, if groups are present, assignment is predetermined based on naturally occurring subject characteristics or activities.[6]

Peer review: A process by which research is appraised by one or more content experts; commonly utilized when articles are submitted to journals for publication and when grant proposals are submitted for funding.[1]

Physiologic study: A study that focuses on the cellular or physiologic systems levels of the subjects; often performed in a laboratory.[6]

Prospective design: A research design that follows subjects forward over a specified period of time.

Quasi-experimental design: A research design in which there is only one subject group or in which randomization to more than one subject group is lacking; controlled manipulation of the subjects is preserved.[11]

Randomized clinical trial (also referred to as a *randomized controlled trial* and a *randomized controlled clinical trial*) [RCT]: A clinical study that uses a randomization process to assign subjects to either an experimental group(s) or a control (or comparison) group. Subjects in the experimental group receive the intervention or preventive measure of interest and then are compared to the subjects in the control (or comparison) group who did not receive the experimental manipulation.[8]

Retrospective design: A research design that uses historical (past) data from sources such as medical records, insurance claims, or outcomes databases.

Single-system design: A quasi-experimental research design in which one subject receives in an alternating fashion both the experimental and control (or comparison) condition.[8]

Synopsis: "A succinct description of selected individual studies or systematic reviews."[5]

Systematic review: A method by which a collection of individual research studies is gathered and critically appraised in an effort to reach an unbiased conclusion about the cumulative weight of the evidence on a particular topic[6]; also referred to as "syntheses."[5]

Systems: "Individual patient characteristics are automatically linked to the current best evidence that matches the patient's specific circumstances and the clinician is provided with key aspects of management (e.g., computerized decision support systems)."[5]

CLINICAL SCENARIO

Relevant Patient Characteristics

Anne's case history contains information about her that may influence your search for evidence and your judgment about its relevance. Examples include age and fitness level.

What other characteristics can you identify that may influence your search for and application of evidence in Anne's situation?

Introduction

The case has been made that physical therapists should use *evidence to inform their decision* making during the patient/client management process. This claim raises the question "What qualifies as evidence?" In their original work, Guyatt and Rennie stated, "any empirical observation about the apparent relation between events constitutes potential evidence."[7] This observation acknowledged that a variety of information types exist that may be integrated with clinical decisions. Options include, but are not limited to, published research articles, clinical practice guidelines, patient or client records, and recall of prior patient or client cases. As these authors acknowledged, however, clinical research is the preferred source of information. Sackett et al. put a finer point on it with their use of the modifier "best available" clinical evidence. They proposed that a method of prioritizing the evidence according to its merits is required to guide the clinician's selection of relevant information.[12] This chapter discusses the forms and general characteristics of evidence available, as well as the hierarchies that have been developed to rank them.

General Characteristics of Desirable Evidence

In light of the variety of evidence potentially available to physical therapists, it is helpful to have some general characteristics to consider during the initial search. Desirable attributes relate both to content as well as to procedural considerations that serve as preliminary indicators of quality.

The first content criterion pertains to the type of question a physical therapist wants to answer. The patient/client management elements of examination, diagnosis, prognosis, intervention (including preventive measures), and outcomes provide potential focus areas for evidence development and application. Ideally, the evidence located will address specifically the test, measure, classification system, prognostic factor, treatment technique, clinical prediction rule, or outcome that the physical therapist is considering relative to an individual patient or client.

The second content criterion pertains to the individuals studied. Desirable evidence includes subjects whose personal and/or clinical characteristics are similar to the patient or client in order to increase the therapist's ability to apply the research findings to this individual. Common attributes of interest include, but are not limited to, the subjects' age, gender, race/ethnicity, education level, occupation, diagnosis(es), stage of illness, duration of the problem(s), functional status, level of disability, and clinical setting in which patient/client management occurs. Subjects in a research study whose personal and/or clinical characteristics differ markedly from those of a patient or client may have different therapeutic experiences than can be achieved by the individual with whom the physical therapist wishes to use the evidence located.

Two basic procedural characteristics have relevance in the evidence selection process as well. The period in time during which the evidence was developed is often of interest given the rapid evolution of medical technology and pharmaceutical agents. This is particularly relevant for research publications given that articles often appear in journals a year or more after the completion of the project.[7] Early release on the Internet ahead of the printed version undoubtedly has reduced this time line in many cases. Nevertheless, older evidence may not reflect current patient management. A hypothetical example might be a 15-year-old study evaluating the effectiveness of an aerobic training program for individuals with multiple sclerosis that has limited relevance now that a variety of disease-modifying drugs are available.[13] However, evidence should not be rejected only because of its age if the techniques in question, and the context in which they were evaluated, have remained relatively unchanged since the data were collected.

A procedural characteristic specific to scientific journals is the application of peer review. *Peer review* is the process by which manuscripts are evaluated by identified content experts to determine their merit for publication. Evaluation criteria usually include the credibility of a research study in terms of its design and execution, relevance of the findings for the field and/or the specific journal, contribution to the body of knowledge about the topic, and, to a lesser degree, writing style.[1] Peer review acts as an initial screening process to weed out lower quality efforts.

Table 2-1 summarizes the four general characteristics of evidence that are preferable. Note that these attributes are labeled "desirable," not "mandatory." This word choice is purposeful because there is much work to be done to expand the depth and breadth of evidence related to physical therapist practice. Many of the clinical questions physical therapists have about their patients or clients have not been explored or have been addressed in a limited fashion. A search for the "best available clinical evidence" may result in the identification of studies that are not peer reviewed or do not include subjects that look like a therapist's individual patient or client. Similarly, studies may not exist that include a test or technique of interest in the clinical setting. The evidence-based physical therapist (EBPT) practice challenge is to decide whether and how to use evidence that is limited in these ways when it is the only evidence available.

TABLE 2-1	Four Desirable Characteristics of Research Identified During a Search for Evidence
1. The evidence addresses the specific clinical question the physical therapist is trying to answer.
2. The subjects studied have characteristics similar to the patient or client about whom the physical therapist has a clinical question.
3. The context of the evidence and/or the technique of interest are consistent with contemporary health care.
4. The evidence was published in a peer-reviewed medium (paper, electronic).

Forms of Evidence

As noted previously, forms of evidence may include anything from patient records and clinical re-call to published research. Evidence-based practice in health care emphasizes the use of research to inform clinical decisions because of the systematic way in which data are gathered and because of its potential to provide objective results that minimize bias. A variety of research design options exist. A key point is that different research designs are suited to answering different types of clinical questions therapists may have about their patients or clients. The usefulness of a diagnostic test must be evaluated with methods that are different from those used to determine whether an intervention works. As a result, therapists should anticipate looking for evidence with different research designs depending on what they want to know. The remainder of this chapter provides highlights of these different designs and their relative merits.

Research Designs: Overview

Forms of evidence fall along a continuum that is dictated by the presence and strength of a research design that was established prior to data collection (**Figure 2-1**). At one end of the continuum is research that attempts to impose maximum control within the design in order to reduce the chance that bias will influence the study's results. *Bias* is a systematic deviation from the truth that occurs as a result of uncontrolled (and unwanted) influences during the study.[1] Various authors refer to research designs with the best features to minimize bias as *randomized clinical trials, randomized controlled tri-als,* or *randomized controlled clinical trials.*[1,6,8] The acronym used for all three is "RCT." These studies also are categorized as *experimental designs.* Irrespective of the label, the researchers' intention is the same: to reduce unwanted influences in the study through random assignment of study participants to two or more groups *and* through controlled manipulation of the experimental intervention. A variant of this approach is the *single-system design* in which only one person is studied who receives, on an alternating basis, both the experimental and control (or comparison) conditions.[8]

An RCT or single-system design is best suited to answer questions about whether an experimental intervention has an effect and whether that effect is beneficial or harmful to the subjects. When con-ducted under ideal conditions—that is, when a high degree of control is achieved—these studies are focused on treatment *efficacy.* An example might be a study in which some individuals with traumatic brain injuries are randomized to an experimental balance-training program that is performed in a quiet research laboratory. Such an environment is free of distractions that may interfere with their ability to pay attention to directions and focus on the required activities. Alternatively, if the same subjects perform the experimental balance-training program during their regular physical therapy appointment

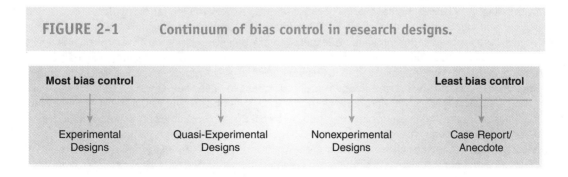

FIGURE 2-1   Continuum of bias control in research designs.

in the outpatient rehabilitation center, then the RCT is focused on treatment *effectiveness*.[14] Investigators in this version of the study want to know if the balance program works in a natural clinical environment full of noise and activity.

Randomized clinical trials and single-system designs are approaches used to conduct an original research project focusing on one or more persons. These individual studies themselves may serve as the focus of another type of controlled research design referred to as a systematic review. *Systematic reviews*, or "syntheses," comprise original evidence that has been selected and critically appraised according to pre-established criteria.[6] The goal of this research design is to draw conclusions from the cumulative weight of studies that, individually, may not be sufficient to provide a definitive answer. The pre-established criteria are used to minimize bias that may be introduced when investigators make decisions about which prior studies to include and when judgments are made about their quality. Systematic reviews may address any type of clinical question; however, most commonly they focus on well-controlled studies of interventions—in other words, on RCTs.

At the other end of the evidence continuum is the unsystematic collection of patient or client data that occurs in daily physical therapist practice. The term *unsystematic* is not meant to imply substandard care; rather, it is an indication that clinical practice is focused on the individual patient or client rather than on groups of subjects on whom behavioral and data collection controls are imposed to ensure research integrity. This type of evidence often is labeled "anecdotal"[11] and frequently put to use when therapists recall from memory prior experiences with patients or clients similar to the person with whom they are currently dealing. In response to regulatory and payment pressures, many clinical settings are creating a degree of consistency in data collection with their implementation of standardized assessment and outcomes instruments, electronic health records, and databases to capture patient or client outcomes. As a result, physical therapists working in these settings may find some evidence that is useful to inform their practice.

In between the two ends of the evidence continuum are study designs that lack one or more of the following characteristics:

1. Randomization techniques to distribute subjects into groups;
2. The use of more than one group in order to make a comparison;
3. Controlled experimental manipulation of the subjects;
4. Measures at the patient or client level (e.g., impairment in body functions and structure, activity limitations, participation restrictions); and/or
5. A systematic method for collecting and analyzing information.

These designs have fewer features with which to minimize bias and/or shift their focus away from patient- or client-centered outcomes. For example, *quasi-experimental designs* maintain the purposeful manipulation of the experimental technique, but they may not randomize subjects to groups or may have only one subject group to evaluate.[11] *Nonexperimental* (or *observational*) *designs* have even less control than quasi-experimental studies because they have the same limitations with respect to their group(s) and they do not include experimental manipulation of subjects.[8] In spite of their less rigorous designs, both quasi-experimental and nonexperimental studies are used to evaluate the effectiveness of interventions, often due to ethical or pragmatic reasons related to the use of patients in research. In addition, observational designs are used to answer questions about diagnostic tests, clinical measures, prognostic indicators, clinical prediction rules, and patient or client outcomes.

Below quasi-experimental and nonexperimental designs on the continuum are research efforts that focus only on cellular, anatomic, or physiologic systems. These studies often have a high degree of control because they are grounded in the scientific method that is the hallmark of good bench research. They are lower on the continuum not because of their potential for bias, but because they do not focus on person-level function. For this reason, they are referred to as *physiologic studies*.[7]

Even lower on the continuum are case reports and narrative reviews. These study approaches have different purposes. *Case reports* simply describe what occurred with a patient or client, whereas *narrative reviews* summarize prior research.[2,3,10] In spite of these differences, these designs have one common element that puts them both at the bottom of the continuum: they lack the kind of systematic approach necessary to reduce bias. It is important to note, however, that the content of a case report or narrative review may provide a stimulus to conduct a more rigorous research project. **Table 2-2** provides a list of citations from physical therapy literature that represent each type of study design described here.

Research Designs: Timing

Research designs also may be categorized according to the time line used in the study. For example, physical therapist researchers may want to know the relationship between the number of visits to an outpatient orthopedic clinic and the workers' compensation insurance status of patients treated over a 3-year period. Such a question may be answered through an analysis of 3 years of historical patient records from the clinic. This *retrospective design* has as an opposite form—a *prospective design*—in which the investigators collect information from new patients that are admitted to the clinic. As **Figure 2-2**

TABLE 2-2	Citations from Physical Therapy Research Illustrating Different Study Designs
Study Design	**Citation**
Systemic Review	Vanti C, et al. Effect of taping on spinal pain and disability: systematic review and meta-analysis of randomized trials. *Phys Ther.* 2015;95(4):493–506.
Randomized Clinical Trial	Fox EE, et al. Effect of Pilates-based core stability training on ambulant people with multiple sclerosis: multi-center, assessor blinded randomized controlled trial. *Phys Ther.* 2016;96(8):1170–1178.
Single-System Design	Chen YP, et al. Use of virtual reality to improve upper-extremity control in children with cerebral palsy: a single subject design. *Phys Ther.* 2007;87(11):1441–1457.
Quasi-Experimental Study	Drolett A, et al. Move to improve: the feasibility of using an early mobility protocol to increase ambulation in the intensive and intermediate care settings. *Phys Ther.* 2013;93(2):197–207.
Observational Study	Farley MK, et al. Clinical markers of the intensity of balance challenge: observational study of older adult responses to balance tasks. *Phys Ther.* 2016;96(3):313–323.
Physiologic Study	Chung JI, et al. Effect of continuous-wave low-intensity ultrasound in inflammatory resolution of arthritis-associated synovitis. *Phys Ther.* 2016;96(6):808–817.
Case Report	Parkitny L, et al. Interdisciplinary management of complex regional pain syndrome of the face. *Phys Ther.* 2016;96(7):1067–1073.
Summary	Barr AE, et al. Pathophysiologic tissue changes associated with repetitive movement: a review of the evidence. *Phys Ther.* 2002;82(2):173–187.

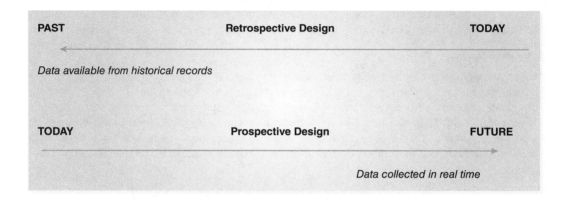

FIGURE 2-2 Graphic depiction of retrospective and prospective research designs.

PAST   Retrospective Design   TODAY

Data available from historical records

TODAY   Prospective Design   FUTURE

Data collected in real time

illustrates, a retrospective approach takes advantage of data that already exist, whereas a prospective approach requires that new data be collected in real time.

In a similar fashion, researchers may be interested in a single point in time or a limited time interval (e.g., *cross-sectional study*), or they may wish to study a phenomenon over an extended period of time (e.g., *longitudinal study*). In the cross-sectional approach, investigators may have an interest in the functional outcome at discharge (a single point in time) from the hospital of patients receiving physical therapist services following total hip replacement. In contrast, a longitudinal approach would include follow-up of these patients to assess outcomes at discharge and at a specified point or points in time in the future (e.g., 3 months, 6 months, 1 year). **Figure 2-3** illustrates these design options.

The sequence of events across time in a study is important, particularly when an investigator is trying to determine whether a change in the patient or client's condition was the direct result of the intervention or preventive measure applied. Specifically, the intervention must have occurred before the outcome was measured to increase one's confidence that it was the technique of interest that made a difference in the subject's status or performance.

Research Designs: What Is the Question?

Remember that the clinical question the physical therapist wants to answer will determine which of these forms of evidence to seek. For example, a question about the best clinical test to identify a rotator cuff tear (diagnosis) is likely to be addressed by a cross-sectional nonexperimental study of patients who are suspected to have the problem based on results from the physical examination. However, a question about risk factors for falls in the elderly may be answered in one of two ways: (1) a longitudinal study in which two groups of elderly subjects are followed in real time (i.e., prospectively) to determine who falls and who does not, or (2) a retrospective study that starts with subjects with documented falls and evaluates possible precipitating characteristics (e.g., visual deficits) in comparison to non-fallers. Finally, a question about the effectiveness of joint mobilization in the management of cervical spine disorders is best answered by a prospective RCT of patients classified with neck pain. Physical therapists should anticipate these differences when planning their search strategies to increase the efficiency of the evidence identification process.

FIGURE 2-3   Graphic depiction of cross-sectional and longitudinal research designs.

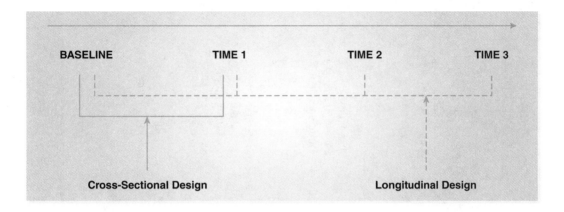

One must also recall that a search for the "best available clinical evidence" may result in the discovery of research that is limited in content and/or quality. In other words, the current state of knowledge in an area may be such that the "best" (and only) evidence available is from studies (or unpublished clinical data) in which the chance of bias is higher because of weaknesses in the research designs. Physical therapists will find this scenario to be true for many of the clinical questions they pose in practice. This reality is not a reason to reject EBPT practice; rather, it is a reaffirmation that clinical judgment and expertise are required to decide whether and how to use evidence that is limited in form.

Hierarchies of Evidence

Previous research has identified a number of barriers to using evidence in physical therapist practice, one of which is the lack of time available to search for, select, and read professional literature.[15] The selection process may be eased somewhat by ranking research designs based on their ability to minimize bias. Proponents of evidence-based medicine have attempted to make the study selection process more efficient for busy clinicians by developing hierarchies, or levels, of evidence. In 2011, Howick et al. at the Oxford Centre for Evidence-Based Medicine (OCEBM) in England consolidated previously developed individual hierarchies for evidence about diagnostic tests, prognostic indicators, and treatment techniques into one reference table for easier use (reprinted in **Table 2-3**).[16-18] The variety of hierarchies is necessary because of the point made previously: different research designs are required to answer different types of clinical questions. Understanding the nuances of each hierarchy is an important skill to develop in order to use them appropriately.

These ranking schemes are similar to one another in that they place systematic reviews at the top of each list. Systematic reviews are valued because they may produce conclusions based on a critical appraisal of a number of individual studies that have been selected according to preestablished criteria. Ideally, the studies reviewed have research designs that minimize the chance of bias (i.e., "high-quality evidence"), are pertinent to the therapist's question, and provide a more definitive answer to the question. This ideal is akin to the "holy grail" in evidence-based practice; however, systematic reviews also have their limitations. As a result, individual studies may provide stronger

TABLE 2-3   Oxford Centre for Evidence-Based Medicine 2011 Levels of Evidence

Question	Step 1 (Level 1*)	Step 2 (Level 2*)	Step 3 (Level 3*)	Step 4 (Level 4*)	Step 5 (Level 5)
How common is the problem?	Local and current random sample surveys (or censuses)	Systematic review of surveys that allow matching to local circumstances**	Local nonrandom sample**	Case-series**	n/a
Is this diagnostic or monitoring test accurate? (Diagnosis)	Systematic review of cross-sectional studies with consistently applied reference standard and blinding	Individual cross-sectional studies with consistently applied reference standard and blinding	Nonconsecutive studies, or studies without consistently applied reference standards**	Case-control studies, or "poor or nonindependent reference standard**	Mechanism-based reasoning
What will happen if we do not add a therapy? (Prognosis)	Systematic review of inception cohort studies	Inception cohort studies	Cohort study or control arm of randomized trial*	Case-series or case-control studies, or poor quality prognostic cohort study**	n/a
Does this intervention help? (Treatment Benefits)	Systematic review of randomized trials or n-of-1 trials	Randomized trial or observational study with dramatic effect	Nonrandomized controlled cohort/follow-up study**	Case-series, case-control studies, or historically controlled studies**	Mechanism-based reasoning

Question	Step 1 (Level 1*)	Step 2 (Level 2*)	Step 3 (Level 3*)	Step 4 (Level 4*)	Step 5 (Level 5)
What are the COMMON harms? (Treatment Harms)	Systematic review of randomized trials, systematic review of nested case-control studies, n-of-1 trial with the patient you are raising the question about, or observational study with dramatic effect	Individual randomized trial or (exceptionally) observational study with dramatic effect	Nonrandomized controlled cohort/follow-up study (post-marketing surveillance) provided there are sufficient numbers to rule out a common harm. (For long-term harms the duration of follow-up must be sufficient.)**	Case-series, case-control, or historically controlled studies**	Mechanism-based reasoning
What are the RARE harms? (Treatment Harms)	Systematic review of randomized trials or n-of-1 trial	Randomized trial or (exceptionally) observational study with dramatic effect			
Is this (early detection) test worthwhile? (Screening)	Systematic review of randomized trials	Randomized trial	Nonrandomized controlled cohort/follow-up study**	Case-series, case-control, or historically controlled studies**	Mechanism-based reasoning

*Level may be graded down on the basis of study quality, imprecision, indirectness (study PICO does not match questions PICO), because of inconsistency between studies, or because the absolute effect size is very small; level may be graded up if there is a large or very large effect size.

** As always, a systematic review is generally better than an individual study.

Reproduced with permission from Oxford Center for Evidence-Based Medicine—www.cebm.net.

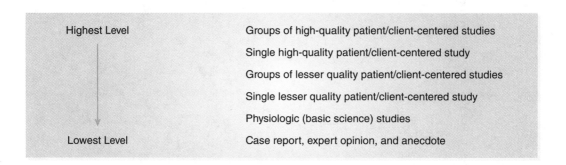

FIGURE 2-4   General ranking of evidence within hierarchies.

Highest Level	Groups of high-quality patient/client-centered studies
	Single high-quality patient/client-centered study
	Groups of lesser quality patient/client-centered studies
	Single lesser quality patient/client-centered study
	Physiologic (basic science) studies
Lowest Level	Case report, expert opinion, and anecdote

evidence in answer to a clinical question. At the lowest end of each OCEBM hierarchy are physiologic studies and research based on *biologic plausibility*. These studies are classified as such because of their focus on the anatomic and/or physiologic mechanisms underlying a pathologic condition or treatment technique. Clinicians who locate studies that fall into this level of evidence must consider the extent to which they can reasonably apply the findings at the person level for an individual patient.

Details about each evidence level between these end points vary because of the types of questions being addressed; however, some common themes regarding use of the hierarchies can be identified. First, level of rank depends on the strength of the study design. For example, an RCT is highly ranked because it is a more rigorous research design than an observational study for investigation of the therapeutic effects of an intervention such as joint mobilization in people with neck pain. Second, individual studies with strong designs should be "graded up" above systematic reviews of studies with weaker designs. For example, a single prospective study of fall risk in the elderly that includes a comprehensive list of predisposing factors for falls in a large number of subjects is more valuable than a systematic review of retrospective studies that failed to include medications, living environment, and mental status as potential contributors to fall risk. Third, systematic reviews of studies with similar directions and degrees of results (e.g., subjects improved in most studies) make a stronger case as a result of this homogeneity than systematic reviews of studies with significant variation in their individual findings (e.g., subjects improved in some studies and not others). **Figure 2-4** summarizes the commonalities among the OCEBM evidence hierarchies. Howick et al. also acknowledged some preliminary findings regarding the potential value of individual patient cases and anecdotes in evidence-based decision making.[16] Although not included in the current edition of the OCEBM hierarchies, these sources of information are reflected in the figure here to illustrate their rank relative to planned, systematic research efforts.

Selection of studies through the use of hierarchies may improve the efficiency of the search process for busy clinicians. These schemas also are used regularly to grade evidence to facilitate the decision-making process about which information to use. This strategy is most apparent in published *clinical practice guidelines*. National and international government agencies and professional associations produce guidelines in an effort to promote effective and efficient health care. A few examples relevant to physical therapist practice include the following:

- VA/DoD Clinical Practice Guideline: Management of Concussion/Mild Traumatic Brain Injury (2016)[19];
- British Thoracic Society's "The BTS Guideline on Pulmonary Rehabilitation in Adults" (2013)[20]; and
- Orthopedic Section – APTA's "Nonarthritic Hip Joint Pain" (2014).[21]

TABLE 2-4	Evidence Grades in a Clinical Practice Guideline about Nonarthritic Hip Joint Pain
Grades Of Recommendation Based On	**Strength of Evidence**
A. Strong evidence	A preponderance of level I and/or level II studies support the recommendation. This must include at least 1 level I study
B. Moderate evidence	A single high-quality randomized controlled trial or a preponderance of level II studies support the recommendation
C. Weak evidence	A single level II study or a preponderance of level III and IV studies, including statements of consensus by content experts, support the recommendation
D. Conflicting evidence	Higher-quality studies conducted on this topic disagree with respect to their conclusions. The recommendation is based on these conflicting studies
E. Theoretical/foundational evidence	A preponderance of evidence from animal or cadaver studies, from conceptual models/principles, or from basic science/bench research supports this conclusion
F. Expert opinion	Best practice based on the clinical experience of the guidelines development team

Reprinted with permission from Enseki K, Harris-Hayes M, White DM, et al. Nonarthritic hip joint pain. *J Orthop Sports Phys Ther.* 2014;44:A1-A32. https://doi.org/10.2519/jospt.2014.0302. ©Journal of Orthopaedic & Sports Physical Therapy®

Each of these documents, as well as numerous other similar publications, contain recommendations based on a review and ranking of available evidence. Grading schemes are described in the guidelines and used to qualify the recommendations made. For example, the Orthopedic Section – APTA assigned the letter grades A, B, C, D, E, and F to rate the strength of the evidence supporting the guideline's recommendations (**Table 2-4**). On the other hand, the Department of Veterans Affairs/ Department of Defense (VA/DoD) used the categories "strong for," "weak for," "weak against," "strong against" based on the quality of the evidence and the balance between desirable and undesirable outcomes of the intervention(s) recommended.

In theory, physical therapists using any of these guidelines could go straight to the recommendations and make decisions about how to change their practice based on these evidence grades. However, clinical practice guidelines should be assessed for quality in their own right before a clinician blindly adopts the practice behaviors they address.

DiCenso and colleagues developed the "6S model" to aid in the selection of "pre-appraised" evidence such as clinical practice guidelines (**Figure 2-5**).[5] In recognition of the value of a cumulative body of evidence, this hierarchy places all individual studies on the lowest level of the continuum. Computerized decision support *systems* that provide clinicians with the ability to integrate a specific patient's characteristics with synthesized evidence sit at the top of the hierarchy. The levels in between comprise progressively greater degrees of abstraction from collections of studies previously evaluated for their quality. Robeson and colleagues explored the availability of these

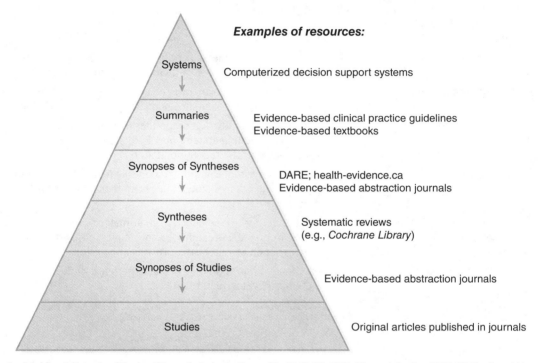

FIGURE 2-5   The 6S hierarchy of pre-appraised evidence.

Examples of resources:

Systems — Computerized decision support systems

Summaries — Evidence-based clinical practice guidelines
Evidence-based textbooks

Synopses of Syntheses — DARE; health-evidence.ca
Evidence-based abstraction journals

Syntheses — Systematic reviews
(e.g., *Cochrane Library*)

Synopses of Studies — Evidence-based abstraction journals

Studies — Original articles published in journals

Reprinted from Evidence Based Nursing, DiCenso, A., Bayley, L., Haynes, RB., 12, 99-101, 2009 with permission from BMJ Publishing Group Ltd.

different forms of preprocessed evidence for questions related to effectiveness of public health.[22] As **Figure 2-6** suggests, the number of research products in each category varies considerably with a predictably higher volume of traditional evidence formats (i.e., individual studies, systematic reviews, and meta-analyses). Development of *synopses, syntheses, summaries,* and *systems* is dependent upon groups with sufficient expertise and resources to locate, critically appraise, write, and publish cohesive analyses and practice recommendations based on the evidence gathered. As such, physical therapists may find it challenging to locate pre-appraised evidence that addresses their clinical questions.

The Quality of Evidence Generated from Words

The research designs described above and the hierarchies used to rank them are consistent with an investigative paradigm that emphasizes objectivity, faithfulness to rules of engagement with subjects, and use of quantitative data to describe clinical phenomena. Even the subjective perspectives of patients or clients are standardized into controlled survey responses through questions with

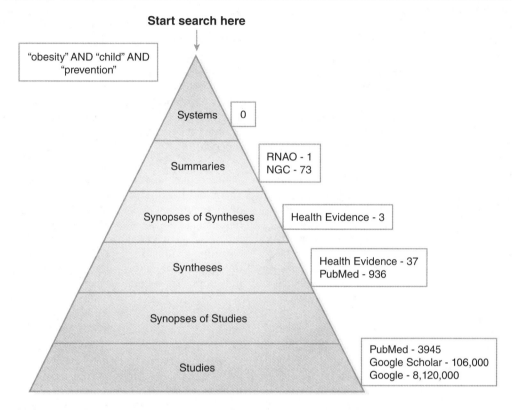

FIGURE 2-6   Search results mapped to 6S pyramid.

Modified from Accessing pre-appraised evidence: fine-tuning the 5S model into a 6S model, DiCenso, Bayley, & Haynes, 2009, 12, 99-101, 2010 with permission from BMJ Publishing Group Ltd.

a limited set of options of known value. The evidence-based practice movement is solidly built on these scientific traditions.

More recently, research generated by thematic analysis of the words people use to describe their experiences, beliefs, opinions, and attitudes has gained legitimacy as a contributor to evidence-based practice in the health care professions. As these qualitative studies have proliferated and their potential value been embraced, a limited effort has been made to help clinicians understand what makes a strong qualitative research design. Daly et al. proposed the four-level hierarchy depicted in **Table 2-5**.[23] Consistent with evidence hierarchies constructed for use with quantitative studies, these authors suggest a progression of increasingly rigorous designs that follow established methods for subject recruitment, data gathering, and analysis. This hierarchy has not been universally adopted by academics, research groups, journal publishers, or professional societies but may be useful to readers unfamiliar with the research methods implemented in this body of work.

			Evidence for
Study Type	**Features**	**Limitations**	**Practice**
Generalizable studies (level I)	Sampling focused by theory and literature, extended as a result of analysis to capture diversity of experience. Analytic procedures comprehensive and clear. Located in literature to assess relevance to other settings.	Main limitations are in reporting when the word length of articles does not allow a comprehensive account of complex procedures.	Clear indications for practice or policy may offer support for current practice, or critique with indicated directions for change.
Conceptual studies (level II)	Theoretical concepts guide sample selection, based on analysis of literature. May be limited to one group about which little is known or a number of important subgroups. Conceptual analysis recognizes diversity in participants' views.	Theoretical concepts and minority or divergent views that emerge during analysis do not lead to further sampling. Categories for analysis may not be saturated.	Weaker designs identify the need for further research on other groups, or urge caution in practice. Well-developed studies can provide good evidence if residual uncertainties are clearly identified.
Descriptive studies (level III)	Sample selected to illustrate practical rather than theoretical issues. Record a range of illustrative quotes including themes from the accounts of "many," "most," or "some" study participants.	Do not report full range of responses. Sample not diversified to analyze how or why differences occur.	Demonstrate that a phenomenon exists in a defined group. Identify practice issues for further consideration.
Single case study (level IV)	Provides rich data on the views or experiences of one person. Can provide insights in unexplored contexts.	Does not analyze applicability to other contexts.	Alerts practitioners to the existence of an unusual phenomenon.

TABLE 2-5   A Hierarchy of Evidence for Practice in Qualitative Research—Summary Features

Reprinted from *Journal of Clinical Epidemiology*, 60(1), Daley J, Willis K, Small R et al., A hierarchy of evidence assessing qualitative health research, 43-49, Copyright 2007, with permission from Elsevier.

Limitations of Evidence Hierarchies

In 2002, the Agency for Healthcare Research and Quality (formerly known as the Agency for Healthcare Policy and Research) published an evidence report entitled "Systems to Rate the Strength of Scientific Evidence."[24] The authors of this report performed an extensive literature review to identify quality assessment methods used to assess the strength of evidence for systematic reviews and meta-analyses, RCTs, observational studies, and diagnostic studies, as well as methods for evaluating the strength of an entire body of evidence on a particular topic. In addition, they examined evidence evaluation methods used by agency-sponsored Evidence-Based Practice Centers and other organizations focused on evidence-based medicine, such as the Cochrane Collaboration.

Of the 121 systems reviewed, only 26 fully addressed quality criteria established by the authors for each type of study. Many of these lengthy systems required an inconvenient amount of time to complete. Also noted was the greater number of quality assessment methods for RCTs as compared with other types of research. The other 95 assessment methods that the authors reviewed were limited in the quality domains addressed, by a "one-size-fits-all" approach that did not distinguish among critical features of different study designs, or by lack of validation. Few of the methods had been tested for reliability or validity. Katrak and colleagues reported similar findings from their investigation into the utility of critical appraisal tools for evaluation of literature relevant to the allied health professions.[25] In an effort to address some of these limitations, Atkins and colleagues conducted a pilot study to refine one of the established grading systems. These authors discovered that statistical agreement among raters on evidence quality ranged from zero to a nearly perfect score (kappa = 0 to 0.82).[26] The take-home message from these reports is that the strength of evidence depends, in part, on the scale against which it is being rated. In response to the potential misuse of evidence grading systems, Glasziou et al. suggested that quality ratings or scales should address different types of research and would be improved by the addition of qualitative statements, as well as more information regarding ratings criteria.[27] More recently, Gugiu and Gugiu proposed a new grading system intended to be more inclusive of treatment studies that are not RCTs.[28, 29]

Understanding the details and bases for evidence hierarchies will help physical therapists select evidence to answer clinical questions about patients or clients. However, a hierarchy is only a tool to facilitate the process; it should not be used to make a final judgment about a study's value and relevance. Physical therapists must still read and critically appraise the evidence they find, whether it is a single study or a filtered synthesis of a collection of studies, before incorporating any results into their clinical decisions. This point is emphasized by an ongoing debate about the relative merits of RCTs versus quasi-experimental and observational studies. Some evidence indicates that the bias in the latter study designs results in overestimations of treatment effects, whereas other authors have reported that none of the study designs consistently estimate an intervention's impact.[30-32] Clinical judgment and expertise are essential to EBPT practice. The variability in research quality requires that physical therapists use their knowledge and skills to determine whether the evidence they find, no matter how high or low on a hierarchy, is useful for an individual patient or client.

Summary

EBPT practice requires clinicians to select the "best available clinical evidence" from studies whose quality depends on their relevance to the question asked, their timeliness, and the level of prior scrutiny of their merits, as well as on their research design and execution. Evidence hierarchies may facilitate study selection because of the ranking structure they create based on important research attributes. Different hierarchies have been designed to address evidence about diagnostic tests, prognostic indicators, and interventions. Producers of clinical practice guidelines also have defined various levels of evidence to demonstrate the degree to which their recommendations are supported by research. No matter what form a hierarchy takes, it is only a tool to facilitate the process; it should not be used to make a final judgment about a study's value and relevance. Physical therapists must still read and critically appraise the evidence they find before incorporating any results into their clinical decisions.

Exercises

1. What does the phrase "best available clinical evidence" mean with respect to a physical therapist's selection and use of studies?
2. Discuss the differences between a randomized controlled trial and an observational study. Under which circumstances might each study design be appropriate? Provide examples of each relevant to physical therapist practice to illustrate your points.
3. Discuss the difference between a retrospective and prospective research design and give an example of each that reflects a study question relevant to physical therapist practice.
4. Discuss the difference between a cross-sectional research design and a longitudinal research design and give an example of each that reflects a study question relevant to physical therapist practice.
5. Explain the importance of similarities between an individual patient or client and subjects in a research study. Provide three examples of personal or clinical characteristics from a patient with whom you have worked recently to illustrate your points.
6. Describe the common organizational characteristics of evidence hierarchies.
7. Discuss the rationale behind the creation of different hierarchies for evidence about diagnostic tests, prognostic factors, and interventions.
8. Discuss the potential difference in value between preappraised collections of individual studies and individual research reports. Why is the hierarchy for preappraised collections structured the way that it is?
9. Discuss the limitations of evidence hierarchies. Why is a hierarchy only a starting point in EBPT practice?

References

1. Helewa A, Walker JM. *Critical Evaluation of Research in Physical Rehabilitation: Towards Evidence-Based Practice.* Philadelphia, PA: W.B. Saunders; 2000.
2. McEwen I. *Writing Case Reports: A How-to Manual for Clinicians.* 3rd ed. Alexandria, VA: American Physical Therapy Association; 2009.
3. Information for Authors: "Full" Traditional Case Reports. Available at: http://ptjournal.apta.org/content /information-authors-full-traditional-case-reports. Accessed July 31, 2016.
4. Graham R, Mancher M, Wolman DM, Greenfield S, Steinberg E, eds. *Clinical Practice Guidelines We Can Trust.* Available at: http://www.nap.edu/catalog/13058/clinical-practice-guidelines-we-can-trust. Accessed July 31, 2016.
5. DiCenso A, Bayley L, Haynes RB. Accessing pre-appraised evidence: fine-tuning the 5S model into a 6S model. *Evid Based Nurs.* 2009;12(4):99–101.
6. Straus SE, Richardson WS, Glaziou P, Haynes RB. *Evidence-Based Medicine: How to Practice and Teach EBM.* 3rd ed. Edinburgh, Scotland: Elsevier Churchill Livingstone; 2005.
7. Guyatt G, Rennie D. *Users' Guides to the Medical Literature: A Manual for Evidence-Based Clinical Practice.* Chicago, IL: AMA Press; 2002.
8. Carter RE, Lubinsky J, Domholdt E. *Rehabilitation Research: Principles and Applications.* 4th ed. St Louis, MO: Elsevier Saunders; 2011.
9. Campbell DT, Stanley JC. *Experimental and Quasi-Experimental Designs for Research.* Boston, MA: Houghton Mifflin; 1963.

10. Herbert R, Jamtvedt G, Hagen KB, Mead J. *Practical Evidence-Based Physiotherapy*. 2nd ed. Edinburgh, Scotland: Elsevier Butterworth-Heinemann; 2011.

11. Cook TD, Campbell DT. *Quasi-Experimentation: Design and Analysis Issues for Field Settings*. Boston, MA: Houghton Mifflin; 1979.

12. Sackett DL, Rosenberg WMC, Gray JAM, Haynes RB, Richardson WS. Evidence-based medicine: what it is and what it isn't. *BMJ*. 1996;312(7023):71–72.

13. Disease Modification. National Multiple Sclerosis Society website. Available at: http://www.nationalmssociety .org/For-Professionals/Clinical-Care/Managing-MS/Disease-Modification. Accessed August 1, 2016.

14. Winstein CJ, Lewthwaite R. Efficacy and Effectiveness: Issues for Physical Therapy Practice and Research. Examples from PTClinResNet. Eugene Michels Forum. Combined Sections Meeting. American Physical Therapy Association. 2004. Available at: http://www.ptresearch.org/members/Weinstein.pdf. Accessed August 1, 2016.

15. Jette DU, Bacon K, Batty C, et al. Evidence-based practice: beliefs, attitudes, knowledge, and behaviors of physical therapists. *Phys Ther*. 2003;83(9):786–805.

16. Howick J, Chalmers I, Glasziou P, et al. Explanation of the 2011 Oxford Centre for Evidence-Based Medicine (OCEBM) Levels of Evidence (Background Document). Oxford Centre for Evidence-Based Medicine. Available at: www.cebm.net/index.aspx?o=5653. Accessed August 1, 2016.

17. Howick J, Chalmers I, Glasziou P, et al. The 2011 Oxford CEBM Levels of Evidence (Introductory Document). Oxford Centre for Evidence-Based Medicine. Available at: www.cebm.net/index.aspx?o=5653. Accessed August 1, 2016.

18. OCEBM Levels of Evidence Working Group. The Oxford Levels of Evidence 2. Oxford Centre for Evidence-Based Medicine. Available at: http://www.cebm.net/wp-content/uploads/2014/06/CEBM-Levels-of-Evidence -2.1.pdf. Accessed August 1, 2016.

19. Department of Veterans Affairs, Department of Defense. VA/DoD Clinical Practice Guideline: Management of Concussion/Mild Traumatic Brain Injury. Washington, DC: Department of Veterans Affairs, Department of Defense; 2016. Available at: http://www.healthquality.va.gov/guidelines/Rehab/mtbi/. Accessed August 8, 2016.

20. Bolton CE, Brevin-Smith EF, Blakey JD, et al. The BTS guideline on pulmonary rehabilitation in adults. *Thorax*. 2013;68(S2):ii1–ii30.

21. Enseki K, Harris-Hayes M, White DM, et al. Nonarthritic hip joint pain. *JOSPT*. 2014;44(6):A1–A32.

22. Robeson P, Dobbins M, DeCorby K, et al. Facilitating access to pre-processed research evidence in public health. *BMC Public Health*. 2010;95.

23. Daley J, Willis K, Small R, et al. A hierarchy of evidence assessing qualitative health research. *J Clin Epidemiol*. 2007;60(1):43–49.

24. West S, King V, Carey TS, et al. Systems to Rate the Strength of Scientific Evidence. Evidence Report/ Technology Assessment Number 47. (Prepared by the Research Triangle Institute–University of North Carolina Evidence-Based Practice Center under Contract No. 290-97-0011.) AHRQ Publication No. 02-E016. Rockville, MD: Agency for Health Care Research and Quality; April 2002.

25. Katrak P, Bialocerkowski AE, Massy-Westropp N, et al. A systematic review of the content of critical appraisal tools. *BMC Med Res Methodol*. 2004;4(22).

26. Atkins D, Briss PA, Eccles M, et al. Systems for grading the quality of evidence and strength of recommendations II: pilot study of a new system. *BMC Health Serv Res*. 2005;5(1):25.

27. Glasziou P, Vandenbroucke J, Chalmer I. Assessing the quality of research. *BMJ*. 2004;328(7430):39–41.

28. Gugiu PC, Gugiu MR. A critical appraisal of standard guidelines for grading levels of evidence. *Eval Health Prof*. 2010;33(3):233–255.

29. Gugiu PC. Hierarchy of evidence and appraisal limitations (HEAL) grading system. *Eval Program Plann*. 2015;48:149–159.

30. Britton A, McKee M, Black N, McPherson K, Sanderson C, Bain C. Choosing between randomised and non-randomised studies: a systematic review. *Health Technol Assess*. 1998;2(13):i–iv,1–124.

31. MacLehose RR, Reeves BC, Harvey IM, Sheldon TA, Russell IT, Black AM. A systematic review of comparisons of effect sizes derived from randomised and non-randomised studies. *Health Technol Assess*. 2000;4(34):1–154.

32. Glasziou P, Chalmers I, Rawlins M, McCulloch P. When are randomised trials unnecessary? Picking signal from noise. *BMJ*. 2007;334(7589):349–351.

CHAPTER 3

THE QUEST FOR EVIDENCE: GETTING STARTED

OBJECTIVES

Upon completion of this chapter, the student/practitioner will be able to do the following:

1. Distinguish between, and provide examples of, background and foreground clinical questions.

2. Write questions pertaining to each of these aspects of physical therapist practice:

   a. Diagnostic tests and clinical measures;

   b. Prognostic factors;

   c. Interventions;

   d. Clinical prediction rules;

   e. Outcomes;

   f. Self-report outcomes measures; and,

   g. Patient or client perspectives or experiences.

3. Use electronic databases reviewed in this chapter to search for evidence about a clinical question.

4. Identify research review services that may be helpful in physical therapist practice.

TERMS IN THIS CHAPTER

Boolean operators: Words such as "and," "or," "not," and "near" that are used to combine search terms in electronic evidence databases and other search engines.

Clinical practice guidelines: ". . . statements that include recommendations intended to optimize patient care. They are informed by a systematic review of evidence and an assessment of the benefits and harms of alternative care options."[1]; also referred to as "summaries."[2]

Database: A structured set of information (data) used for rapid search and retrieval purposes.

Diagnosis: A process of "integrating and evaluating the data that are obtained during the examination to describe the individual condition in terms that will guide the physical therapist in determining the prognosis and developing a plan of care."[3]

Examination: "Physical therapists conduct a history, perform a systems review, and use tests and measures in order to describe and/or quantify an individual's need for services."[3]

Hits: A term used to indicate the records retrieved by an electronic search engine that meet the criteria entered into the search function.

Intervention: "Physical therapists purposefully interact with the individual and, when appropriate, with other people involved in his or her care, using various" procedures or techniques "to produce changes in the condition."[3]

Keyword(s): The word(s) or term(s) that is/are entered into an electronic database search function to locate evidence pertaining to a clinical question.

Measurement reliability: The extent to which repeated measurements agree with one another. Also referred to as "stability," "consistency," and "reproducibility."[4]

Measurement validity: The degree to which a measure captures what it is intended to measure.[4]

MeSH: Abbreviation for "Medical Subject Heading"; the term used to describe approved search vocabulary in the U.S. National Library of Medicine electronic database (PubMed); the MeSH vocabulary also may be used by other electronic evidence databases.

Outcome: "The actual results of implementing the plan of care that indicate the impact on functioning"; may be measured by the physical therapist or determined by self-report from the patient or client.[3]

Primary sources: Original research reports such as articles in peer-reviewed journals or on websites, theses and dissertations, and proceedings from professional meetings.[5]

Prognosis: "The determination of the predicted optimal level of improvement in function and the amount of time needed to reach that level and also may include a prediction of levels of improvement that may be reached at various intervals during the course of therapy."[3]

Responsiveness: The ability of a measure to detect change in the phenomenon of interest.

Search engine: A computer software program used to search and identify records in a database or on the World Wide Web (the Web) using characteristics such as words, phrases, numbers, and dates.

Search string: A combination of keywords, phrases, names, or other information that is entered into an electronic database search function to locate evidence pertaining to a clinical question.

Secondary sources: Textbooks, summaries on websites, and review papers that contain information based on primary sources of information.[5]

Synopsis: "A succinct description of selected individual studies or systematic reviews."[2]

Systematic review: A method by which a collection of individual research studies is gathered and critically appraised in an effort to reach an unbiased conclusion about the cumulative weight of the evidence on a particular topic[6]; also referred to as "syntheses."[2]

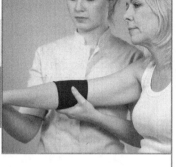

© Photographee.eu/Shutterstock

CLINICAL SCENARIO

Searching for Evidence Relevant to Anne's Situation

Anne searched the Internet trying to learn more about her condition and the options available for treating it. She reported that she located several websites from medical associations, a few from nationally recognized hospitals, and some medically oriented consumer information portals. She learned that her problem is due to overuse and that it could go away on its own but that waiting for a natural resolution could take months. She wants to recover more quickly than that but could not discern which of the treatment techniques available would do the trick.

How will you describe your efforts to locate evidence to guide your collaborative decision making?

Introduction

The first step toward evidence-based physical therapist (EBPT) practice is a professional commitment to make the attempt as best one can, given individual work environments and resource constraints. Once that commitment is made, the next step is to consider the questions that arise during the daily management of a patient or client's problems or needs. These questions direct the search for evidence that may inform clinical decision making. This chapter focuses on the types of questions physical therapists and their patients or clients might ask. Several electronic databases and search techniques that are available to support the quest for evidence are described in this chapter.

Formulating Clinical Questions

EBPT practice starts and ends with a physical therapist's patient or client. As the therapeutic relationship develops, questions naturally arise regarding the individual's problems and concerns and the best course of action with which to address them. Questions may pertain to (1) the anatomic, physiologic, or pathophysiologic nature of the problem or issue; (2) the medical and surgical management options; (3) the usefulness of diagnostic tests and clinical measures to identify, classify, and/or quantify the problem; (4) which factors will predict the patient or client's future health status; (5) the benefits and risks of potential interventions; (6) the utility of clinical prediction rules; (7) the nature of the outcomes themselves and how to measure them; and/or (8) the perspectives and experiences of others with similar problems or issues. Any of these questions may prompt a search for evidence to help inform the answer.

When formulating a clinical question, it is important to consider how that question is phrased. Questions designed to increase understanding about a situation (numbers 1 and 2 above) are different than questions used to facilitate clinical decision making (numbers 3 to 8). These different forms are referred to as "background questions" and "foreground questions," respectively.[6,7]

Background Questions

Background questions reflect a desire to understand the nature of an individual's problem or need. Often these questions focus on the natural evolution of a condition and its medical or surgical management rather than on the physical therapy component. Here are some examples:

- "What are the side effects of steroid treatment for asthma?"
- "How long will it take for a total knee arthroplasty incision to heal?"
- "What are the signs and symptoms of an exacerbation of multiple sclerosis?"
- "Will it be possible to play baseball again after elbow surgery?"

Understandably, these are the most common types of questions that patients or clients and their families will ask. In addition, these questions are typical of professional physical therapy students and new graduates who are still learning about the many clinical scenarios they may encounter in practice. Experienced clinicians, in contrast, will use background questions when a new or unusual situation is encountered (e.g., functional consequences of acquired immune deficiency syndrome [AIDS]), when entering a new practice area (e.g., transferring from the acute hospital orthopedic team to the oncology team), or when returning to practice after a significant absence. Answers to background questions help therapists to understand the clinical context of their patient or client's situation so that an individual's needs can be anticipated and planned for accordingly. Precautions, contraindications, exercise limits, and other parameters may be determined based on evidence gathered to answer background questions.

Research articles often contain information relevant to background questions in their introductory paragraphs. However, searching for original evidence pertaining to these types of questions generally is not the most efficient approach to take. Government agencies, professional societies, and national patient advocacy groups often vet this type of information and publish it for clinicians and consumers in written and electronic formats. **Table 3-1** provides some representative examples. Content posted on the web often is updated more frequently than content in printed materials. However, textbooks also may provide answers to background questions. Readers are cautioned to consider a book's publication date and the likelihood that knowledge will have evolved since that time before accepting information from these sources at face value.

Foreground Questions

Foreground questions are the heart of EBPT practice. These questions help clinicians and their patients or clients make decisions about the specific physical therapist management of their problem or concern. Foreground questions contain four key elements originally referred to with the acronym "PICO" (population, intervention, comparison, outcome).[6-8] Given the full scope of physical therapist practice elements that may prompt a search for relevant evidence, a modification to the acronym suggested by Hoffman et al. is adopted for this text:[9]

- P = person, problem, or population (i.e., relevant personal and/or clinical details such as age, gender, diagnosis, acuity, severity, and/or preferences);
- I = issue (i.e., diagnostic test, clinical measure, prognostic factor, intervention, clinical prediction rule, outcome, self-report outcome measure of interest, patient or client perspective);
- C = comparison (i.e., a comparison test, measure, predictive factor, intervention, clinical prediction rule, outcome, or self-report outcome measure);] and,
- O = outcome (i.e., the consequence[s] of applying or including the issue of interest).

TABLE 3-1	Examples of Potential Sources of Answers to Background Questions	

Name	Type of Source	Helpful Links
Centers for Disease Control and Prevention	Government	www.cdc.gov/Diseases Conditions/
		www.cdc.gov/HealthyLiving/
		www.cdc.gov/DataStatistics/
National Institutes of Health	Government	http://health.nih.gov/
American Heart Association	Professional Society	www.heart.org/HEARTORG /Conditions/Conditions_UCM _001087_SubHomePage.jsp
American Physical Therapy Association	Professional Society	www.moveforwardpt.com /Default.aspx
National Coalition for Cancer Survivorship	Patient Advocacy	https://www.canceradvocacy .org
National Down Syndrome Society	Patient Advocacy	www.ndss.org/Resources /Health-Care/

The first and second components are included because a good foreground question has sufficient detail to search for answers that are specific to the individual about whom the question is asked. The third component, a comparison, is in brackets because there may be times when a simpler question is indicated or when a comparison simply is not available. Clinicians with more expertise in a particular content area may find it easier to ask comparative questions by virtue of their knowledge about a variety of options for diagnostic tests, clinical measures, predictive factors, interventions, clinical prediction rules, outcomes, self-report outcomes measures and patient or client perspectives. Finally, the fourth component of a foreground question refers to what the therapist and patient or client hopes to achieve during the management step about which the question is raised.

Although questions about diagnostic tests, clinical measures, prognostic factors, interventions, clinical prediction rules, outcomes, self-report outcomes measures and patient or client perspectives have this basic structure in common, they also have unique features that are important to recognize. The following sections outline details about each type of question. **Table 3-2** provides examples of simple and comparative questions for each content area. Each element of the foreground question acronym is noted in parentheses.

Questions About Diagnostic Tests

Diagnosis is a process by which physical therapists label and classify an individual's problem or need.[3,] Tests used during the physical therapist's *examination* provide the objective data for the diagnostic process. Foreground questions about diagnostic tests usually focus on which tests will provide the most accurate and persuasive information (e.g., the likelihood that an individual has the condition of interest) in a timely manner with the least amount of risk, cost, or both.

TABLE 3-2	Foreground Questions Physical Therapists Might Ask About Diagnostic Tests, Clinical Measures, Prognostic Factors, Interventions, Clinical Prediction Rules, Outcomes, Self-Report Outcomes Measures and Patient or Client Perspectives	
	Foreground Questions: Simple	**Foreground Questions: Comparative**
Diagnostic Test	Will the Neer's test (I) help me to detect rotator cuff impingement (O) in a 35-year-old male tennis player with shoulder pain (P)?	Is the Neer's test (I) more accurate than the lift-off test (C) for detecting rotator cuff impingement (O) in a 35-year-old male tennis player with shoulder pain (P)?
Clinical Measure	Is a manual muscle test (I) a reliable and valid measure of quadriceps strength (O) in a 42-year-old woman with multiple sclerosis (P)?	Is a manual muscle test (I) as reliable and valid as a handheld dynamometer (C) for measuring quadriceps strength (O) in a 42-year-old woman with multiple sclerosis (P)?
Prognostic Factor	Is lower extremity muscle strength (I) a predictor of fall risk (O) in a 76-year-old woman with diabetes (P)?	Which is a more accurate predictor of fall risk (O), lower extremity muscle strength (I) or proprioception (C), in a 76-year-old woman with diabetes (P)?
Intervention	Is proprioceptive neuromuscular facilitation (PNF) (I) an effective treatment technique for restoring core trunk stability (O) in a 7-year-old child with right hemiparesis due to stroke (P)?	Is PNF (I) more effective than the neurodevelopmental technique (NDT) (C) for restoring core trunk stability (O) in a 7-year-old child with right hemiparesis due to stroke (P)?
Clinical Prediction Rule	Are the Ottawa Ankle Rules (I) a valid clinical prediction rule to determine the need for a radiograph (O) in an 11-year-old child with ankle pain after a fall on an icy surface (P)?	Which is a more valid clinical prediction rule to determine the need for a radiograph (O) in an 11-year-old child with ankle pain after a fall on an icy surface (P): the Ottawa Ankle Rules (I) or the Malleolar Zone Algorithm (C)?
Outcomes	Does participation in a cardiac rehabilitation program (I) increase the chance that a 58-year-old man who has had a myocardial infarction (P) will return to work (O)?	Does participation in a cardiac rehabilitation program (I) increase the chance of returning to work (O) more than a home walking program (C) for a 58-year-old man following a myocardial infarction (P)?

	Foreground Questions: Simple	**Foreground Questions: Comparative**
Self-Report Outcomes Measure	Will the Minnesota Living with Heart Failure Questionnaire (ML-HFQ) (I) detect change following rehabilitation (O) in an 82-year-old woman with chronic heart failure (P)?	Which instrument is more sensitive to change following rehabilitation (O) for an 82-year-old woman with chronic heart failure (P): the MLHFQ (I) or the Chronic Heart Failure Questionnaire (CHFQ) (C)?
Patient or Client Perspective	Will a 66-year-old homeless man (P) perceive as helpful (O) the implementation of a physical activity program at a local shelter (I)?	When considering homeless individuals (P), do perceptions about the helpfulness (O) of a physical activity program (I) differ between males and females (C)?

Questions About Clinical Measures

Clinical measures are distinct from diagnostic tests in that they are not used to detect the presence of, or put a label on, a suspected condition per se. Instead, they are used to quantify and/ or describe in a standardized fashion a person's impairments in body functions and structures as well as activity limitations and participation restrictions. Foreground questions about clinical measures usually focus on assessments of *measurement reliability*, *measurement validity*, and *responsiveness*.

Questions About Prognostic Factors

Prognosis is the process by which therapists make predictions about an individual's future health status.[3] Foreground questions about prognostic factors arise because therapists and patients or clients want to know which pieces of information—collectively referred to as indicators, predictors, or factors—are most important to consider when predicting the outcomes of preventive activities, interventions, or inaction. Predictors often take the form of demographic information such as age, gender, race/ethnicity, income, education, and social support; disorder-related information such as stage, severity, time since onset, recurrence, and compliance with a treatment program; and/or the presence of comorbid conditions.[7]

Questions About Interventions

Interventions are the techniques and procedures physical therapists use to produce a change in an individual's body structures and functions, activity limitations, and/or participation restrictions.[3] Foreground questions about interventions may focus on the benefits or risks of a treatment technique, or both. The goal is to identify which treatment approaches will provide the desired effect in a safe manner consistent with an individual's preferences and values. Additional objectives may include a desire to expedite the treatment process and minimize costs.

Questions About Clinical Prediction Rules

Clinical prediction rules are systematically derived and statistically tested combinations of clinical findings that provide meaningful predictions about an outcome of interest. An outcome of interest may be classification in a diagnostic category, calculation of a prognostic estimate, or anticipation of a treatment response.[10-12] Foreground questions about these algorithms focus on the accuracy of their predictions and the circumstances in which their performance is most useful.

Questions About Outcomes and Self-Report Outcomes Measures

Outcomes are the end results of the patient or client management process.[3] Questions about outcomes may focus on the type of end point(s) possible in response to a particular treatment or on the methods by which the end point can be measured. Outcomes are likely to have the most relevance for an individual when they pertain to activities and participation as performed in the context of the individual's daily life.

Of particular clinical interest is the usefulness of self-report instruments that measure outcomes from an individual's point of view. These tools usually focus on the impact of a disorder or condition on a patient's health-related quality of life. Foreground questions about these instruments focus on their ability to capture relevant information, their responsiveness to change in a patient or client's status, and their ease of administration and processing.

Questions About the Meaning of the Health Care Experience

The experience of health, illness, and disability is personal to each individual and is shaped by his or her unique perspectives, beliefs, attitudes, and opinions as well as by cultural context. Understanding how a person perceives and interprets what is happening to him or her is central to the therapeutic relationship physical therapists develop with their patients or clients. Questions directed toward exploring these subjective constructions of the health care experience can help physical therapists anticipate the potential appropriateness, practicality, and acceptance of options being considered for a plan of care.

Searching for Evidence

Once a person-centered clinical question is formulated, it is important to plan a general search strategy before diving into the various sources of evidence available. The following five steps are recommended as a starting point.

Determine Which Database Will Be Most Useful

An enormous variety of sources is available through which a physical therapist may search for evidence, many of which are available through the Internet. As these electronic *databases* have proliferated, their focus areas have evolved. Some are broad based and cover any type of background or foreground question (e.g., Medline/PubMed); others only focus on specific elements of patient or client management such as interventions (e.g., Physiotherapy Evidence Database [PEDro]). Most databases list citations of individual original works (e.g., Cumulative Index to Nursing and Allied Health Literature [CINAHL]), whereas others provide syntheses or reviews of collections of research articles (e.g., National Guideline Clearinghouse). Some only address questions specific to physical therapist patient/client management (e.g., PTNow); others cover a wider range of medical and allied health topics (e.g., Cochrane Library). Familiarity with the options will help a physical therapist select the database that will provide citations for evidence about the clinical question in an efficient manner.

Readers may be tempted to use more general Web-based *search engines* such as Google Scholar (http://scholar.google.com) or Yahoo Education (http://education.yahoo.com) because they are familiar to frequent Web users. These types of services have a user-friendly feel to them and have evolved over the last several years to mimic traditional scholarly databases. In addition, recent studies have demonstrated that citation identification accuracy is comparable or better than that of more traditional biomedical search engines.[13,14] However, because they are general search engines, Google Scholar and other similar services are not designed to search efficiently through a designated collection of resources devoted to medical or physical therapist practice. In addition, they do not have clinically relevant search features, such as the ability to restrict the search according to patient characteristics or type of research design. They also often rank articles according to the frequency with which they have been cited by other authors, which may provide inconsistent results and bias the information provided away from contemporary works with newer information.[15] These limitations mean that evidence to answer a question may be missed or that irrelevant information may be returned. Finally, they may or may not provide access to the online journals in which the evidence is published. As a result, evidence-based physical therapists should spend the time necessary to learn the features of the databases described in this chapter and save Google and Yahoo for other types of searches.

Identify Search Terms to Enter into the Database

All electronic databases and search engines require input from the user to start the search. The most common form of input is a *keyword*, or search term that will be used to identify relevant information. In EBPT practice, the keywords are derived directly from the clinical question of interest. Consider the following example:

> *"Does age and prior functional status (I) predict discharge to home following inpatient rehabilitation (O) for a fractured hip in a 92-year-old woman (P)?"*

Possible keywords from this question include "age," "functional status," "predict," "discharge," "home," "inpatient," "rehabilitation," "fracture," "hip," and "woman." Additional terms may be used to reflect concepts in the question such as "function" instead of "functional status" and "elderly" in place of "92-year-old." Finally, some of the words may be combined into phrases, such as "inpatient rehabilitation" and "hip fracture," to provide a more accurate representation of the question's content.

The challenge is to determine which combination of these keywords and phrases will produce the most efficient *search string*. One option is to start simply by using a few words or phrases, such as "predict," "discharge," and "hip fracture." This approach may improve the chances of identifying a wide variety of evidence because of the general nature of the terms. However, the question addresses specific predictive factors, namely age and prior functional status, in an elderly woman. The second option, therefore, is to include more keywords or phrases to narrow the search to evidence directly addressing the question.

In addition to these decisions, therapists also should consider other synonyms that may be useful or necessary to enhance the search. Relevant synonyms in this example include "femur" for "hip" and "female" for "woman." Synonyms come in handy when a search for evidence returns no citations. Evidence-based health care databases usually have specific keyword vocabularies, or "index terms," that are used to build queries. Familiarity with these vocabularies is essential to optimize the efficiency of the search.

Use Search Configuration Options to Streamline the Process

Every electronic database and search engine has rules that determine which keywords it will recognize and what letter size (case) and punctuation must be used when entering search terms. Words such as "and," "or," "not," and "near"—collectively referred to as *Boolean operators*—are used universally to create search term combinations. Configuration options also include methods to limit or to expand the search. Search filters may include the language in which the evidence was written, publication date, type of research design, and search basis, such as keyword, author, or journal name. Choices might also be available regarding subject characteristics, such as age and gender. Selecting from these options allows the user to keep the number of search terms to a minimum because the search function is "programmed" to work within the specified parameters. Finally, a method for including synonyms or related terms (referred to as "exploding" the search term) usually is available. Some electronic databases and search engines make these rules and choices apparent by the way that they format their search pages. Others require some effort to hunt for the information through the "search help" features. In either case, spending some time on the front end learning these details will save time and frustration during the search.

Be Prepared to Reformulate the Question

A common problem during an evidence search is either an excessive number of citations (or *hits*) or none at all. When this situation happens, the first thing to do is go back to the database features and determine if there are additional options to narrow or expand the search. Keyword and phrase substitutions also may be required. If these approaches are unsuccessful, then it may be time to revise the question. Consider the following example:

> "Which is more effective for symptom management (O), aquatic (I) or land-based (C) exercise, in a middle-aged man with joint pain (P)?"

Too many hits using keywords from this question likely indicates that the question is too broad. There are several options for revising the question into a more precise form, including:

1. Using a more specific diagnostic label such as "degenerative joint disease" or "rheumatoid arthritis" instead of the general phrase "joint pain";
2. Adding more specific details about the individual, such as his age; and/or
3. Using a more specific outcome, such as "pain relief" instead of "symptom management."

A revised question might read

> "Which is more effective for pain relief, aquatic or land-based exercise, in a 58-year-old man diagnosed with rheumatoid arthritis?"

In contrast, too few hits may indicate that the question is too specific or that no evidence is yet available to answer it. In that case a broader question may be useful, such as

> "Is exercise effective for pain relief in a man with arthritis?"

Keep in mind that as questions become more general, there is a greater chance the evidence located will contain information that is not directly related to the current situation. For example, subjects in a study may be older than the patient or the intervention may be a home walking program rather than a program supervised in the clinic. In these situations, physical therapists must use their clinical expertise and judgment to determine whether the study is relevant and whether there is enough in common between the patient or client and the subjects studied to extrapolate the results to this specific situation.

In extreme cases there may be difficulty finding any physical therapy–related evidence for a patient or client's disease, disorder, or need. Physical therapist management of the sequelae of heart disease is a common example of such a situation. In these instances, it may be helpful to search for evidence that includes providers other than physical therapists (e.g., exercise physiologists, nurses). Once again, clinical expertise and judgment will be required to determine if it is safe and appropriate to extrapolate and apply any findings from this general evidence to the physical therapist management of an individual patient or client.

Aim for the Highest Quality Evidence Available

The two general sources of evidence are described as primary and secondary. *Primary sources* provide individual original research reports via peer-reviewed journals and websites, theses and dissertations, and proceedings from professional meetings. *Secondary sources*, such as textbooks, summaries on websites, and review papers, contain information based on primary sources.[5] Traditionally, primary sources of evidence have been preferred because they provide the original works about which the physical therapist can make an independent critical appraisal. As evidence about clinical questions has expanded, however, the ability to draw more accurate and precise conclusions based on a collection of individual studies has become possible. Individual and collaborative groups of researchers, as well as professional societies, have developed summaries and *systematic reviews* of individual literature. These secondary sources of evidence are valued because of the comprehensive and rigorous methodology used to search for, select, and appraise original works about a particular topic. They have the added benefit of reducing the time a busy clinician may spend trying to locate the best available evidence. Evidence hierarchies have been developed to expedite the process of identifying high-quality evidence from primary and secondary sources.

Electronic Databases for Evidence-Based Physical Therapist Practice

As mentioned earlier, a variety of electronic databases are available to search for evidence. This section reviews important features of five that are likely to be most relevant to physical therapists. An entire textbook could be devoted to all of the details required to master searches in each database! Fortunately, numerous "help" and tutorial functions are available to guide a user through the process. You should plan to spend time on the computer using these functions to learn more about each database and to explore the features highlighted here.

U.S. National Library of Medicine: PubMed

The U.S. National Library of Medicine has developed a bibliographic database of basic and applied research citations dating back to the late 1800s. The electronic version, PubMed, contains over 26 million citations starting from the 1950s (**Figure 3-1**).[16]

This search engine has several advantages because it:

- Is free to the public;
- Is comprehensive;
- Contains links to online journals that provide full text versions of articles; and
- Has rigorous standards for determining which journals will be listed (i.e., indexed).

Challenges with the database include its size, the complexity of keyword searches, and its exclusion of several physical therapy and other allied health journals due to its indexing standards.

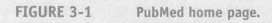

FIGURE 3-1   PubMed home page.

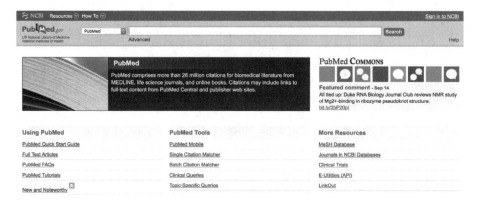

Screenshot from PubMed (www.pubmed.gov), National Center for Biotechnology Information, U.S. National Library of Medicine, Bethesda, MD, USA, and the National Institutes of Health. Accessed September 1, 2016.

Medical Subject Headings (MeSH)

The complexity of searches in PubMed relates in part to the database's use of the Medical Subject Heading (*MeSH*) vocabulary to determine which keywords will be recognized in the indexing process. As explained on the National Network of Libraries of Medicine website, "MeSH provides a consistent way to retrieve information where different terms are used by authors for the same concept."[17] The MeSH database can be accessed through a link on the right-hand side of the PubMed home page (Figure 3-1). Key features to understand include the ability to select subheadings under a MeSH term, as well as the ability to expand the search to include subcategories of MeSH terms.

Recall the hypothetical clinical question:

"Which is more effective for pain relief (O), aquatic (I) or land-based (C) exercise, in a 58-year-old man diagnosed with rheumatoid arthritis (P)?"

A search for the words "rheumatoid arthritis" reveals that the condition is listed in the MeSH vocabulary. The word "aquatic" is primarily related to organisms that live in water. The synonym "water" is associated with 82 MeSH terms, all of which relate to the chemical composition and properties of the substance. A term for the clinical use of water—"hydrotherapy"—is located in the MeSH database and defined as the "external application of water for therapeutic purposes." The word "exercise" as intended in the clinical question is most accurately characterized by the MeSH term "exercise therapy." Situations like these reinforce the need to think of synonyms for keywords before starting a search so that roadblocks to the process can be addressed efficiently. **Figure 3-2** illustrates MeSH term search results as well as the PubMed query field with the selected MeSH vocabulary terms combined in a search string. Note that when using the MeSH search box Boolean operators are entered automatically and do not need to be typed in by the user. Once the MeSH terms are selected, a search can be executed along with any limits the physical therapist chooses.

FIGURE 3-2 **PubMed MeSH terms results page.**

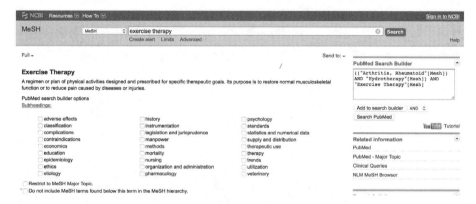

Screenshot from PubMed (www.pubmed.gov), National Center for Biotechnology Information, U.S. National Library of Medicine, Bethesda, MD, USA, and the National Institutes of Health. Accessed September 1, 2016.

General Keyword Search

An alternative to using the MeSH vocabulary is to type keywords or phrases directly into the search box on the PubMed home page. Users may create various combinations of terms with this freestyle approach; however, keyword choice becomes more challenging because the database does not provide definitions of terms it recognizes through this general search feature. **Figure 3-3** illustrates an example using the general keyword search field. Note that the word "AND" must be typed using uppercase, or capital, letters to be recognized as a Boolean operator in PubMed. This example also demonstrates what can happen when an ineffective keyword combination is selected without use of additional parameters with which to limit the search. The terms "arthritis" and "exercise" are so broad that 5,964 hits are returned—too many citations to read through efficiently.

Search Filters

One method available to enhance the efficiency of a search in PubMed is to use the "Filters" function. This feature provides a variety of menus to help direct a search. Because EBPT practice is a person-centered endeavor, it is often practical to select "human" for study subjects. Selection of the language choice "English" is helpful to avoid retrievals of evidence written in a foreign language in which the therapist is not fluent. Users may choose to restrict where the search engine looks for the keywords or phrases by selecting an option such as "title" or "title/abstract" so that only the most relevant hits will be identified. However, this tactic may result in missed citations because abstracts are limited in length and simply may not contain the keywords of interest.

A search also may be restricted to author name or journal. Other filter options include specifying the age range and gender of the subjects studied, the type of article desired (e.g., clinical trial, practice guideline), the date the citation was entered into PubMed, and the article's publication date. Keep in mind that numerous limits may result in too few or no citations. If that is the case, then filters should be changed or removed one at a time and the search repeated.

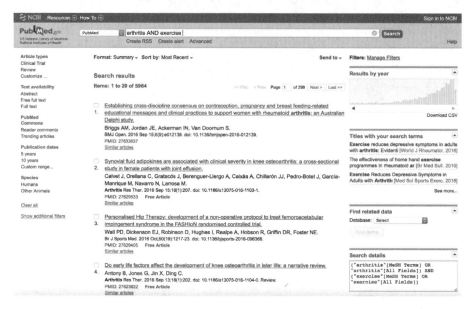

FIGURE 3-3   Search results using general keyword terms without filters in PubMed.

Screenshot from PubMed (www.pubmed.gov), National Center for Biotechnology Information, U.S. National Library of Medicine, Bethesda, MD, USA, and the National Institutes of Health. Accessed September 1, 2016.

Figure 3-4 illustrates an example of a keyword search using the limits "clinical trials," "systematic reviews," "English," "humans," "male," and "middle-aged: 45–64." Note that the keywords used are more specific to the clinical question posed.

Two of the articles returned appear specific to the clinical question based on their titles. However, it is possible that the search limits were too restrictive given the small number of hits overall. The results of searches performed with fewer limits are depicted in **Table 3-3**; the progressive increase in the number of hits bears out this assessment of the initial search parameters. Interestingly, three of the citations were not directly relevant to the clinical question, a reminder about the value of using the MeSH vocabulary in the PubMed system. Other titles are related to the search terms but appear to include subjects whose characteristics are different from the patient about whom the clinical question was posed. Filter options also can be applied when searches are conducted using the MeSH vocabulary feature (**Table 3-4**). Note that using the MeSH vocabulary with all of the filters used in the previous examples results in fewer hits but only returns titles that are clearly related to the clinical question in some fashion.

Search History

The search history function in PubMed is accessed via the "Advanced Search" link on the top of the home page (Figure 3-1). This feature is useful for two reasons: (1) it keeps a record of your search strings, and (2) it can be used to combine search strings with each other or with other keywords. Keeping track of the different search terms and combinations is important in situations when limits

FIGURE 3-4   Search results using more specific keywords and filters in PubMed.

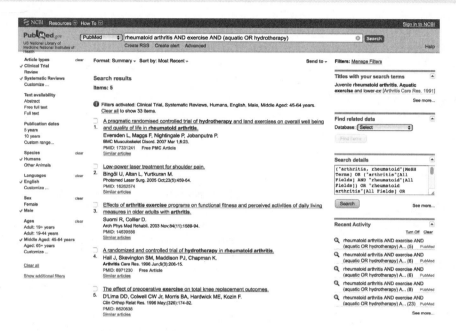

Screenshot from PubMed (www.pubmed.gov), National Center for Biotechnology Information, U.S. National Library of Medicine, Bethesda, MD, USA, and the National Institutes of Health. Accessed September 1, 2016.

TABLE 3-3   Results Using Keywords Other Than MeSH Vocabulary with Different Filter Combinations in PubMed

Search Method	Number of Hits	Titles
Search Terms* plus limits: • Clinical trials • Systematic reviews • Humans • English language • Male • Middle-aged: 45–64	5	• A pragmatic randomized controlled trial of hydrotherapy and land exercises on overall well-being and quality of life in rheumatoid arthritis • Low-power laser treatment for shoulder pain • Effects of arthritis exercise programs on functional fitness and perceived activities of daily living measures in older adults with arthritis • A randomized and controlled trial of hydrotherapy in rheumatoid arthritis • The effect of preoperative exercise on total knee replacement outcomes

(continues)

TABLE 3-3	**Results Using Keywords Other Than MeSH Vocabulary with Different Filter Combinations in PubMed (*Continued*)**	

Search Method	Number of Hits	Titles
Search Terms* plus limits: • Clinical trials • Systematic reviews • Humans • English language • Middle-aged: 45–64	6	Five titles from previous search plus: • Postural sway characteristics in women with lower extremity arthritis before and after an aquatic exercise intervention
Search Terms* plus limits: • Clinical trials • Systematic reviews • Humans • English language	12	Six titles from previous search plus: • Aquatic exercise and balneotherapy in musculo-skeletal conditions • Effectiveness of aquatic exercise and balneotherapy: a summary of systematic reviews based on randomized controlled trials of water immersion therapies • Aquatic fitness training for children with juvenile idiopathic arthritis • Cardiorespiratory responses of patients with rheumatoid arthritis during bicycle riding and running in water • The way forward for hydrotherapy • Juvenile rheumatoid arthritis. Aquatic exercise and lower extremity function

*Search Terms: rheumatoid arthritis AND exercise AND (aquatic OR hydrotherapy)

are added or subtracted and when multiple synonyms are exchanged in response to unsuccessful searches. Combining search strings often narrows the search and reduces the number of hits obtained; however, the citations retrieved may be more relevant to the question of interest. **Figure 3-5** depicts the history for the search using the string [rheumatoid arthritis AND exercise AND (aquatic OR hydrotherapy)] along with different filter options. The last search string also is entered in the advanced search builder above and a new search term—"outcomes"—is entered for a different query in PubMed.

Clinical Queries

"Clinical Queries," PubMed's version of an evidence-based practice search function, is accessible via a link in the middle of the home page (Figure 3-1). This feature allows a more tailored search for studies pertaining to etiology, diagnosis, prognosis, therapy, or clinical prediction rules. Depending on which topic area is selected, this feature automatically adds terms that focus the search on the most useful forms of evidence for that practice element. In addition, the user can direct the search engine

TABLE 3-4   Results from Search Using MeSH Terms and Different Filter Options in PubMed

Search Method	Number of Hits	Titles
Search Terms* plus limits: • Clinical trials • Systematic reviews • Humans • English language • Male • Middle-aged: 45–64	2	• A pragmatic randomized controlled trial of hydrotherapy and land exercises on overall well-being and quality of life in rheumatoid arthritis • A randomized and controlled trial of hydrotherapy in rheumatoid arthritis
Search Terms* plus limits: • Clinical trials • Systematic reviews • Humans • English language • Middle-aged: 45–64	2	• Same titles from previous search
Search Terms* plus limits: • Clinical trials • Systematic reviews • Humans • English language	3	Same titles from previous search plus: • The way forward for hydrotherapy

*MeSH Terms: "Arthritis, Rheumatoid" AND "Exercise Therapy" AND Hydrotherapy

to narrow or expand the search with filters that are programmed to reflect the highest quality forms of evidence in each content area. Selecting "systematic reviews," for example, may reduce the need to search further if a high-quality relevant example of this comprehensive form of evidence is located.

Figure 3-6 illustrates the results for the search string [rheumatoid arthritis AND exercise AND (aquatic OR hydrotherapy)] entered through the "Clinical Queries" function. This approach yielded several of the same citations obtained during the search with MeSH terms (Table 3-4). As noted earlier, the goal is to find the highest quality evidence available; therefore, using the "Clinical Queries" feature is the more efficient option in this example because of its automatic search for the best research design for intervention studies.

Similar Articles

The "Similar Articles" function in PubMed is another feature that may enhance the efficiency of a search. **Figure 3-7** illustrates how this feature works. The abstract for one of the articles located during the search with MeSH terms has been accessed by clicking its citation link. To the right of the abstract is a list of titles related to this one under the label "Similar Articles." Users have the option of viewing all comparable citations or only viewing review articles about similar topics.

FIGURE 3-5   Using search history in the advanced search builder in Pubmed.

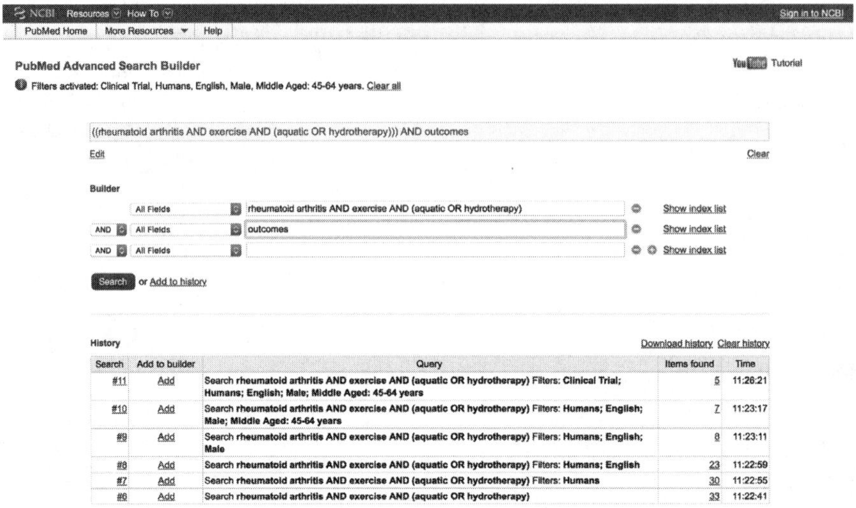

Screenshot from PubMed (www.pubmed.gov), National Center for Biotechnology Information, U.S. National Library of Medicine, Bethesda, MD, USA, and the National Institutes of Health. Accessed September 1, 2016.

FIGURE 3-6   PubMed search results using clinical queries.

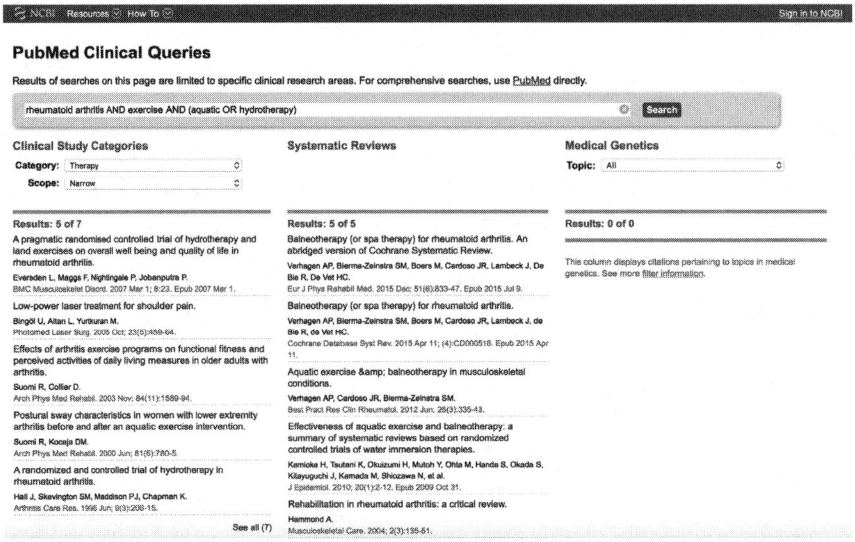

Screenshot from PubMed (www.pubmed.gov), National Center for Biotechnology Information, U.S. National Library of Medicine, Bethesda, MD, USA, and the National Institutes of Health. Accessed September 1, 2016.

FIGURE 3-7   PubMed article abstract display and similar articles feature.

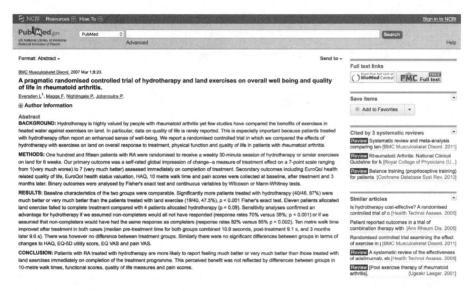

Screenshot from PubMed (www.pubmed.gov), National Center for Biotechnology Information, U.S. National Library of Medicine, Bethesda, MD, USA, and the National Institutes of Health. Accessed September 1, 2016.

The challenge in using this feature is that citations will be returned that relate to any of the keywords or concepts in the originally selected title. As a result, physical therapists may find additional evidence specific to the original clinical question as well as articles pertaining to other interventions for rheumatoid arthritis or to the effectiveness of aquatic exercise or land-based exercise for other conditions. As it turns out, 208 individual citations were identified when the "See All" link was selected, an outcome that suggests numerous irrelevant hits.

"My NCBI"

"My NCBI" (National Center for Biotechnology Information) allows therapists to individualize a free account on the PubMed website that will save search parameters, perform automatic searches for new studies, and email updates about the results of these searches. Registration with a password is required via a link in the top right corner of the PubMed home page (Figure 3-1). This is a particularly useful feature for therapists who anticipate routine exploration of a particular topic area (e.g., "shoulder pain" or "multiple sclerosis").

PubMed Tutorials

PubMed has a variety of instructional materials that can be accessed via a link on the left-hand side of the home page (Figure 3-1). They cover a wide range of topics, including use of the MeSH database. Brief animated audio productions are an easy way to learn the nuances of this comprehensive search engine beyond what is described here. Supplemental written information also is available. **Figure 3-8** provides a sample of the topics covered.

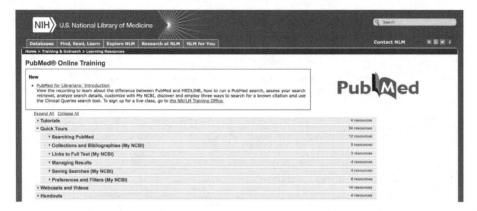

FIGURE 3-8   PubMed tutorial page.

Screenshot from PubMed (www.pubmed.gov), National Center for Biotechnology Information, U.S. National Library of Medicine, Bethesda, MD, USA, and the National Institutes of Health. Accessed September 1, 2016.

Cumulative Index of Nursing and Allied Health Literature (CINAHL) Complete

As its name suggests, CINAHL Complete is a database of citations from journals pertaining to nursing and the allied health professions (**Figure 3-9**).[18] Some of these journals are not indexed through the U.S. National Library of Medicine because they do not meet the inclusion criteria. For example, studies published in the *Physical Therapy Journal of Policy, Administration, and Leadership* are not listed in PubMed because the journal is both a research dissemination vehicle and a format for providing information to members of the Health Policy and Administration Section of the American Physical Therapy Association. However, this journal's articles are cited by CINAHL Complete. As a result of this differential in indexing rules, physical therapists may find it useful to start a search with CINAHL Complete rather than with PubMed.

Additional characteristics of this database include

- Links to online journals and full-text articles;
- Easy-to-understand search pages;
- The ability to limit or expand the search by specifying
  - Characteristics of the subjects studied (e.g., age, gender);
  - Characteristics of the article or publication (e.g., publication date, journal type);
  - Treatment setting (e.g., inpatient, outpatient);
  - Special interest areas (e.g., physical therapy, complementary medicine);
- Automated suggestions for additional limits returned with search results;
- The ability to view the retrieved hits by citation only, citation plus additional details about the study's characteristics, or citation plus the abstract (available through the "Preferences" function toward the top of the search page);

FIGURE 3-9   **CINAHL Complete home page.**

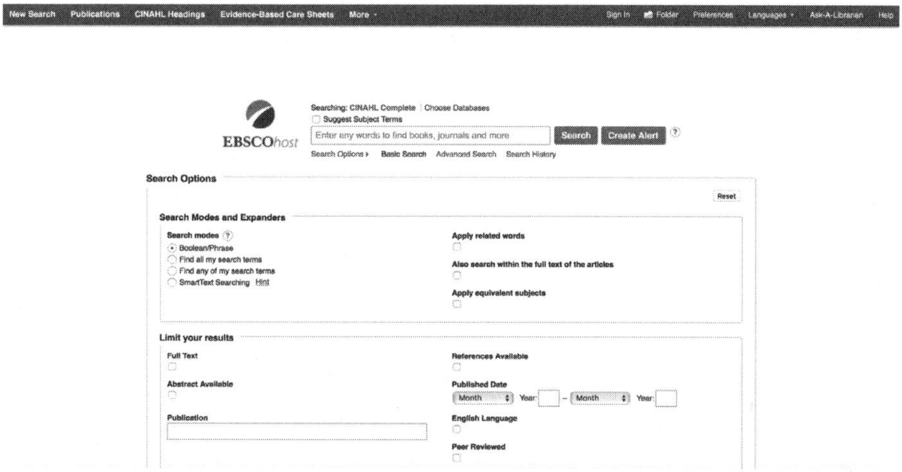

Courtesy of EBSCO*host*. EBSCO Industries, Inc. Accessed September 1, 2016.

- Easy-to-view search history;
- Weekly updates of the database;
- A non-MeSH–based search vocabulary that focuses on terms considered to be more relevant or specific to nursing and allied health; and
- A subscription fee required through EBSCO Industries, Inc. EBSCO*host* for individual users who do not have access through an institutional (i.e., university or hospital) site license. The database is available to members of the American Physical Therapy Association through its PTNow evidence portal.

CINAHL Complete has two search page options: basic and advanced. The basic option contains a search box similar to the one used in PubMed that requires the user to type in the search terms along with any Boolean operators. Boolean operators must be entered in uppercase letters. Several filter options are available related primarily to characteristics of the article or of the journal in which it is published. The advanced search page includes more features to limit or expand the search (**Figure 3-10**). Alternatively, CINAHL Complete vocabulary can be searched via the CINAHL Headings function, a feature analogous to the PubMed MeSH function.

Figure 3-11 illustrates the results of a search using the search string [rheumatoid arthritis AND exercise AND (aquatic OR hydrotherapy)] with the limits "humans," "English," "male," and "middle-aged: 45–64." Results were returned in the brief *synopsis* format. Only three citations were identified, two of which also were retrieved by PubMed. This differential is a reflection of the different indexing methods used by each database.

FIGURE 3-10   CINAHL Complete advanced search page.

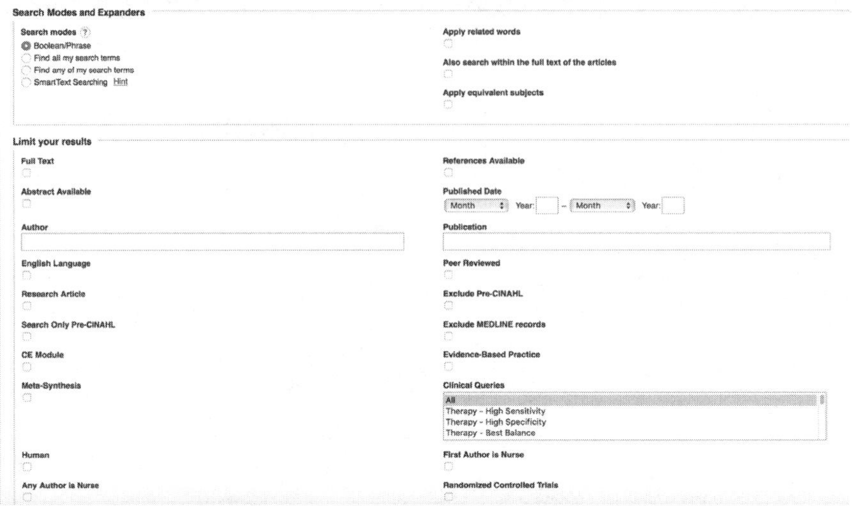

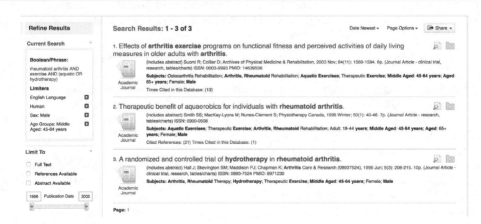

Courtesy of EBSCO*host*. EBSCO Industries, Inc. Accessed September 1, 2016.

FIGURE 3-11   CINAHL Complete search results using the brief citation format.

Courtesy of EBSCO*host*. EBSCO Industries, Inc. Accessed September 1, 2016.

The Cochrane Library

The Cochrane Library, developed and maintained by an international organization, the Cochrane Collaboration,[19] offers a potentially more efficient means of searching for evidence (**Figure 3-12**). The Cochrane Library is actually a collection of six databases and registries:

- The Cochrane Database of Systematic Reviews (Cochrane Reviews);
- The Database of Abstracts of Reviews of Effects (Other Reviews);
- The Cochrane Central Register of Controlled Trials (Trials);
- The Cochrane Methodology Register (Methods Studies);
- Health Technology Assessment Database (Technology Assessments);
- The National Health Service Economic Evaluation Database (Economic Evaluations).

The Cochrane Reviews database contains systematic reviews and meta-analyses developed according to rigorous methodology established and executed by members of the Cochrane Collaboration. Systematic reviews of empirical methodologic studies also are included. "Other Reviews" (DARE) is a collection of citations and abstracts of systematic reviews and meta-analyses performed by other researchers who are not members of the collaboration. Similarly, "Trials" (CENTRAL) is a database of citations and abstracts of individual randomized controlled trials performed by other investigators.

FIGURE 3-12   **The Cochrane Library home page.**

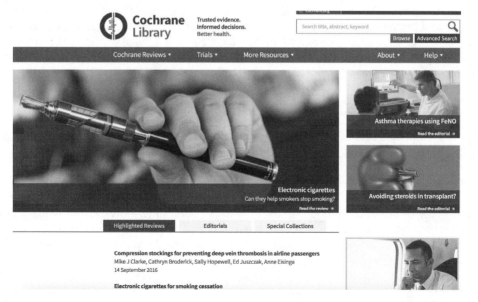

Screenshot from John Wiley & Sons, Inc.'s World Wide website. Copyright © 1999–2006, John Wiley & Sons, Inc. Accessed September 1, 2016. Reproduced with permission.

These three databases are the most useful for searching for evidence to answer clinical questions. Characteristics of the Cochrane Reviews database include the following:

- Reviews about interventions limited to randomized clinical trials;
- Use of the same MeSH search vocabulary used in PubMed;
- The availability of full-text versions of the reviews that include complete details of the process and results;
- Fewer reviews pertaining to etiology, diagnostic tests, clinical measures, prognostic factors, clinical prediction rules, outcomes, and self-report outcomes measures;
- A limited online overview of the system; however, detailed user guides in Adobe Acrobat PDF format are available for downloading and printing; and
- A subscription fee required for individual users who do not have access through an institutional (i.e., university or hospital) site license. The database is available to members of the American Physical Therapy Association through its PTNow evidence portal.

The remaining databases in the Cochrane Library contain citations pertaining to research methods (Methods Studies), health technology appraisals (Technology Assessments) conducted by other investigators or agencies (such as the Agency for Healthcare Research and Quality), and health economics topics (Economic Evaluations). Users may search all of the databases simultaneously or select specific databases.

The Cochrane Library has both a basic and an advanced search page, although neither has nearly the number of options to expand or limit the search as compared with PubMed and CINAHL Complete. **Figure 3-13** illustrates the results obtained searching titles, abstracts, and keywords with the search string ["rheumatoid arthritis" AND exercise AND aquatic OR hydrotherapy] via the advanced search page. The number of hits is indicated in parentheses next to the names of each of the relevant databases: two in the Cochrane Reviews, zero in Other Reviews, and 16 in Trials. Unfortunately, the citation title that is specific to aquatic exercise for rheumatoid arthritis is a protocol for a systematic review that dates back to 2001. The completed review is about the effectiveness of mineral baths and is unrelated to the clinical question. However, four of the citations in the Clinical Trials database are the same as those identified in the PubMed and CINAHL Complete search.

Physiotherapy Evidence Database (PEDro)

PEDro is an initiative of the Centre for Evidence-Based Physiotherapy (**Figure 3-14**) in Sydney, Australia, that provides citations "of over 34,000 randomized trials, systematic reviews, and *clinical practice guidelines* in physiotherapy."[20] Individual trials are rated for quality on a 0 to 10 scale based on their internal validity and statistical interpretability. The reliability of the total rating score was determined to be "fair" to "good" based on a study by Maher et al.[21] De Morton used a sophisticated statistical method (Rasch analysis) to determine the extent to which the score measured methodologic quality of studies cited in the database. Her work confirmed the validity of the scale items as well as an ability to treat the scores as real numbers (i.e., as an interval scale).[22] Preliminary evidence of construct and convergent validity of the PEDro scale with other established rating scales also was reported by Macedo et al.[23] The rating scores appear next to citations in the search results to help the user prioritize which studies to review first. Reviews and practice guidelines are not rated.

FIGURE 3-13 The Cochrane Library search results for the Cochrane Database of Systematic Reviews.

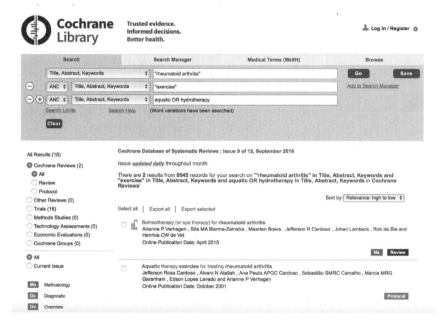

Screenshot from John Wiley & Sons, Inc.'s World Wide Website. Copyright 1999–2006, John Wiley & Sons, Inc. Accessed September 1, 2016. Reproduced with permission.

The primary reason to use PEDro is its focus on physical therapy research, although access to other allied health citations is now available through the site. Like CINAHL Complete and the Cochrane Library, this database has simple and advanced search pages. Additional features include:

- An ability to search by
  - Therapeutic approach
  - Clinical problem
  - Body part
  - Physical therapy subspecialty
- Written and video tutorials related to searching the site, using the PEDro rating scale and determining the usefulness of the evidence located
- Downloads to facilitate
  - Citation import into bibliography management software products
  - Calculation of confidence intervals
- An opportunity for readers to submit feedback when they disagree with a rating score

FIGURE 3-14   PEDro home page.

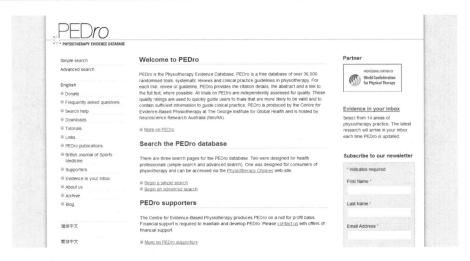

Screenshot from PEDro (http://www.pedro.org.au), Musculoskeletal Health Sydney, School of Public Health, Sydney Medical School, University of Sydney, Australia. Accessed September 1, 2016.

Figure 3-15 illustrates use of the keyword search box in combination with search parameter drop-down menu options that focus the search on the type of treatment provided (therapy) and the type of clinical issue addressed (problem) as well as the evidence format (method).

The primary limitation of the PEDro database is the lack of citations pertaining to diagnostic tests, clinical measures, prognostic factors, clinical prediction rules, outcomes, and self-report outcomes measures. In addition, the options available to tailor the search are limited to characteristics of the study; more specific details about the subjects are unavailable. Unlike CINAHL Complete or the Cochrane Library, PEDro is free and updated once per month. In addition, the database does not have a specific search vocabulary to learn.

Figure 3-16 illustrates the results returned from a search using the combination of terms and fields depicted in Figure 3-15. The quality ratings for each trial are displayed in descending order from highest to lowest quality. One option is to select only those articles that meet a minimum threshold score, such as "greater than or equal to 5/10." There is no evidence to support the selection of a threshold, however, so the target value is arbitrary and should be acknowledged as such. Quality rankings of individual studies should be treated as screening tools in much the same way that evidence hierarchies are used. Therapists are best served by reviewing a citation on its own merits rather than solely relying on a quality score to a make a decision about the relevance and utility of the evidence.

Other Databases and Services

The search engines discussed in this chapter do not comprise an exhaustive list of options. Additional databases such as ClinicalTrials.gov[24] and ProQuest[25] may be useful depending on the type and

FIGURE 3-15   PEDro advanced search page.

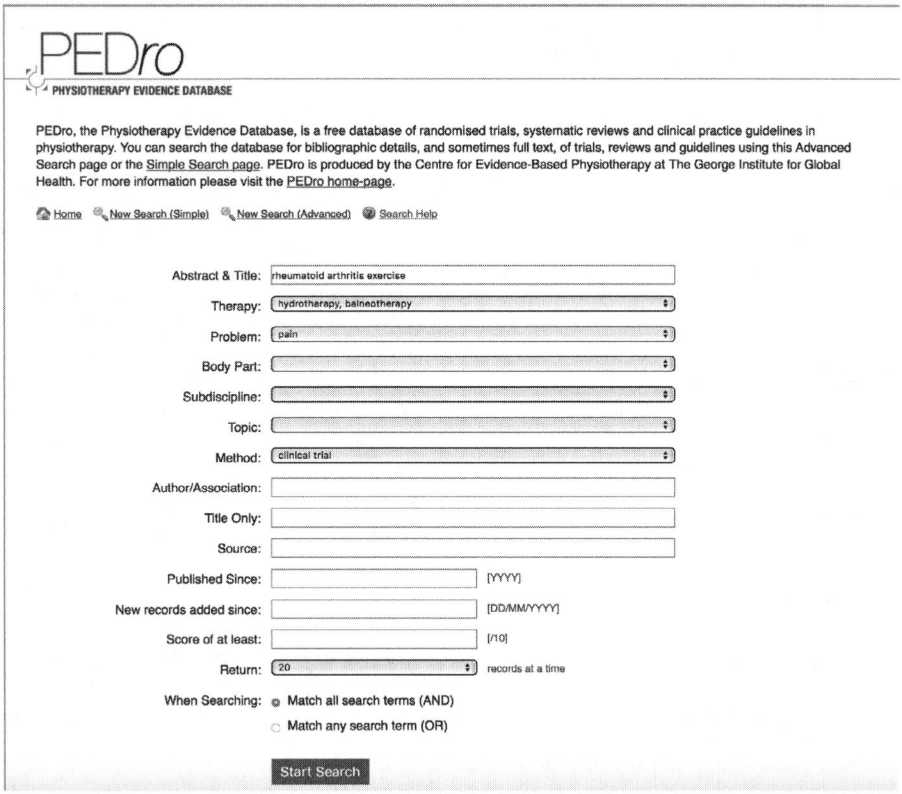

Screenshot from PEDro (http://www.pedro.org.au/), Musculoskeletal Health Sydney, School of Public Health, Sydney Medical School, University of Sydney, Australia. Accessed September 1, 2016.

content of the questions asked. In addition, services are available that evaluate studies and provide brief synopses regarding content and quality for subscribers who do not have time to read original material. Examples include Evidence-Based Medicine[26] and ACP Journal Club.[27] These services are oriented primarily toward physicians, but they are excellent resources regarding the principles and methods of evidence-based practice. Other services, such as Medscape[28] and WebMD,[29] allow users to sign up for periodic emails announcing the publication of new studies, similar to the "My NCBI" function in PubMed. Users of these alert services will still have to obtain and read the articles to determine their usefulness.

The rapidly increasing volume of research publications challenges busy clinicians to keep up with current developments. That logistical challenge is compounded by the potential to draw inaccurate conclusions based on limited data. Therefore, there is a greater emphasis on the use of "preappraised" collections of evidence (e.g., systematic reviews, clinical practice guidelines) to inform clinical decision

FIGURE 3-16 PEDro search results.

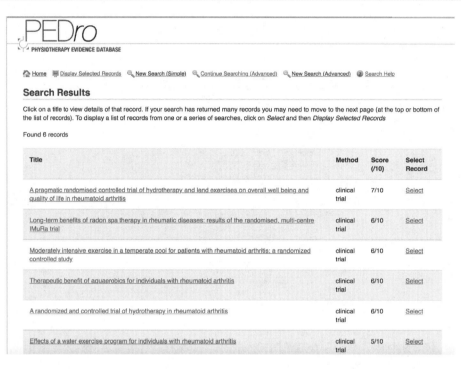

Screenshot from PEDro (http://www.pedro.org.au/), Musculoskeletal Health Sydney, School of Public Health, Sydney Medical School, University of Sydney, Australia. Accessed September 1, 2016.

making. Databases that focus on these types of research products are becoming more prevalent. In addition to the Cochrane Library, physical therapists may find the following resources useful:

- Turning Research into Practice (TRIP):[30] This is a commercial search engine that has a no-cost level of service and a subscription service with more sophisticated features. What makes this search engine unique is the method by which it filters citations that are returned. Instead of classifying the returns by type of article, TRIP classifies by publisher based on the output they produce. Citations from the Cochrane Library are categorized as systematic reviews as would be expected. Research from journals that publish mostly individual studies are categorized as key primary research. The formatting of results is similar to that illustrated by Robeson and colleagues in that it is visually easy to spot synthesized research products.[31] **Figure 3-17** depicts results for the search string "rheumatoid arthritis" AND "exercise" AND "aquatic OR hydrotherapy." The pyramid icons next to each citation provide a quick visual indication of their quality level with preappraised evidence at the top of the hierarchy.
- National Guideline Clearinghouse:[32] This initiative by the U.S. Agency for Healthcare Research and Quality is a database that provides a searchable mechanism for locating clinical practice guidelines that meet inclusion criteria related to content and quality.

FIGURE 3-17   TRIP results.

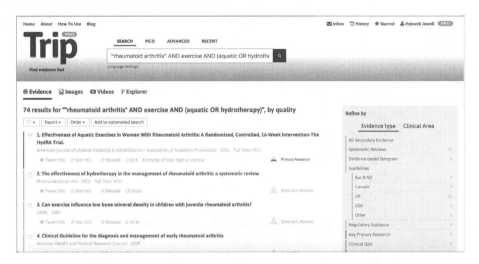

TRIP Database. Turning Research into Practice. Available at: www.tripdatabase.com. Accessed September 1, 2016.

FIGURE 3-18   National guideline clearinghouse.

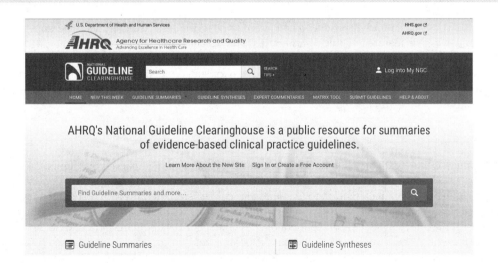

Reproduced from National Guideline Clearinghouse. Available at: https://www.guideline.gov. Accessed September 1, 2016.

FIGURE 3-19   PTNow home page.

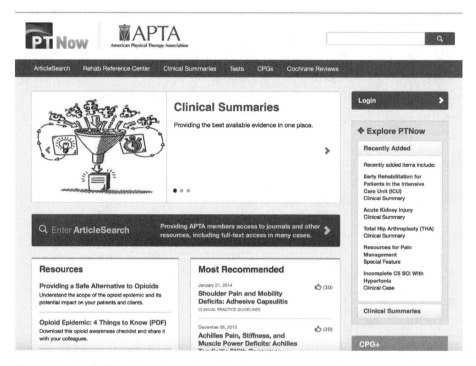

- PTNow:[33] This platform is produced and maintained by the American Physical Therapy Association. Two of its features, "clinical summaries" and "CPG+," allow association members to access evidence syntheses with a focus on physical therapist patient or client management. The content in these areas is developed based on member and/or staff interest and updates occur as time and resources allow, a limitation that may force physical therapists to rely on the larger commercial and government-run databases.

Summary

EBPT practice starts with the formulation of a clinical question about a patient or client. Background questions seek information to increase understanding about the individual's clinical context. Foreground questions seek information to facilitate clinical decision making with respect to diagnostic tests, clinical measures, prognostic factors, interventions, clinical prediction rules, outcomes, self-report outcomes measures, and patient or client perspectives about his or her health and health care experience. The acronym PICO (Person/Problem/Population, Issue, Comparison, Outcome) can be used as a guide to develop searchable foreground questions relevant to the individual with whom the physical therapist is working. Once the question is formulated, therapists should plan their search strategy and include identification of search terms and databases that will be used.

The four electronic databases commonly accessed by physical therapists are PubMed, CINAHL Complete, the Cochrane Library, and PEDro. APTA's PTNow portal provides association members with access to these databases as well as to clinical practice guidelines. Each database has specific search features with which users should be familiar to enhance the efficiency of the process. Research synthesis and alert services also are available to facilitate identification of relevant evidence; however, therapists will want to review the evidence for themselves to judge its quality and relevance for a specific patient or client.

Exercises

1. Think about a patient or client scenario in which you have an interest and consider what you would like to know about it.
   - Practice writing "background" questions to increase your understanding of the scenario.
   - Using the PICO format, write one "foreground" question each pertaining to diagnostic tests, clinical measures, prognostic factors, interventions, clinical prediction rules, outcomes, self-report outcomes measures, and patient or client perceptions/experiences for this scenario.
2. Review the MeSH database online tutorials on the PubMed website.
3. Upon completion of the tutorials, choose one of your foreground questions and identify the search terms you might use. Look for these terms in the MeSH database.
4. Perform a PubMed search for evidence about your clinical question using the MeSH terms you identified and any other "Limits" you prefer.
5. Answer the following questions about your PubMed search:
   - What were your initial search term choices? Why?
   - Were your keywords in the MeSH database?
   - If not, what keywords did you choose from the MeSH vocabulary instead? Why?
   - What limits did you select? Why?
   - What were your search results?
     - Number of hits
     - Number of articles that looked promising based on their titles
     - What search strategy changes did you need to make? Why?
     - What was the outcome of your revised search strategies (more hits, fewer hits)?
6. Try your search with one other database (CINAHL Complete, Cochrane, or PEDro) that you think would best help you answer the question.
   - Which electronic database did you choose? Why?
   - Which keywords did you use in this database? Why?
   - Which limits did you use in this database? Why?
   - What were your results?
     - Number of hits
     - Number of articles that look promising based on their titles
   - How would you compare this database with PubMed in helping you to answer this question?
7. Now try your search with the TRIP search engine and compare your results with the prior two efforts. Which of the three search methods was most efficient with respect to the time and effort required to return citations relevant to your search?

References

1. Graham R, Mancher M, Wolman DM, Greenfield S, Steinberg E, eds. *Clinical Practice Guidelines We Can Trust.* Available at: http://www.nap.edu/catalog/13058/clinical-practice-guidelines-we-can-trust. Accessed July 31, 2016.

2. DiCenso A, Bayley L, Haynes RB. Accessing pre-appraised evidence: fine-tuning the 5S model into a 6S model. *Evid Based Nurs.* 2009;12(4):99–101.

3. American Physical Therapy Association, Guide to Physical Therapist Practice. *3.0.* Available at: http://guidetoptpractice.apta.org. Accessed July 16, 2016.

4. Portney LG, Watkins MP. *Foundations of Clinical Research: Applications to Practice.* 3rd ed. Upper Saddle River, NJ: Prentice Hall Health; 2009.

5. Helewa A, Walker JM. *Critical Evaluation of Research in Physical Rehabilitation: Towards Evidence-Based Practice.* Philadelphia, PA: W.B. Saunders; 2000.

6. Straus SE, Richardson WS, Glaziou P, Haynes RB. *Evidence-Based Medicine: How to Practice and Teach EBM.* 3rd ed. Edinburgh, Scotland: Elsevier Churchill Livingstone; 2005.

7. Guyatt G, Rennie D. *Users' Guides to the Medical Literature: A Manual for Evidence-Based Clinical Practice.* Chicago, IL: AMA Press; 2002.

8. Centre for Evidence-Based Medicine. *Asking Focused Questions.* Available at: http://www.cebm.net/asking-focused-questions/ Accessed July 31, 2016.

9. Hoffman T, Bennett S, Del Mar C. *Evidence-based Practice Across the Health Professions.* Chatswood, NSW, Australia: Churchill Livingstone; 2010.

10. Beattie P, Nelson N. Clinical prediction rules: what are they and what do they tell us? *Aust J Physiother.* 2006;52(3):157–163.

11. Childs JD, Cleland JA. Development and application of clinical prediction rules to improve decision-making in physical therapist practice. *Phys Ther.* 2006;86(1):122–131.

12. McGinn TG, Guyatt GH, Wyer PC, et al. Users' guides to the medical literature XXII: how to use articles about clinical decision rules. *JAMA.* 2000;284(1):79–84.

13. Jean-Francois G, Laetitia R, Stefan D. Is the coverage of Google Scholar enough to be used alone for systematic reviews. *BMC Med Inform Decis Mak.* 2013;13(7):1–5.

14. Nourbakhsh E, Nugent R, Wang H, et al. Medical literature searches: a comparison of PubMed and Google Scholar. *Health Info Libr J.* 2012;29(3):214–222.

15. Bramer WM. Variation in the number of hits for complex searches in Google Scholar. *J Med Libr Assoc.* 2016;104(2):143-145.

16. PubMed. U.S. National Library of Medicine website. Available at: http://www.ncbi.nlm.nih.gov/pubmed. Accessed September 1, 2016.

17. Searching PubMed with MeSH. National Network of Libraries of Medicine. U.S. National Library of Medicine website. Available at: https://nnlm.gov/sites/default/files/atoms/files/meshtri.pdf? Accessed September 1, 2016.

18. Cumulative Index of Nursing and Allied Health Literature. Available via EBSCO*host* website at: https://health.ebsco.com/products/cinahl-complete. Accessed September 1, 2016.

19. The Cochrane Library. The Cochrane Collaboration website. Available via Wiley Interscience at: http://www.cochranelibrary.com. Accessed September 1, 2016.

20. Physiotherapy Evidence Database. Center for Evidence-Based Physiotherapy website. Available at: http://www.pedro.org.au. Accessed September 1, 2016.

21. Maher CG, Sherrington C, Herbert RD, et al. Reliability of the PEDro scale for rating quality of randomized controlled trials. *Phys Ther.* 2003;83(8):713–721.

22. de Morton NA. The PEDro scale is a valid measure of methodological quality of clinical trials: a demographic study. *Aust J Physiother.* 2009;55(2):129-133.

23. Macedo LG, Elkins MR, Maher CG, et al. There was evidence of convergent and construct validity of Physio-therapy Evidence Database quality scale for physiotherapy trials. *J Clin Epidemiol*. 2010;63(8):920-925.

24. ClinicalTrials.gov. Available at: https://clinicaltrials.gov. Accessed September 1, 2016.

25. ProQuest. Available at: www.proquest.com. Accessed September 1, 2016.

26. Evidence-Based Medicine. Available at: http://ebm.bmj.com. Accessed September 1, 2016.

27. ACP Journal Club. Available at: http://annals.org/journalclub.aspx. Accessed September 1, 2016.

28. Medscape. Available at: www.medscape.com. Accessed September 1, 2016.

29. WebMD. Available at: www.webmd.com. Accessed September 1, 2016.

30. TRIP Database. Turning Research into Practice. Available at: www.tripdatabase.com. Accessed September 1, 2016.

31. Robeson P, Dobbins M, DeCorby K, Tirilis D. Facilitating access to pre-processed research evidence in public health. *BMC Public Health*. 2010;95.

32. National Guideline Clearinghouse. Available at: https://www.guideline.gov. Accessed September 1, 2016.

33. PTNow. Available at: http://www.ptnow.org/Default.aspx. Accessed September 1, 2016

ELEMENTS OF EVIDENCE

CHAPTER 4

QUESTIONS, THEORIES, AND HYPOTHESES

OBJECTIVES

Upon completion of this chapter, the student/practitioner will be able to do the following:

1. Discuss the purpose and characteristics of a well-worded research question or problem statement.

2. Discuss the purpose and characteristics of background information used to support the need for a study, including literature reviews and publicly available epidemiologic data.

3. Differentiate among the terms *theory*, *concept*, and *construct*.

4. Explain the use of theories and conceptual frameworks in clinical research.

5. Discuss the concept of biologic plausibility and explain its role in clinical research.

6. Differentiate between the form and uses of the null and research hypotheses.

TERMS IN THIS CHAPTER

Biologic plausibility: The reasonable expectation that the human body could behave in the manner predicted.

Concept: A mental image of an observable phenomenon that is expressed in words.[1]

Conceptual framework: A collection of interrelated concepts or constructs that reflect a common theme; may be the basis of a more formal theory; usually depicted in schematic form.[2]

Construct: A nonobservable abstraction created for a specific research purpose; defined by observable measures such as events or behaviors.[2]

Null hypothesis: Also referred to as the "statistical hypothesis"; a prediction that the outcome of an investigation will demonstrate "no difference" or "no relationship" between groups (or variables) in the study other than what chance alone might create.[3]

Research hypothesis: Also referred to as the "alternative hypothesis"; a prediction that the outcome of an investigation will demonstrate a difference or relationship between groups (or variables) in the study that is the result of more than chance alone (e.g., statistically significant). May be written using directional language such as "more than," "less than," "positive," or "negative."[3]

Theory: An organized set of relationships among concepts or constructs; proposed to describe and/or explain systematically a phenomenon of interest, as well as to predict future behaviors or outcomes.[1,2]

CLINICAL SCENARIO

How Did I Develop This Problem?

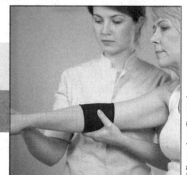

© Photographee.eu/Shutterstock

Anne wants to understand better how she developed her elbow pain. One of the websites she located indicated that this problem was typically the result of overuse. The background literature you have read suggests symptoms are due to changes in the tissue structure of the affected tendons that appear more degenerative in nature rather than due to acute inflammation.

How might you link together these pathologic findings with excessive use of the upper extremity so that you can provide Anne with a clearer picture of how she may have ended up in this situation?

Introduction

In the broadest sense, research is a quest for answers about the way the world works. Depending on one's perspective, these answers are viewed either as absolute truths that are waiting to be revealed (the quantitative research view) or as constructions of reality that are relevant only to those involved (the qualitative research view).[1] Either way, a plan for obtaining the desired knowledge usually is developed and implemented by individuals or groups who have the motivation and resources to embark on the research journey. This plan, and its outcome, is documented in a variety of forms, the most common of which is the research article. Although the articles themselves may have different formats dictated by publishers' preferences, they usually contain information pertaining to a study's essential elements:

- Research question(s) or purpose statement(s);
- Background information;
- Theoretical or conceptual basis of the study;
- Hypothesis(es) about the study's outcome;
- Subjects used in the study;
- Research design;

- Variables and their measures;
- Method(s) of statistical analysis;
- Study results; and
- Implications and importance of the study's findings.

Additional details may be provided related to limitations of the researchers' efforts, as well as suggestions for future research. This chapter reviews the purpose, key features, and practical issues surrounding the first four bulleted items.

The Research Question

Research is a serious and potentially complex endeavor that requires time and resources in support of the quest for answers. The desire to conduct a study may be stimulated by clinical experience and observation, a curious nature, or an interest in advancing knowledge for its own sake. To plan appropriately, an investigator must start with a specific objective toward which his or her research efforts will be directed. This objective may be expressed in the form of a question, a purpose statement, or a problem statement.[4] The content is more important than the form; in other words, the researcher should be clear about what he or she wants to know. **Table 4-1** lists general questions that may serve as a study's objective, any of which can be tailored to address specific clinical concerns. Washington et al. used these research questions to describe their objectives in their study of neurologically impaired infants:[5(p.1066)]

1. "What are the effects of a CFS (contoured foam support) on postural alignment for infants with neuromotor impairments?"
2. "What are the effects of a CFS on the infants' ability to engage with toys?"
3. "How do parents perceive the use and effects of a CFS when used at home?"

TABLE 4-1   General Research Questions and Their Clinical Focus

Questions for Research to Answer	Clinical Focus
How does this work?	Background about a clinical technique or instrument
What does that look like?	Background about a clinical problem
How do I quantify or classify . . . ?	Development of a clinical measure
Which is the best analytic technique to determine if . . . ?	Usefulness of a diagnostic test
What is the risk of . . . ?	Prediction about a future outcome
How does the body respond when I do . . . ?	Evaluation of treatment effects
How does my patient's or client's performance change when . . . ?	Evaluation of outcomes
How do I measure a patient's or client's perspective . . . ?	Development of a self-report outcomes measure
What is my patient's or client's perception of . . .?	Exploration of the subjective meaning of an experience

The first two questions address the treatment effects of a specific intervention—contoured foam support—and the third question considers the impact of the device from the parents' point of view. Other authors have expressed their research objectives in purpose statement format, as illustrated in **Table 4-2**.[6-13] Whether formulated as a question or as a purpose statement, the research objective should be articulated clearly so that anyone reading will understand immediately

TABLE 4-2	Purpose Statements from Physical Therapy Research
Citation	**Purpose Statement**
Systematic Review Lau B, et al. *Phys Ther.* 2016;96(9):1317–1332.	"The purpose of this study was to investigate the experiences of physical therapists working in acute hospitals."
Randomized Clinical Trial Fox EE, et al. *Phys Ther.* 2016;96(8):1170–1178.	"The primary aim of the study was to compare the effects of 12 weeks of Pilates exercises with relaxation on balance and mobility. Secondary aims were: (1) to compare standardized exercises with relaxation and (2) to compare Pilates exercises with standardized exercises."
Quasi-Experimental Study Bhatt T, et al. *Phys Ther.* 2013;93(4):492–503.	"The purpose of this study was to examine differences in the control of dynamic stability in people with PD and people who were healthy and the extent to which externally cued training can improve such control during the sit-to-stand task in people with PD."
Observational Study Farlie MK, et al. *Phys Ther.* 2016;96(3):313–323.	"The aim of this study was to explore verbal and nonverbal markers that differentiated tasks of high, medium, and low balance intensity to inform the development of an instrument to measure the intensity of balance challenge."
Physiologic Study Chung JI, et al. *Phys Ther.* 2016;96(6):808–817.	"This study aimed to investigate the effect of LIUS on synovial inflammation and its resolution via neutrophil clearance." LUIS stands for low intensity ultrasound.
Case Report Lee AWC, et al. *Phys Ther.* 2016;96(2):252–259.	"The purposes of this case report are: (1) to describe the development, implementation, and evaluation of a telehealth approach for meeting physical therapist supervision requirements in a skilled nursing facility (SNF) in Washington and (2) to explore clinical and human factors of physical therapist practice in an SNF delivered via telehealth."
Summary Yamato TP, et al. *Phys Ther.* 2016;96(10):1508–1513.	"This article focuses on the effectiveness of virtual reality for stroke rehabilitation."
Qualitative Inquiry Lloyd A, et al. *Physiother Res Int.* 2014;19:147–157.	"The purpose of this study was to investigate physiotherapists' perceptions about their experiences of collaborative goal setting with patients in the sub-acute stages after stroke, in the hospital setting."

what the study was about. The challenge for the investigators is to construct a research question or purpose statement so that it is not too broad to answer in a reasonable fashion but not so small as to be insignificant.

Background

A well-worded research question or purpose statement is necessary but not sufficient by itself to define a useful study. Although knowledge may be important for its own sake to some individuals, evidence-based practice is best supported by research that is relevant and advances knowledge in the professional field. These criteria also are used as part of the article review process required for publication in most scientific journals.[1] As a result, investigators are obligated to demonstrate

- Why the question or purpose statement is important to answer; and
- How the results obtained will increase understanding of a particular phenomenon or situation.

In other words, they must provide sufficient background information to justify the need for their study. This background material usually comes in two forms: (1) a literature review and (2) citations of publicly available epidemiologic data. Either or both may be used to support the relevance of the research question or purpose statement.

Literature Review

Investigators often summarize and critique prior studies to clarify what is currently known and what remains to be answered about the research topic in which they are interested. These literature reviews may be brief in form and generally focus on previous works that have the closest relationship to the research question or purpose statement. Occasionally these reviews indicate the need to explore new frontiers in practice altogether, as may be the case when innovative technology is introduced to treat an established clinical problem in a new and different way. More often, limitations of prior research, such as insufficient numbers or types of subjects, supply the rationale for the current study.

For example, an earlier work that evaluated a physical therapy intervention in 5 adult men may be offered as an argument for repeating the research with 200 adult men to verify that the first study's results were not a fluke related to such a small group. Similarly, the study of 200 men may be cited as justification for conducting the same research on a large group of adult women to evaluate potential gender differences in response to the experimental intervention. Other design problems related to measurement techniques, management of subjects during the study, and statistical analysis also may be identified as reasons for further study of a phenomenon or problem. In the end, the goal is to build a logical case supporting the necessity and importance of the current project.

A literature review must be comprehensive, but it often must conform to the space restrictions a publisher imposes. As a result, investigators must select wisely the previous works they will include as part of their justification for their study. Evidence-based physical therapists then must decide whether the investigators considered, and accurately evaluated, the most relevant studies. A therapist with experience and/or expertise in a particular subject area usually can recognize whether a literature review is thorough and accurate. Less experienced practitioners, however, may rely on more superficial indicators such as (1) the age of the prior studies reviewed, (2) whether the review flows in a logical sequence toward the current research question, and (3) whether the articles reviewed are related to the research question.

This last point is tricky, however, because there are many occasions when an investigator has a question because there is no prior evidence available. In these cases, researchers may review studies from other disciplines (e.g., medicine, nursing, occupational therapy) or other practice settings (e.g., skilled nursing facilities, outpatient rehabilitation, home health). Alternatively, they may consider studies that look at diagnoses or clinical problems that have similar characteristics to the disease or disorder in which the researchers are interested. For example, if investigators want to study an exercise technique in patients with Guillain-Barré syndrome, they may consider prior research on other remitting paralyzing diseases, such as multiple sclerosis or polio, because there is a limited body of evidence about rehabilitation for Guillain-Barré. Any of these tactics is reasonable as long as the researcher is able to use the information to demonstrate the relevance and significance of the current project.

Citations of Epidemiologic Data

In addition to, or in lieu of, a literature review, researchers may cite routinely collected data about the phenomenon and/or about its impact on society. Commonly used data in clinical research include health statistics[4] from (1) federal agencies, such as the Centers for Disease Control and Prevention,[14] the Occupational Health and Safety Administration,[15] the Department of Health and Human Services,[16] and the U.S. Census Bureau;[17] (2) state agencies, such as departments of health and disability services, workers' compensation boards, and health care regulatory agencies; and (3) private organizations, such as the Pew Charitable Trusts,[18] and the Robert Wood Johnson Foundation.[19] Academic centers also may collect and provide data about health-related issues in their community or data for which they have dedicated practice or research resources. Examples of data that physical therapy researchers might use include, but are not limited to

- The incidence or prevalence of an impairment in body structures and functions (e.g., joint stiffness after total knee arthroplasty), activity limitations (e.g., impact of stroke on self-care), or participation restrictions (e.g., involvement of individuals with disabilities in organized sport);
- The loss in productive work time due to injury;
- The cost of health care services provided to treat a problem that could have been prevented; and
- Which segments of the population have the least access to rehabilitation services.

In rare instances, the need for a study is justified by the identification of a previously undiscovered clinical phenomenon. These events are more likely to be medical in nature, as was the case with polio, human immunodeficiency virus (HIV), and sudden acute respiratory syndrome (SARS). However, the onset of these events may stimulate the need for physical therapy research into examination and treatment techniques to manage their functional consequences. Data in these situations may be incomplete at best, but they still may provide support for pilot studies that explore the impact of physical therapy on these phenomena.

Theories, Concepts, and Constructs

In addition to its clinical origins, a research study also may have a theoretical or conceptual basis that incorporates relevant concepts or constructs. A *concept* is a mental image of an observable phenomenon described in words.[2] For example, the concept "fatigue" refers to a collection of observable behaviors or states such as falling asleep in class, dark circles under one's eyes, and complaints of low energy. In contrast, a *construct* is a nonobservable abstraction created for a specific research purpose that is defined by observable measures.[2] For example, the construct "readiness to change" describes an individual's openness to adopting a different behavior.[20] "Readiness" is not directly observable in the same way that one can detect an expression of fatigue. However, "readiness" can be inferred

TABLE 4-3	Examples of Concepts and Constructs Used in Physical Therapy Research	
Element	**Example**	**Potential Measure**
Concept	Age	Years since birth
	Pain	Visual scale with progressively grimacing faces
	Flexibility	Degrees of joint motion
Construct	Patient satisfaction	Ratings of care and the clinical environment
	Health-related quality of life	Ability to engage in physical, emotional, and social functions and roles
	Motivation	Attendance and active participation in a program

from behaviors, such as gathering information about the proposed lifestyle changes, discussing the change with people from whom an individual will need support or guidance, and writing out a plan for implementing the change. **Table 4-3** provides several examples of concepts and constructs used in physical therapy research.

A *theory* is an organized set of relationships among concepts or constructs that is proposed to systematically describe and/or explain a phenomenon of interest. A successful theory is one that is consistent with empirical observations and that, through repeated testing under various conditions, is able to predict future behavior or outcomes.[1,4] Comprehensive theoretical models, such as Einstein's theory of relativity and Darwin's theory of evolution, are referred to as "grand theories" because of their scope and complexity.[1] As the title implies, grand theories seek to explain as much as possible related to their focus areas.

Jean Piaget's theory of cognitive development in children is an example of a grand theory relevant to physical therapy.[21] Based on numerous empirical observations, Piaget proposed that children progress through four stages during which their understanding of the world develops from concrete perceptions and reflex-driven actions to abstract conceptualizations and purposeful choices. A child's interactions with his or her environment and social context, as well as the natural maturation of his or her physical and linguistic abilities, fuel the progression from one stage to another. Together these experiences result in the creation of new knowledge and understanding about the world that serves as the foundation for the next developmental stage. **Figure 4-1** depicts Piaget's theory in schematic form. The diagram illustrates an important point about grand theories: they are comprehensive in detail but often impractical to test in their entirety. The accumulation of evidence about various aspects of these theories usually is required to demonstrate their overall usefulness.

Smaller-scale theories often are referred to as conceptual frameworks. *Conceptual frameworks* also describe relationships among concepts and constructs from which predictions may be made, but they are not elaborate enough to explain all of the intricacies of the phenomenon of interest. An example of a conceptual framework relevant to physical therapist practice is Nagi's model of the disablement process.[22] As **Figure 4-2** illustrates, the concepts in the model are active pathology,

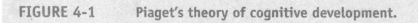

FIGURE 4-1   Piaget's theory of cognitive development.

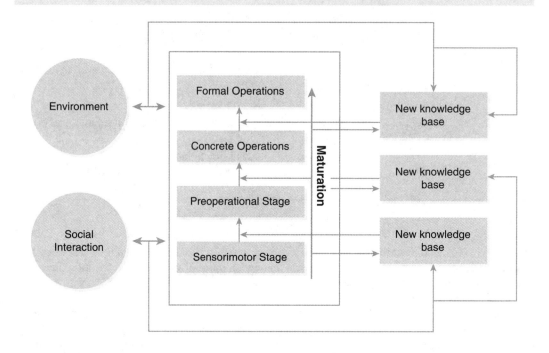

FIGURE 4-2   Nagi's model of disablement.

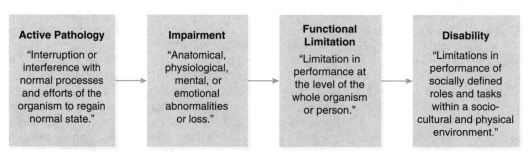

Active Pathology	**Impairment**	**Functional Limitation**	**Disability**
"Interruption or interference with normal processes and efforts of the organism to regain normal state."	"Anatomical, physiological, mental, or emotional abnormalities or loss."	"Limitation in performance at the level of the whole organism or person."	"Limitations in performance of socially defined roles and tasks within a socio-cultural and physical environment."

Potential Observable Measures:

Active Pathology: Data from lab tests, cell biopsies, radiographs, surgical exploration, etc.
Impairment: Limited degrees of motion in a joint, reduced torque in a muscle group, change in structure due to amputation or defect, etc.
Functional Limitation: Inability to move in and out of bed, rise from a chair, walk across a room, climb stairs, etc.
Disability: Inability to attend school, work, care for family, participate in leisure and social activities, etc.

Reprinted from Jette AM. Physical disablement concepts for physical therapy research and practice. *Phys Ther*. 1994;74(5):380–386 with permission from the American Physical Therapy Association. Copyright 1994 American Physical Therapy Association.

impairment, functional limitation, and disability. They are related to one another in a unidirectional sequential fashion; in other words, an impairment may be predicted as the result of active pathology, a functional limitation may be predicted as the result of an impairment, and a disability may be predicted as a result of a functional limitation. In comparison to Figure 4-1, this model is simple and easy to interpret. Conceptual frameworks usually do not have the complexity of grand theories, making them easier to test in clinical research. However, frameworks with little detail may be criticized for their lack of sensitivity to environmental influences and individual subject variability. The World Health Organization's International Classification of Functioning, Disability and Health (ICF) model is an example of a framework that addresses the limited information in Nagi's model but that is not as elaborate as a grand theory (**Figure 4-3**).[23]

Whether a clinical study of human behavior is based on a theory or conceptual framework, it must also meet the test of *biologic plausibility*—that is, the reasonable expectation that the human body could behave in the manner predicted. For example, a research question about the effect of a new therapeutic exercise technique on restoration of normal movement in adults following stroke might

FIGURE 4-3   World Health Organization's disablement model for the International classification of functioning, disability, and health.

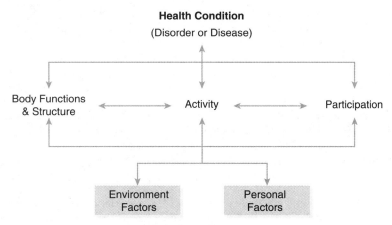

Body Functions: "Physiological functions of body systems (including psychological functions)."
Body Structures: "Anatomical parts of the body such as organs, limbs, and their components."
Impairments: "Problems in body functions or structure such as a significant deviation or loss."
Activity: "Execution of a task or action by an individual."
Participation: "Involvement in a life situation."
Activity Limitations: "Difficulties an individual may have in executing activities."
Participation Restrictions: "Problems an individual may experience in involvement in life situations."
Environmental Factors: "Make up the physical, social, and attitudinal environment in which people live and conduct their lives."

reasonably be based on observations about the developmental sequence of motor patterns in infants and children. Conversely, a study that examined the strengthening effects of a 3-day active-assisted exercise program fails to meet the biologic plausibility test because of the insufficient time frame and intensity implemented for skeletal muscle adaptation to increased workloads. As revealed by national hormone replacement trials, approaches based on biologic plausibility also must be tested by empirical research to avoid potentially harmful misdirection.[24]

Many clinical studies do not have a formally stated theoretical or conceptual framework to test. Their focus is much more pragmatic in terms of identifying the usefulness of a diagnostic test, clinical measure, prognostic factor, intervention, clinical prediction rule, or outcome. These studies are not intended to explain a phenomenon in an abstract way by developing or testing a theory. Nevertheless, researchers may "theorize" about phenomena they wish to study. Unless the investigators are proposing a formal theory of their own, their use of the term "theorize" is meant to indicate informed speculation and nothing more. Similarly, authors interchange the terms *theory*, *concept*, and *construct*, as well as *theoretical model* and *conceptual model*. The key is to avoid being distracted by the terminology and focus on the content of what is proposed so that the remainder of the study may be evaluated based on this information.

Hypotheses

In addition to proposing a basis for the study, researchers also may offer predictions about its outcomes. When these statements are derived from theoretical or conceptual models they are called "hypotheses." They usually are written as stand-alone statements that are structured in one of two ways. One version is the *null hypothesis* (H_0), the phrasing of which indicates that the researchers anticipate that "no difference" or "no relationship" between groups or variables will be demonstrated by their study's results. This approach is also referred to as the "statistical hypothesis" because statistical tests are designed specifically to challenge the "no difference (no relationship)" statement.[1-4] The premise behind this approach is that a study's results may be due to chance rather than due to the experiment or phenomenon of interest. Jones et al. used a null hypothesis in their study of lung sound intensities recorded when subjects were placed in different positions:[25(pp.683-684)]

> We hypothesized that there would be no differences in the data recorded in corresponding regions between (1) the left and right lungs in the sitting position, (2) the dependent and nondependent lungs in the side-lying position (in side-lying positions, the upper hemithorax is "nondependent," and the side in contact with the bed is "dependent"), (3) the sitting position and the dependent position, or (4) the sitting position and the nondependent position.

In other words, these authors anticipated that values for lung sounds would be the same, on average, regardless of the position in which the subjects were placed. Any differences among the sounds would be due to chance—that is, these differences could not be reproduced systematically through repeated study. If the statistical tests that investigators perform confirm their expectations, then the null hypothesis is "accepted." Researchers identify this situation with phrases such as "we found no statistically significant difference (or relationship) between. . . ." However, if the tests indicate that the study's results are not due to chance, then the null hypothesis is "rejected." Researchers indicate this situation with phrases such as "we found a statistically significant difference (or relationship) between. . . ."

The second form of hypothesis statement is referred to as a *research hypothesis* or "alternate hypothesis" (H_A). These statements predict that a difference or relationship between the groups or variables will be demonstrated by the study's results. Researchers even may provide directional language, such as "more than," "less than," "positive," or "negative," to make their predictions more specific.[1-4] Henry et al. used directional research hypotheses in their study of the effect of the number of exercises assigned on performance and compliance with a home program for older adults:[26(p.273)]

> *Three hypotheses were formulated prior to this study: (1) Subjects who are prescribed two exercises will perform better than subjects who are prescribed eight exercises, (2) Subjects who are prescribed two exercises will comply on their self-report exercise log more than subjects who are prescribed eight exercises, and (3) Self-report percentage rates will highly correlate with performance assessment tool scores.*

In other words, these authors predicted that a lower number of exercises would be related to greater success with the home program. In this example, if a statistical test demonstrates a significant difference or relationship, then the research hypothesis is "accepted." If the test indicates that the results likely occurred due to chance, then the research hypothesis is "rejected." It is important to note that, regardless of the form, hypotheses are tested as stated such that the statements are either accepted or rejected. Researchers may speculate about another possible outcome when their original hypothesis is rejected, but it would be inappropriate for them to claim that this alternate prediction has been "proven."

As is true with theories and conceptual frameworks, researchers may "hypothesize" about a result without stating their intentions in a formal way. An additional challenge for readers is that authors of physical therapy research often do not present any hypotheses at all. The presence or absence of hypothesis statements may be driven by publishers' formatting preferences, by the manner in which the researchers were trained to develop and communicate about their research, or by the nature of the research itself. The lack of formal hypothesis statements does not reduce the quality of the research in and of itself; rather, it is the manner in which the authors interpret their results relative to these statements that may cause the reader to question the research quality.

Summary

Research is a quest for answers about a question or purpose statement that investigators have identified through a variety of methods. The relevance and importance of the quest may be demonstrated through a review of prior literature, as well as by other data about the impact of a phenomenon on individuals or society. The quest may be guided or based on formally stated relationships among ideas and observations that may be as elaborate as a grand theory or as simple as a conceptual framework. In all cases, proposals about human behavior must be based on biologic plausibility.

Researchers may predict the outcome of their study using formal null or research hypotheses. Statistical tests are used to determine whether these hypotheses should be accepted or rejected as written; however, rejection does not prove that other possible explanations are true.

Finally, the use of theories, models, or hypotheses will depend on the investigator's research purpose and intent. Clinical studies may not have any of these elements, but authors may use the terminology in an informal way to convey their speculations or predictions. Readers should focus on the content of the material presented to determine the success with which the investigators have justified the need for their study and described the foundation on which the project will be conducted.

Exercises

1. Think about a patient scenario or clinical situation in which you have been involved, and ask yourself what more you would like to know about that situation.
   a. Write that thought in the form of a research question.
   b. Write that thought in the form of a purpose statement.
   c. Rewrite your statement from (a) or (b) to make it broader.
   d. Rewrite your statement from (a) or (b) to make it narrower.
2. Write a brief rationale justifying why your idea is relevant and important to study. Remember the issue of biologic plausibility.
3. Describe a plan for a literature review you would conduct to determine what is known about your research question or purpose statement. Include alternative strategies in case your first search attempt reveals no prior studies.
4. Identify sources of epidemiologic data you would include (assuming they are available) to justify the need for your study.
5. Differentiate between a theory and a conceptual framework. Provide a clinical example relevant to physical therapist practice to illustrate your points.
6. Differentiate between a concept and a construct. Provide a clinical example relevant to physical therapist practice of each.
7. Differentiate between the null and the research hypotheses. Give an example of each based on your research question or purpose statement from question 1.

References

1. Carter RE, Lubinsky J, Domholdt E. *Rehabilitation Research. Principles and Applications.* 4th ed. St Louis, MO: Elsevier Saunders; 2011.
2. Polit DF, Beck CT. *Nursing Research: Principles and Methods.* 7th ed. Philadelphia, PA: Lippincott Williams & Wilkins; 2003.
3. Portney LG, Watkins MP. *Foundations of Clinical Research. Applications to Practice.* 3rd ed. Upper Saddle River, NJ: Prentice Hall Health; 2009.
4. Batavia M. *Clinical Research for Health Professionals: A User-Friendly Guide.* Boston, MA: Butterworth-Heinemann; 2001.
5. Washington K, Deitz JC, White OR, Schwartz IS. The effects of a contoured foam seat on postural alignment and upper-extremity function in infants with neuromotor impairments. *Phys Ther.* 2002;82(11):1064–1076.
6. Lau B, Skinner EH, Lo K, Bearman M. Experiences of physical therapists working in the acute hospital setting: systematic review. *Phys Ther.* 2016;96(9):1317–1332.
7. Fox EE, Hough AD, Creanor S, Gear M, Freeman JA. Effect of Pilates-based core stability training in ambulant people with multiple sclerosis: multi-center, assessor-blinded, randomized controlled trial. *Phys Ther.* 2016;96(8):1170–1178.

8. Bhatt T, Yang F, Mak MKY, et al. Effect of externally cued training on dynamic stability control during the sit-to-stand task in people with Parkinson disease. *Phys Ther.* 2013;93(4):492–503.

9. Farlie MK, Molloy E, Keating JL, Haines TP. Clinical markers of the intensity of balance challenge: observational study of older adult responses to balance tasks. *Phys Ther.* 2016;96(3):313–323.

10. Chung JI, Min BH, Baik EJ. Effect of continuous-wave low-intensity ultrasound in inflammatory resolution of arthritis-associated synovitis. *Phys Ther.* 2016;96(6):808–817.

11. Lee ACW, Billings M. Telehealth implementation in a skilled nursing facility: case report for physical therapist practice in Washington. *Phys Ther.* 2016;96(2):252–259.

12. Yamato TP, Pompeu JE, Pompeu SMAA, Hassett L. Virtual reality for stroke rehabilitation. *Phys Ther.* 2016;96(10):1508–1513.

13. Lloyd A. Roberts AR, Freeman JA. 'Finding a balance' involving patients in goal setting early after stroke: a physiotherapy perspective. *Physiother Res Int.* 2014;19:147–157.

14. Data & Statistics. Centers for Disease Control and Prevention website. Available at: www.cdc.gov/datastatistics. Accessed September 1, 2016.

15. Statistics & Data. Occupational Health and Safety Administration website. Available at: www.osha.gov/oshstats. Accessed September 1, 2016.

16. Reference Collections. U.S. Department of Health and Human Services website. Available at: https://datawarehouse.hrsa.gov. Accessed September 1, 2016.

17. U.S. Census Bureau website. Available at: www.census.gov. Accessed September 1, 2016.

18. The Pew Charitable Trusts website. Available at: http://www.pewtrusts.org/en/topics/health. Accessed September 1, 2016.

19. Robert Wood Johnson Foundation website. Available at: www.rwjf.org. Accessed September 1, 2016.

20. DiClemente CC, Schlundt D, Gemmell L. Readiness and stages of change in addiction treatment. *Am J Addict.* 2004;13(2):103–119.

21. Jean Piaget's Stage Theory. ChangingMinds.org website. Available at: http://changingminds.org/explanations/learning/piaget_stage. Accessed September 1, 2016.

22. Jette AM. Physical disablement concepts for physical therapy research and practice. *Phys Ther.* 1994;74(5):380–386.

23. World Health Organization. *Towards a Common Language of Functioning, Disability and Health. ICF.* Geneva, Switzerland: World Health Organization; 2002.

24. Women's Health Information Participant Information. Women's Health Initiative website. Available at: https://www.nhlbi.nih.gov/whi/. Accessed July 16, 2016.

25. Jones A, Jones RD, Kwong K, Burns Y. Effect of positioning on recorded lung sound intensities in subjects without pulmonary dysfunction. *Phys Ther.* 1999;79(7):682–690.

26. Henry KD, Rosemond C, Eckert LB. Effect of number of home exercises on compliance and performance in adults over 65 years of age. *Phys Ther.* 1999;79(3):270–277.

CHAPTER 5

RESEARCH DESIGN

OBJECTIVES

Upon completion of this chapter, the student/practitioner will be able to do the following:

1. Differentiate between quantitative and qualitative research paradigms.

2. Differentiate among experimental, quasi-experimental, and nonexperimental research designs.

3. Discuss methods by which control may be imposed in the research process.

4. Describe research designs used for questions about diagnostic tests, clinical measures, prognostic factors, interventions, clinical prediction rules, outcomes, and self-report outcomes measures.

5. Describe research designs for secondary analyses and qualitative studies.

TERMS IN THIS CHAPTER

Between-subjects design: A research design that compares outcomes between two or more groups of subjects.[1]

Bias: Results or inferences that systematically deviate from the truth "or the processes leading to such deviation."[2(p.251)]

Biologic plausibility: The reasonable expectation that the human body could behave in the manner predicted.

Case-control design: A retrospective epidemiologic research design used to evaluate the relationship between a potential exposure (e.g., risk factor) and an outcome (e.g., disease or disorder); two groups of subjects—one of which has the outcome (the case) and one that does not (the control)—are compared to determine which group has a greater proportion of individuals with the exposure.[3]

Case report: A detailed description of the management of a patient or client that may serve as a basis for future research,[4] and describes the overall management of an unusual case or a condition that is infrequently encountered in practice or poorly described in the literature.[5]

Case series: A description of the management of several patients or clients for the same purposes as a case report; the use of multiple individuals increases the potential importance of the observations as the basis for future research.[6]

Cohort: A group of individuals in a study who are followed over a period of time; often the group is defined by a particular characteristic, such as age.[7]

Cohort design: A prospective epidemiologic research design used to evaluate the relationship between a potential exposure (e.g., risk factor) and an outcome (e.g., disease or disorder); two groups of subjects—one of which has the exposure and one of which does not—are monitored over time to determine who develops the outcome and who does not.[3]

Cross-sectional study: A study that collects data about a phenomenon during a single point in time or once within a defined time interval.[8]

Dose-response relationship: The magnitude of an outcome increases as the magnitude of an exposure or intervention increases.[3,8]

Effectiveness: The extent to which an intervention or service produces a desired outcome under usual clinical conditions.[2]

Efficacy: The extent to which an intervention or service produces a desired outcome under ideal conditions.[2]

Experimental design: A research design in which the behavior of randomly assigned groups of subjects is measured following the purposeful manipulation of an independent variable(s) in at least one of the groups; used to examine cause-and-effect relationships between an independent variable(s) and an outcome(s).[1,9]

Longitudinal study: A study that looks at a phenomenon occurring over time.[2]

Masked (also referred to as *blinded*): (1) In diagnostic test and clinical measure papers, the lack of knowledge about previous test/measure results; (2) in prognostic factor papers, the lack of knowledge about exposure status; and (3) in intervention papers, the lack of knowledge about to which group a subject has been assigned.

Measurement reliability: The extent to which repeated measurements agree with one another. Also referred to as "stability," "consistency," and "reproducibility."[7]

Measurement validity: The degree to which a measure captures what it is intended to measure.[7(p.77)]

Meta-analysis: A statistical method used to pool data from individual studies included in a systematic review.[10]

Narrative review (also referred to as a *literature review*): A description of prior research without a systematic search and selection strategy or critical appraisal of the study's merits.[10]

Nonexperimental design (also referred to as an *observational study*): A research design in which controlled manipulation of the subjects is lacking[1]; in addition, if groups are present, assignment is predetermined based on naturally occurring subject characteristics or activities.[8]

Patient-centered care: Health care that "customizes treatment recommendations and decision making in response to patients' preferences and beliefs . . . This partnership also is characterized by informed, shared decision making, development of patient knowledge, skills needed for self-management of illness, and preventive behaviors."[11(p.3)]

Placebo: "An intervention without biologically active ingredients."[3(p.682)]

Posttest: Application of an outcome measure at the conclusion of a study to determine whether a change occurred in response to manipulation of the independent variable.[9]

Power: The probability that a statistical test will detect, if it is present, a relationship between two or more variables (or scores) or a difference between two or more groups (or scores).[1,7]

Pretest: Application of an outcome measure at the start of a study for the purposes of obtaining baseline performance of the subjects prior to manipulation of the independent variable.[9]

Prospective design: A research design that follows subjects forward over a specified period of time.

Qualitative research paradigm: A research model that seeks to understand the nature of a phenomenon from the perspective and social context of the subjects who are studied, with the assumption that multiple realities may be possible and may evolve as the subjects interact with the researchers.[1,12]

Quantitative research paradigm: A research model that assumes an objective reality exists that is observable and can be measured through systematic, bias-free methods.[1,12]

Quasi-experimental design: A research design in which there is only one subject group or in which randomization to more than one subject group is lacking; controlled manipulation of the subjects is preserved.[13]

Randomized clinical trial (also referred to as a *randomized controlled trial* and a *randomized controlled clinical trial*) [RCT]: A clinical study that uses a randomization process to assign subjects to either an experimental group(s) or a control (or comparison) group. Subjects in the experimental group receive the intervention or preventive measure of interest and then are compared to the subjects in the control (or comparison) group who did not receive the experimental manipulation.[1]

Research design: The plan for conducting a research study.

Retrospective design: A study that uses previously collected information to answer a research question.

Sample: A collection of individuals (or units of analysis, such as organizations) selected from the population for the purposes of a research study.

Single-system design: A quasi-experimental research design in which one subject receives in an alternating fashion both the experimental and control (or comparison) condition.[1]

Subjects: Individuals, organizations, or other units of analysis about whom information is gathered for the purposes of a research study.

Systematic review: A method by which a collection of individual research studies is gathered and critically appraised in an effort to reach a conclusion about the cumulative weight of the evidence on a particular topic[9]; also referred to as a "synthesis."[14]

Within-subjects design: A research design that compares repeated measures of an outcome within the same individuals.[1]

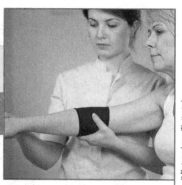

© Photographee.eu/Shutterstock

CLINICAL SCENARIO

Help Me Understand What I'm Reading

Anne majored in chemistry in college and completed an honors thesis under the direction of a faculty mentor. She understands the traditional scientific method and read numerous journal articles as part of her studies that described meticulously controlled experiments in the lab. She is perplexed by the format of some of the studies she was able to access in full text online and is concerned about the apparent subjectivity in many of them.

How will you explain the similarities and differences between the "bench research" she is used to and the clinical research you will use to inform decision making?

Introduction

Research is a purposeful effort to answer a question or explore a phenomenon. In clinical care those questions most often relate to (1) the human body and its responses to disease and injury; (2) the methods by which providers attempt to prevent, reverse, or minimize any harmful consequences resulting from these problems; and (3) the experiences of those engaged in the health care enterprise. To answer these questions in a meaningful and believable way, investigators should plan each step of the research process in careful detail. This plan is referred to as the *research design*. Research designs are analogous to the plans of care physical therapists develop for their patients or clients. Both include details about the methods by which the investigator (therapist) will interact with research *subjects* (patients or clients), the timing of these interactions, the length of time of the entire effort, and the type of outcomes that will be measured. In addition, research designs and plans of care are crafted to meet the needs of a specific research question or a specific individual. Research designs and plans of care also may attempt to minimize the influence of unwanted factors or events that will interfere with the outcomes. This last point is more nuanced, however, because the real-life circumstances of research subjects and patients or clients may be a central, purposeful theme in research designs and plans of care, respectively.

Physical therapists using evidence to inform their practice decisions must evaluate the strength of research designs to determine whether the research question was answered in a believable and useful way. Research designs have been classified in evidence hierarchies to facilitate easier identification of their strengths; however, these hierarchies only serve as an initial screening process. A thorough reading of the research report is needed to identify specific strengths and weaknesses of an individual study before its conclusions can be accepted or rejected for use in patient/client management.

This chapter discusses general approaches to research designs that are used in health care research, along with their purposes, benefits, and limitations. Designs best suited for questions about diagnostic tests, clinical measures, prognostic factors, interventions, clinical prediction rules, outcomes, self-report outcomes measures, and patient or client perspectives and experiences are described in more detail. Methods of controlling unwanted influences within some of these designs also are reviewed.

General Features of Research Designs

The following general features of research designs are important to recognize and understand when reviewing evidence:

- The investigator's research paradigm;
- The overall design format implemented consistent with the research paradigm;
- The number of groups studied;
- The type(s) of data collected;
- The role of time in the study; and
- The type and degree of control imposed, if any.

Research Paradigms

Research designs usually reflect one of two paradigms about how the world is understood—that is, either a quantitative or a qualitative perspective. A *quantitative research paradigm* is based in a positivist philosophy that assumes that there is an objective truth that can be revealed by investigators who attempt to conduct their inquiries in a value-free manner.[1,12] Researchers strive to achieve this objectivity by imposing specific controls to minimize any unwanted (extraneous) influences that may bias the studies' outcomes. This view defines the traditional scientific method that is ubiquitous across many fields of research.

A *qualitative research paradigm*, in contrast, assumes that knowledge and understanding are contextual and relative to each individual studied.[1,12] Investigators and subjects are assumed to influence each other as the researchers gather information about subjects' "lived experiences" and worldviews. Methods of control relative to extraneous environmental influences are irrelevant in this approach because it assumes that cause-and-effect relationships, if present, should be identified as they naturally occur. Instead, an emphasis is placed on description and iterative interpretation of the information that is gathered.

Design Format: Quantitative Research

Quantitative research designs are characterized by whether the investigators actively intervene with the research subjects. *Experimental designs* are those in which the researchers purposefully manipulate some of the subjects and then measure their resulting behavior.[1,9] These designs use at least two groups of subjects for comparison purposes and include a process for randomly allocating individuals into each of these groups. The comparison allows investigators to determine whether there are differences in outcomes between the group(s) that is (are) manipulated and the group(s) that is (are) not. Random assignment to these groups is the method best suited to distributing individuals equally among them.

Quasi-experimental designs also involve purposeful manipulation of the subjects by the investigators, but they lack either a second group for comparison purposes or a random assignment process, or both.[13] These designs often are used when the investigators have difficulty obtaining sufficient numbers of subjects to form groups or when group membership is predetermined by a subject characteristic, such as whether the subject received a particular medical or surgical intervention prior to physical therapy.[13] The inability to randomly assign subjects to groups or to make a comparison to a nontreatment group means that other influences may explain the outcome of the study, thereby potentially reducing the usefulness of its results.

Finally, *nonexperimental designs* are those in which the investigators are simply observers who collect information about the phenomenon of interest; there is no purposeful manipulation of subjects by the researchers to produce a change in behavior or status. Interventions intended to effect a change are simply part of the normal course of care and are applied according to the norms and abilities of the health care providers involved. In addition, if groups are present, assignment is predetermined based on naturally occurring subject characteristics or activities. These designs also are referred to as "observational studies."[3]

Design Format: Qualitative Research

Qualitative studies investigate subjects' thoughts, perceptions, opinions, beliefs, attitudes and/or experiences. The analyses focus on the identification of patterns or themes in the data (i.e., words or descriptive observations) that may be used for further exploration in a subsequent round of data collection. Carter et al. refer to this step as "generating meaning."[1] The final set of verified themes is presented as the results of the study once data collection and analyses are complete. Researchers do not introduce experimental interventions or controls that limit knowledge or behavior in an artificial context (i.e., a clinic or laboratory). Rather, they attempt to capture how subjects construct meaning about naturally occurring phenomena and interactions within their environment.

As illustrated in **Table 5-1**, different qualitative research designs are intended to answer different types of questions researchers may pose.

TABLE 5-1	Types of Questions Answered by Different Qualitative Research Designs	
Qualitative Research Tradition	**General Approach**	**Type of Question Addressed**
Discourse analysis	Analysis of the form, content and rules of conversations	How do individuals in this setting communicate with one another under these circumstances or conditions?
Ethnography	Holistic analysis of a culture	How are individuals' behaviors shaped by the culture of this setting under these circumstances or conditions?
Ethology	Observation of behaviors in a natural context	How do individuals behave in this setting under these circumstances or conditions?
Grounded theory	Analysis of social, psychological and structural processes within a social setting	How do individuals make sense of their experiences in this setting under these circumstances or conditions?
Historical analysis	Analysis and interpretation of historical events	How did individuals behave or interpret their experiences in this setting under these previous circumstances or conditions?
Phenomenology	Analysis of experiences, interpretations, meanings	How do individuals make sense of interactions with others and/or with their setting under these circumstances or conditions?

Qualitative studies related to physical therapist practice often use an ethnographic, grounded theory or phenomenologic format.[1,12]

An ethnographic approach focuses on the observation of cultural patterns and experiences in an attempt to understand "what the subjects' lives are like." Data are collected through observational methods in which the researcher may be (1) removed from the daily interactions of the subjects ("nonparticipant observation") or (2) immersed in the subjects' natural environment ("participant observation"). Investigators using the latter method require a level of acceptance from their subjects that permits intimate access to the cultural components of interest. As a result, a significant amount of time may be required to conduct a study in this manner.

A grounded theory approach seeks to understand individuals' points of view from a theoretical perspective that is based on the empirical data collected. Researchers using this method repeatedly collect and analyze information that may be gathered via interview and/or observation from their subjects within their natural context. Conceptual categories, or themes, reflective of different aspects of the phenomenon of interest are generated and refined through successive cycles of data gathering and analysis until a "saturation point" is reached.

Finally, a phenomenologic approach addresses current or previously "lived experiences" of the individuals studied by gathering data through interview and discussion. Interview formats include semi-structured, in-depth, and narrative approaches that may be applied with each individual subject or during focus group sessions. Questions are posed in an open-ended manner that allows subjects to respond in their own words rather than selecting from a pre-established set of options or being confined to "yes" or "no". The product of these accounts is intended to be a vivid picture that improves our understanding of a phenomenon from the subjects' point of view.

Many qualitative research studies in physical therapy use a combination of these approaches. Additional methods also are available. A more detailed review of these design formats is beyond the scope of this text. Readers with an interest in learning more are encouraged to obtain one of the qualitative research methods resources listed in this chapter.[12,15,16]

Number of Groups

Research designs may be characterized by the number of groups of subjects used in the analysis. In quantitative approaches, the number of groups commonly is of most interest when comparisons between or among data points are intended to answer the research question. A study in which repeated measures of an outcome are compared for a single group of subjects is referred to as a *within-subjects design*.[1] In these designs each individual's baseline measure is compared to any of their own subsequent measures to determine if a change has occurred. Alternatively, a design in which outcomes are compared between two or more independent groups of subjects is referred to as a *between-subjects design*.[1] Typically, the average outcome score for each group is used in these analyses. The number of groups studied also is relevant to investigations in which associations between variables and predictions about outcomes are evaluated.

In qualitative approaches, the number of groups included depends on the extent to which knowledge and experience is distributed across the population of interest as well as the influence of logistical considerations related to access and/or time.

Type of Data

Quantitative designs most commonly use numeric data that may be analyzed by mathematical techniques. However, non-numeric data also may be used, as is often the case with survey responses or classifications into descriptive categories such as gender, race/ethnicity, or religious affiliation. In both situations, the goal typically is to answer the questions "how much?" or "how many?" Qualitative designs, in contrast, focus on the collection of subjects' words or the researchers' descriptions of subject behaviors in order to identify themes that provide insight into the meaning of a phenomenon.

Time Elements

All quantitative and qualitative research designs incorporate a time element that has both duration and direction. With regard to the duration, investigators must decide whether they want data collected once during a single point in time or a limited time interval (a *cross-sectional study*) or whether they will take repeated measures over an extended period of time (a *longitudinal study*).[6] The choice is dictated by the research question to be answered, as well as by logistical issues that may limit the degree to which subject follow-up is possible. The time "direction" is determined by whether the investigators want to use historical information for data (a *retrospective design*) or whether they want to collect their own data in real time (a *prospective design*).

Previously collected data often are attractive because they are readily available and may provide information about large numbers of subjects. However, retrospective approaches have several important disadvantages. First, they lack control over the original measurement processes, a situation that may introduce inaccuracies into the data. Second, they lack control over the method by which variables of interest (e.g., treatment techniques) are manipulated. Uncontrolled manipulation of variables may cause excessive variation in the outcomes, making it difficult to determine if an intervention had a meaningful impact. Third, the lack of randomization to groups in a retrospective intervention study also means that underlying factors pertinent to the individual may influence the outcomes. These consequences make it difficult to identify a cause-and-effect sequence. Prospective data collection allows the researchers to create and implement specific rules and methods by which the data are collected and the variables are manipulated so other factors that may influence the study's outcome are minimized.

Degree of Control

Another design feature is the degree to which controls can be imposed on the behavior of all participants in the study, as well as the conditions under which the project is conducted. As noted previously, the concept of "control" is only relevant to quantitative study formats because the artificial imposition of limitations on human behavior is contrary to the intention of qualitative studies.

The issue of control relates to the need to minimize bias in a study. *Bias* refers to results that systematically deviate from the truth,[2] a situation that is likely to occur when a research project is executed without detailed, thoughtful procedures related to:

- Recruitment, assignment, communication with and management of subjects;
- Calibration and use of necessary equipment;
- Maintenance of the environmental conditions during study activities;
- Administration of testing and/or training activities;
- Collection and recording of data; and
- Communication among investigators and others involved in the project.

Experimental designs are the most restrictive in terms of the amount of control imposed on study participants and conditions. At a minimum this effort starts with randomization of subjects to two or more groups for comparison. This control is necessary to improve the believability of a study whose aim is to demonstrate a cause-and-effect relationship between the variable that is manipulated (e.g., a new treatment technique) and the change in subject behavior (e.g., improvement in function).[7,9] Quasi-experimental designs lack either the control achieved by random placement of subjects into groups or the use of a comparison group, or both; however, they may still include procedures that manage participant behavior and environmental conditions pertinent to the study. Finally, the extent of control in nonexperimental studies is limited to protocols for measurement and collection of data. In all of these designs, additional control (or adjustment) may be achieved statistically.

Research Question

Which characteristics a particular study demonstrates depends on the type of question the investigators want to answer,[17] as well as on the logistical considerations with which each research team must contend. For example, a question about the effectiveness of joint mobilization on low back pain may be answered through an experimental design in which one group of randomly assigned subjects receives specified mobilization techniques plus exercise while another group of randomly assigned subjects receives exercise alone. In this hypothetical study, the researchers are purposefully intervening (providing mobilization to one group and not to the other) and collecting outcome data in a prospective fashion according to the duration of the study. A significant logistical challenge in this design is the need to recruit a sufficient number of patients with low back pain to enhance the strength of subsequent statistical analyses. The availability of such patients often is out of the investigators' control and may result in a lengthy time frame for the execution of the study.

However, a more efficient approach may be to review medical records of patients with low back pain who have completed an episode of physical therapy care during which they received either mobilization plus exercise or exercise alone. A potential advantage of this retrospective, nonexperimental approach is the immediate availability of data for many more subjects than it would be practical to recruit in real time. The disadvantage of this approach is the potential lack of standardized procedures for application of the mobilization techniques, the exercise, or the outcome measures. In this situation, the benefit gained from a large sample size may be undermined by the variability in the interventions and the resulting performance data such that it is difficult to determine the true impact of joint mobilization. Nevertheless, this study may provide information that serves as the basis for a more definitive experimental design.

Table 5-2 summarizes the general features and related options for research designs. Questions about diagnostic tests, clinical measures, prognostic factors, interventions, clinical prediction rules, outcomes, self-report outcomes measures, and patient or client perceptions and experiences are answered best by different research designs. The following sections discuss details of specific designs for each category of questions, as well as designs used to summarize a body of literature and designs used to explore subject experiences and perceptions.

Research Designs for Questions About Diagnostic Tests and Clinical Measures

Studies about diagnostic tests usually are nonexperimental and cross-sectional in design. The goal of these projects is to determine the usefulness of the test of interest (i.e., the "index test") for correctly detecting a pathology or an impairment in body functions and structure. Assignment to groups and purposeful manipulation of a variable is not relevant to these studies. Instead, the strongest research design is one in which individuals who appear to have a particular disorder or condition are evaluated with the index test, as well as with a second test about which the usefulness already has been established.[8] The second test usually is referred to as the "gold standard" or "reference standard" because of its superior ability to correctly identify individuals with, and without, the clinical problem of interest. Comparison of the scores from both tests allows the investigators to determine if the index test provides accurate information about the presence or absence of a suspected condition

TABLE 5-2　　General Features of Research Designs

Feature	Options	Characteristics
Paradigm	• Quantitative	• Objective reality; answers questions such as "how much?" or "how many?"
	• Qualitative	• Subjective reality; answers questions about subjects' perspectives or experiences in the natural context
Design Format: Quantitative	• Experimental	• Purposeful manipulation of a variable(s); random assignment of subjects to two or more groups
	• Quasi-experimental	• Purposeful manipulation of a variable(s); no random assignment to groups; may have only one group
	• Nonexperimental	• Observational without manipulation of a variable(s); no random assignment to groups; may have only one group
Design Format: Qualitative	• Ethnographic	• Observation at a distance or immersed in context
	• Grounded theory	• Iterative analysis of empiric data to generate theory
	• Phenomenologic	• Interview
Number of Groups	• Within-subjects analysis	• One group of subjects available for study; outcome scores compared to baseline scores for each subject
	• Between-subjects analysis	• Two or more groups of subjects available for study; mean scores for each group typically used in statistical analyses
Type of Data	• Numeric	• Used in quantitative studies
	• Non-numeric	• Used in quantitative studies (symbols, words, categories) and qualitative studies (words)
Time Elements: Duration	• Cross-sectional	• Data collected once from one point in time
	• Longitudinal	• Data collected repeatedly over a period of time
Time Elements: Direction	• Retrospective	• Historical data
	• Prospective	• Data collected in real time
Degree of Control	• Maximal	• Experimental design
	• Moderate	• Quasi-experimental design
	• Minimal	• Nonexperimental design
	• None	• Qualitative studies

(i.e., *measurement validity*). Additional information about *measurement reliability*, or the stability of the results over repeated administrations, also can be obtained.

Control of unwanted factors in these studies can be achieved through several strategies. First, investigators can clearly delineate and apply criteria for identifying which individuals are suspected of having the disorder or condition of interest. Second, protocols for performance of the index test and the comparison test can be implemented to ensure that each subject is examined using the same methods in the same sequence. These protocols also should identify criteria for determining a positive or negative result for both tests. Third, verification of the examiner's (or examiners') competence performing the index test and the comparison test will reduce potential inaccuracies in the results. Fourth, criteria for verifying the presence or absence of the condition of interest via the comparison test can be delineated. Finally, investigators can withhold the results of the index test from the examiners responsible for confirming the diagnosis and vice versa. Keeping the examiners *masked* will reduce the chance that they will introduce bias through their expectations about the outcome of the test they are administering.

Cook et al. used many of these methods of control in their study of the usefulness of five clinical examination techniques for identifying individuals with glenoid labrum pathologies (i.e., SLAP lesions).[18] In this study, arthroscopic surgery was used as the "reference standard" test; therefore, individuals with shoulder pain were required to meet established criteria for surgical eligibility in order to participate. The authors also defined the signs used to recognize a positive and negative result for the clinical tests, as well as for diagnosis confirmation during the arthroscopy. However, the authors did not verify whether the examiners consistently performed the clinical tests, so some variation in results may have occurred. In addition, the surgeons conducting the diagnostic arthroscopy were occasionally aware of the clinical tests' results prior to surgery. Overall, the controls these authors implemented improved the credibility of this article's results by decreasing, although not eliminating, the chance that extraneous factors influenced the outcomes.

Methodologic Studies of Clinical Measures

Research about the usefulness of diagnostic tests is complemented by studies in which new instruments are developed or existing instruments are modified and tested for their usefulness. Collectively referred to as "methodologic research,"[7] these studies usually focus on clinical measures used to quantify impairments in body functions and structure, such as limited range of motion,[19] weakness,[20] and loss of balance.[21] Like studies for diagnostic tests, the designs for methodologic studies are nonexperimental. Methodologic studies also tend to be cross-sectional but may use a longitudinal approach when the goal is to determine a clinical measure's ability to detect change in the impairment over time. These studies may evaluate an instrument's measurement reliability through repeated administrations and/or measurement validity through comparison to a superior instrument. The usefulness of the instrument in different patient or client populations also may be explored. Methods of control in these designs focus on the procedures for identification and recruitment of subjects, protocols for the development and administration of the instruments, and statistical adjustment to account for extraneous factors that may influence subject performance or for loss of information due to subject dropout.

Irwin and Sesto evaluated the reliability and validity of a new handheld dynamometer with respect to measurement of strength and other parameters related to grip.[20] Two established grip-strength testing devices were used for comparison. The study data were collected at two points in time to determine the new measure's stability. Protocols for subject positioning and application of force with the handheld devices were implemented. The new handheld device demonstrated reliability as consistently as the established devices as well as concurrent validity for both younger and older subjects. However, the authors did not indicate how many examiners participated or whether they were aware of previous results. These limitations suggest further study is warranted to confirm the findings.

Research Designs for Questions About Prognostic Factors

Studies focusing on prognostic factors commonly have one of the following three research designs used routinely in epidemiologic research: prospective cohort, retrospective cohort, or case control.[10]

All of these designs assess the relationship between a prognostic factor (epidemiologists use the label "exposure") and an outcome. They also are nonexperimental in nature; therefore, control often is limited to methods by which the investigators identify eligible subjects and collect the data. Management of extraneous influences usually occurs through statistical adjustment. An important feature of these designs is that causal links between a prognostic factor and an outcome cannot be established directly. Causality may be inferred, however, when the following conditions are met:

- The prognostic factor clearly preceded the outcome (demonstrated by longitudinal designs);
- The relationship between the prognostic factor and the outcome was strong (as defined by the nature of its measurement);
- A *dose-response relationship* between the prognostic factor and the outcome was demonstrated;
- The findings were consistent with results from previous (preferably well-designed) studies; and
- The results met criteria for *biologic plausibility.*[22]

Inferences about causality based on prognosis studies may be necessary in situations in which it would be inappropriate or unethical to perform an experiment to determine a cause-and-effect relationship. For example, requiring one set of subjects to initiate a smoking habit while another set abstains in order to determine if there is a difference in the incidence of lung cancer between the groups would violate federal and professional obligations related to human subjects' protection. Instead, observational research designs are needed to provide the necessary evidence.

Cohort Designs

The term *cohort* refers to a group of subjects who are followed over time and who usually share a common characteristic such as gender, age, occupation, the presence of a prognostic factor or diagnosis, and so forth.[7] Cohort studies have observational descriptive designs from which results are analyzed statistically to determine the relationship between prognostic factors and outcomes.

A prospective *cohort design* is one in which a group of subjects is identified and then followed over a specified period of time to see if, and when, the outcome of interest occurs.[10] Often more than one group is followed for the purposes of comparison. The second group usually does not have the prognostic factor of interest. Prospective cohort designs are the preferred research designs for questions about prognostic factors because the authors have the best opportunity to control unwanted influences by collecting their own data in real time, rather than using historical information. In addition, starting with the prognostic factor and working toward the outcome is a necessary sequence to make a stronger case for a potential cause-and-effect relationship. An important challenge to this design is the time needed to ensure that the outcome could occur and be measured, as well as the resources necessary to follow subjects over long periods.

Alemdaroglu et al. used a prospective cohort design to determine whether any factors collected on a baseline evaluation prior to hospital discharge would predict future falls in individuals following stroke.[23] Patients from one rehabilitation hospital were followed for 6 months after discharge to determine who fell and who did not. Standardized instruments with established reliability and validity were used to measure balance and mobility in the study, thereby reducing the chances of variation due to instability or inaccuracy of the measures collected at baseline. The 6-month follow-up implemented was consistent with previous evidence regarding the time frame in which falls following acute stroke were most likely to occur.

A retrospective cohort design is one in which data from medical records, outcomes databases, or claims databases are examined and a cohort or cohorts are identified during the review process.[10] This approach addresses the challenge of the prospective cohort design in that the outcomes already have occurred and can be identified. However, control over how the measures were collected during actual encounters with the subjects is lost.

Bland et al. used this design to examine the relationship between clinical data collected on admission and 10-meter walking speed at discharge in individuals following stroke.[24] These authors identified a cohort of patients previously admitted to one inpatient rehabilitation hospital and collected historical data regarding motor and sensory status; performance on standardized function, balance, and gait speed tests; patient age; and time since stroke onset. The tests and measures had established reliability and validity but the investigators could not control how those instruments were applied at the point of patient care. As a result, data accuracy may be affected. In addition, other variables that may have contributed to performance on the walking test were not measured or documented consistently. In the absence of a known research question and protocol, the providers involved collected information they determined to be relevant to individual patient's health care needs. The variability of available historical information is a common limitation to retrospective designs.

Case-Control Designs

A *case-control design* is a retrospective approach in which subjects who are known to have the outcome of interest are compared to a control group known to be free of the outcome.[10] The question investigated is the relative frequency of exposure to the prognostic factor in each group. The quintessential example here is the initial investigation into the relationship between smoking and lung cancer. Lung cancer takes years to develop, so it was impractical to wait and see what happens once someone started smoking. Instead, researchers identified subjects diagnosed with lung cancer and subjects free of the disease and worked backward to determine each individual's exposure to smoking. Eventually, results from both prospective and retrospective designs provided enough convincing evidence to conclude that smoking was a causal factor.[25]

A case-control design also is useful in research of interest to physical therapists. Wang et al. used a case-control design to examine risk factors for the development of idiopathic adhesive capsulitis of the shoulder (IAC).[26] In this study, each of the 87 subjects with IAC were matched according to age and gender with 176 control subjects who did not suffer the condition. Potential risk factors then were measured in both groups and their relative proportions compared. Given that the etiology of adhesive capsulitis is unknown in most cases, it may be logistically impractical to study the development of this disorder in a prospective fashion. Identification of risk factors through a retrospective design may provide useful information to fill the gap in knowledge.

Other Designs for Prognostic Indicators

Prognostic indicators also may be gleaned from intervention papers, including randomized controlled trials. Because prognostic information is not the focus of this type of research, readers will have to do some digging to determine what factors, if any, may be associated with the outcomes measured.[10] In light of the limited information available about prognostic indicators that are useful in physical therapy, any data about prognosis from clinical trials are important to evaluate.

Research Designs for Questions About Interventions

Studies of interventions are used to determine their beneficial effects or harmful consequences, or both. Projects that measure the extent to which an intervention produces a desired outcome under ideal conditions focus on treatment *efficacy*. Studies that measure the impact of an intervention under usual clinical conditions focus on treatment *effectiveness*.[2] In both cases, these studies must be designed so that the treatment clearly precedes the outcome measured. In addition, the design should control or account for extraneous variables so that any treatment effect can be isolated and captured. Experimental research designs are promoted as the "gold standard" for determining the effects of interventions.[2,3,8,10,17] Increasing numbers of research articles pertaining to physical therapy interventions have experimental designs. However, numerous physical therapy research articles also have been published that are quasi-experimental in nature. Details of each of these design types are presented in the following sections.

Experimental Studies

The classic experimental study design used in clinical research is the *randomized clinical (or controlled) trial (RCT)*. An RCT includes two or more groups to which subjects have been randomly assigned. The experimental intervention is provided to one of the groups, and the resulting behavior in all of the groups is then compared. Campbell and Stanley described three experimental research formats that may be adopted for randomized clinical trials: the pretest–posttest control group design, the Solomon four-group design, and the posttest-only control group design.[9] Of these, the pretest–posttest control group design is the most commonly used in RCTs of interest to physical therapists.

In its simplest form the pretest–posttest format is composed of two groups: experimental and control. Performance on the outcome(s) of interest is measured in both groups at the start of the study (the *pretest*[s]). Then the intervention of interest is applied to the experimental group. Finally, subjects are measured again at the conclusion of the experiment (the *posttest*[s]) to determine whether a change has occurred. Repeated posttest measures over time are used for longitudinal versions of this design. **Figure 5-1** illustrates the pretest–posttest format. All else being equal, if the subjects in the experimental group change and the subjects in the control group do not, then it is likely that the intervention of interest was the change agent.

RCTs are valued research designs because of their ability to control a number of unwanted influences that may interfere with a study's results. The typical methods of control in this design are

FIGURE 5-1   **Schematic representation of a pretest-post experimental design.**

R O_1 X O_2
R O_3 O_4

R = Random assignment to the group
O_1 = Pretest for the experimental group
X = Experimental intervention
O_2 = Posttest for the experimental group
O_3 = Pretest for the control group
O_4 = Posttest for the control group

Republished with permission of South-Western College Publishing, a division of Cengage Learning, from Experimental and Quasi-Experimental Designs for Research, Campbell (Ed.), 1, © 1966; permission conveyed through Copyright Clearance Center, Inc.

outlined in **Table 5-3**. Control groups are the primary method by which investigators isolate the effects, if any, of the intervention of interest. A control group is differentiated from the experimental treatment group in one of several ways.[7] Subjects in the control group may receive no treatment at all and be instructed to behave as their usual routines dictate. Alternatively, they may be provided with a *placebo* or sham intervention that looks like the experimental treatment but is inactive or inert. The classic example of the placebo in medical research is the sugar pill provided to control groups in drug trials. A third option commonly used in physical therapy research is to provide both groups with traditional (or "usual") care but also to provide the intervention of interest to the experimental group. Finally, each group may be provided different treatments altogether, a situation that will challenge readers to remember which group is experimental and which is control. Often ethical issues related to withholding treatment from patients will dictate what type of control group is used.

Random assignment of subjects to groups is another method of control in experimental research. Randomization is used in an effort to create groups that are equal in size and composition. Equality of the groups is a necessary condition at the start of a study to protect its outcomes from the influence of extraneous factors inherent to the subjects. Characteristics commonly assessed for balanced distribution among groups in physical therapy research may include, but are not limited to, age, gender, ethnicity, baseline severity or function, and medication use, as well as sociodemographic factors such as education, employment, and social support.

Masking of subjects and investigators helps to control bias by preventing changes in behavior as a result of knowledge of group assignment. Similarly, defined protocols for outcomes measurement and application of the intervention(s), as well as control of environmental conditions, are important

TABLE 5-3 Methods of Control in Experimental Designs

Method of Control	Benefit
Two (or more) groups to compare, one of which is a "control" group that does not receive the experimental treatment	Effects of experimental treatment are isolated.
Random assignment of subjects to groups	Subject characteristics that might influence the outcomes are more likely to be distributed equally among the groups.
Efforts to mask (or "blind") subjects from knowledge of their group assignment	Changes in subject behavior due to knowledge of group assignment are minimized.
Efforts to mask investigators (or test administrators) from knowledge of subject group assignment	Bias introduced because of investigator expectations about behaviors in different groups is minimized.
Carefully delineated and applied protocols for subject testing and subject treatment	Consistency of techniques is ensured so that outcomes can be attributed to experimental intervention, not to procedural variation.
Stable environmental conditions during study activities	Subject performance is unrelated to factors outside of the test or treatment procedure.
Complete and sufficient follow-up to determine the outcomes of treatment	Adequate time is provided for outcomes of interest to develop and be measured.

to avoid unintended variation in the data that is unrelated to the intervention of interest. Finally, the time line for follow-up is important to ensure that an intervention's effects, if any, are not underestimated because they did not have sufficient opportunity to develop.

In addition to numerous methods for control within the study, an ideal RCT enrolls a large representative group of subjects and suffers little attrition along the way. A higher number of subjects enhances the function of statistical tests and the ability to apply the findings to a large group from which the subjects were recruited. That said, clinical research with patients makes a representative selection of numerous subjects difficult except for the most well-funded and logistically supported investigators. These studies are the multiyear investigations financed by large granting institutions, such as the National Institutes of Health and the Agency for Healthcare Research and Quality. Attrition, or loss of subjects during the study, often is out of the researchers' hands, but there are statistical methods with which to deal with the impact from those who drop out or who stop cooperating as the study proceeds.

An article by Cotchett et al. illustrates the use of an RCT to investigate the usefulness of a physical therapy intervention.[27] These authors implemented a randomized pretest–posttest design to evaluate the effectiveness of trigger point dry needling in the management of plantar heel pain. An experimental group of subjects received the actual dry needling intervention while the control group received a sham dry needling technique. The groups were equal in terms of subject age, time since onset and severity of pain, and impact on foot health. The person responsible for executing the random assignment process was masked to the baseline performance of subjects. Similarly, the individuals applying the pre- and posttest measures were blinded to subject group assignment. Masking of subjects was achieved using an opaque current to block their vision; however, therapists providing the intervention could not be blinded to the technique they were implementing. The authors provided details regarding the standardized application of the interventions and outcome measures. Only 81 individuals were enrolled in this study, a sample size that may be considered small but predictable for clinical research. However, the statistical significance of the findings suggests that the number of subjects was sufficient to detect differences in outcomes between the two groups.

Quasi-Experimental Studies

Quasi-experimental studies are projects in which there is a purposeful intervention with research subjects, but a comparison group and/or randomization to groups is missing.[9,13] However, other control methods used in experimental designs still may be imposed. Quasi-experimental research relies on several design options, including the time series design and the nonequivalent control group design. A simple time series format is one in which repeated measures are collected over time before and after the experimental intervention is introduced to a single group. If the baseline measures are stable prior to the intervention but change following its introduction, then a cause-and-effect relationship might be inferred.[9] Unfortunately, the lack of a control group reduces the certainty with which this causal connection can be stated because it is not possible to rule out natural subject improvement.

Bhambhani et al. used a time series design to evaluate the effectiveness of circuit training in patients with traumatic brain injury.[28] The time line for the study was divided into three phases. During the first phase, the stability of the outcome measures was evaluated through repeated measures 1 week apart (T_1 and T_2). Routine rehabilitation was introduced during the second week. The experimental intervention—circuit training—was introduced to all subjects at week 7 and continued for 14 weeks. Outcome measures were repeated at the conclusion of the rehabilitation (T_3), halfway through the circuit training (T_4), and at the conclusion of circuit training (T_5). **Figure 5-2** provides a schematic representation of the design used in this study.

FIGURE 5-2   **Schematic representation of a time series design as performed by Bhambhani et al.**

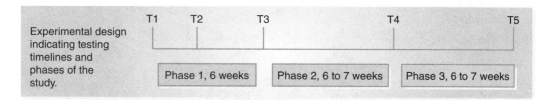

Experimental design indicating testing timelines and phases of the study.

A nonequivalent control group format is similar to the experimental pretest–posttest design except that random assignment to groups is lacking. Instead, naturally occurring groups are identified with only one receiving the experimental intervention. Unlike the time series design, this format has a control group for the purposes of comparison; however, as the name implies, subject characteristics probably are not distributed equally at the start of the study.[13]

Robitaille et al. used a nonequivalent control group design to evaluate the effectiveness of a group exercise program for improving balance in community-dwelling elderly individuals.[29] Two sets of community centers providing services to the elderly recruited potential participants. Subjects in one group of community centers received the experimental treatment, whereas subjects in the other centers had to wait for a period of time until the programs were initiated in their area. Although this study lacked randomized assignment of subjects to groups, it provides an example of a study conducted in typical community settings rather than in research labs or health care facilities.

Single-System Designs

Single-system designs are a type of quasi-experimental study that can be used to investigate the usefulness of an intervention. The distinguishing feature of these designs is their use of only one subject who undergoes, in an alternating fashion, an experimental treatment period and a control or comparison period. All of the controls used in quasi-experimental research can be imposed in this design. Studying only one individual is logistically easier for investigators as well. A single-system design is distinct from a *case report* or *case series* design in which the author simply describes the management of patients or clients

Carter et al. describe five variations of the single-system design, each of which is progressively more complex, as illustrated in **Table 5-4**.[1] Letters are used to represent the different phases of the design. "A-B designs" are the simplest version and reflect a control period (A) followed by the experimental treatment period (B). "Withdrawal designs" add a second control period that is imposed following the withdrawal of the experimental treatment. This approach is preferable to the "A-B design" because it may be easier to detect a true treatment effect if the subject's condition reverts to baseline after the experimental intervention is removed.

A "multiple baseline design" may be used with multiple individuals—each serving as their own single-system study—when investigators want to control for external events that may influence the

TABLE 5-4	Schematic Representations of Single-System Designs
Type of Design	**Schematic Depiction**
A-B Designs	A-B
Withdrawal Designs	A-B-A
Multiple Baseline Designs	A(1)-B-A
	A(2)-B-A
	A(1)-B-A
Alternating Treatment Designs	A-B-A-C-A
Interaction Designs	A-B-A-C-A-BC-A

A = control phase.
A(1) = control phase with one duration.
A(2) = control phase with a different duration.
B = intervention phase with one experimental treatment.
C = intervention phase with a different experimental treatment.
BC = intervention phase with both experimental treatments combined.

outcomes of the study. Each individual may be assigned to baseline control periods that both vary in length and occur at different times, followed by the experimental intervention and subsequent withdrawal periods. Results from all of the individuals then can be compared. This approach reduces the chance that a false conclusion will be drawn based on the response of one patient at one point in time. Finally, "alternating treatment designs" and "interaction designs" may be used to evaluate more than one experimental treatment and, in the latter case, the interaction of the two. In these designs investigators may randomize the order in which these interventions are applied. This approach is referred to as an "n-of-1 randomized controlled trial."[3]

Carr et al. used an alternating treatment design to evaluate the effect of four different interventions on hand range of motion, strength, and edema in a single patient with scleroderma.[30] The subject was a 42-year-old woman who had been diagnosed 3 years prior to the study. The baseline phase lasted 2 weeks and was followed by three treatment phases of 6 weeks' duration each to the right hand. The left hand served as the comparison and was treated in a similar time pattern but with a different sequence of interventions. This approach was used in lieu of withdrawal phases between each intervention type. No statistically significant changes were detected at the conclusion of the study. This result should prompt readers to consider whether the intervention application methods and/or the characteristics of the individual patient may have influenced the outcome.

The focus on one individual in a study may be useful for evidence-based physical therapists if that subject is very similar to the patient or client about whom the therapist has a clinical question. Any treatment effects detected are relevant to that person, not to an aggregate group in which the unique qualities of individuals are washed out in the averages. Guyatt and Rennie even went so far as to place an "n-of-1 randomized controlled trial" at the top of their evidence hierarchy for intervention studies.[3] Unfortunately, the need to withhold or withdraw a potentially beneficial treatment as part of the alternating sequence of the study design poses important ethical challenges that limit the extent to which this approach is used.

Research Designs for Clinical Prediction Rules

Studies about clinical prediction rules are nonexperimental in design; however, their specific features vary depending on the rule's intended use. Studies about clinical prediction rules that focus on diagnostic classification and potential treatment response resemble studies about individual diagnostic tests. In contrast, clinical prediction rules that focus on prognostic estimates may be designed like studies about prognostic factors. All of the same design enhancements and potential weaknesses in studies about diagnostic tests and prognostic factors apply here.

A clinical prediction rule's developmental stage also will influence the study design. Evidence about newly derived prediction rules will emphasize the methods used to identify and select the clinical indicators that provide the most meaningful predictions. Initial validation also will be performed. In these cases, study design elements resemble those used in methodologic research about self-report outcomes instruments (discussed in the next section). Wainner et al. used a prospective research design to develop a clinical prediction rule for diagnosis of carpal tunnel syndrome.[31] These authors explained in careful detail which patient data elements were collected, their methods for obtaining the data, and the analytic approaches used to finalize the list of predictors. They also evaluated the diagnostic accuracy of the rule via comparison to a criterion standard used to identify carpal tunnel syndrome. This study had a small sample size, which should prompt physical therapists using this evidence to consider the potential for inaccuracies in the model.

Alternatively, clinical prediction rules that are in the validation phase of their development will be studied using design features comparable to those used in methodologic research about clinical measures (discussed earlier). Gravel et al. evaluated the diagnostic accuracy of three clinical prediction rules used to identify the likelihood of ankle fracture.[32] In addition to providing readers with comparative performance information about each of the rules, these authors also confirmed the validity of one of them in children. The Ottawa Ankle Rules originally were derived and validated on adult populations.[33] Gravel et al.'s findings demonstrate that the Ottawa Ankle Rules also are useful in pediatric practice.

The bottom line is that evidence-based physical therapists should keep in mind the benefits and drawbacks of methodologic research designs when critically reviewing derivation and validation studies about clinical prediction rules.

Research Designs for Outcomes Research

Outcomes research focuses on the impact of clinical practice as it occurs in the "real world."[1,34] By definition, these studies focus on the "end results" experienced by patients or clients following an episode of care, rather than on the relative efficacy or effectiveness of individual interventions.[35,36] The study designs are nonexperimental (observational).[1] As a result, they lose much of the control that is imposed in experimental and quasi-experimental research. For example, they do not include randomization to groups, assuming there are groups to compare in the first place, and the researchers do not control the interventions applied to the subjects. Nevertheless, the motivation to conduct such studies stems from the desire to capture outcomes based on treatments applied in actual practice. The benefits accrued from an intervention under controlled conditions may be mitigated by factors in the clinical environment, such as variability in medical or surgical management, that also should be considered in physical therapist clinical decision making.[1] Outcomes research often focuses on results that are meaningful to patients or clients in addition to, or in lieu of, pathology or impairment-based measures. Finally, these studies have become the basis for assessing the quality of health care delivered across settings and professional disciplines.[37,38]

Outcomes research commonly is retrospective in its approach; however, studies may be cross-sectional or longitudinal depending on the question to be answered and the nature of the data that are available. Retrospective studies usually rely on large secondary administrative, insurance claims, or commercial outcomes databases for their data. For example, Jewell and Riddle used retrospective data maintained by Focus on Therapeutic Outcomes, Inc., on 2,370 patients with adhesive capsulitis to evaluate the likelihood of improvement in physical health based on the types of interventions provided.[39,40] The large sample size is an important statistical advantage for detecting relationships (if they exist) among the intervention categories and the outcome.

The primary disadvantage is that Jewell and Riddle did not have control over the application of the interventions or the collection and recording of the data. In addition, a true cause-and-effect relationship could not be demonstrated with this study because of its cross-sectional design. Rather, this study provides the foundation for a future experimental design in which similar patients can be randomized into experimental and comparison groups and in which the provision of interventions can be controlled by the investigators in real time. Despite their limitations, retrospective single-group studies may be the only evidence available about outcomes in some physical therapist practice areas; therefore, they should still be evaluated to determine whether there is any information that would be useful during management of the individual patient or client.

Although less common, it is possible to conduct an observational outcomes study with more than one group of subjects. For example, a hypothetical investigator may want to answer the following research question:

> *Which patients achieved normal gait patterns after physical therapy following anterior cruciate ligament reconstruction—those who received resistance training earlier or those who received it later in the rehabilitation program?*

In this study, the investigator could gather data to compare the gait patterns of patients from surgeon A, whose orders include resistance exercises at postoperative week 3, with patients from surgeon B, who does not order resistance exercises until postoperative week 6. This project could be conducted retrospectively through a medical records review or prospectively through standardized data recording methods. Again, the benefit of such a project is that it reflects real-world clinical conditions. However, because individuals are not randomized to the different surgeons there may be any number of inequalities between the two treatment groups (e.g., differences in medical history or preoperative activity levels) that may interfere with the outcomes of the study. In addition, the number of subjects in such a study is likely to be small unless both surgeons perform a high volume of anterior cruciate ligament surgeries over the time period in question. Both situations provide statistical challenges that must be addressed during the study.

Methodologic Studies About Self-Report Outcomes Measures

For the purposes of this text, outcomes measures refer to standardized self-report (i.e., surveys) or performance-based (i.e., balance tests) instruments or procedures that capture person-level end points such as activity limitations, participation restrictions, and quality of life. This distinction between impairment measures and outcomes measures may seem arbitrary to some; after all, remediation of impairments such as weakness in response to a physical therapist's intervention is a worthwhile result (i.e., "outcome"). Philosophically, however, defining outcomes measures in this fashion is more consistent with the concept of *patient-centered care*, as well as with the disablement model on which the American Physical Therapy Association's *Guide to Physical Therapist Practice 3.0* is based.[11,41] Physical therapists also are encouraged by payers to write treatment goals that focus on functional performance meaningful to their patients or clients rather than emphasizing impairment-related targets.

The development of outcomes measures is analogous to the development of impairment measures, as discussed earlier. The designs for methodologic studies about outcomes measures also are nonexperimental in nature. A significant body of methodologic research exists pertaining to the development and usefulness of self-report outcomes measures that are used by patients or clients to provide information about their disability,[42,43] health status,[44,45] satisfaction,[46,47] or quality of life.[48]

Health status, satisfaction, and quality of life are abstractions that cannot be observed in the direct way that we can "see" height or eye color. In addition, these constructs are based on patient or client perceptions and experiences. As a result, these phenomena require operational definitions that are measurable through a format that solicits the patient or client's assessment of his or her situation. The typical design for such an instrument is a survey with questions or statements serving as the direct measure of the phenomenon. For example, health status surveys may include items that ask an individual to indicate the impact of symptoms experienced on his or her physical and social activities, whereas satisfaction surveys may prompt assessments about the interpersonal and technical skill of the physical therapist and the comfort of the clinical environment. Surveys can be as short as one question (e.g., a global rating of change scale) but more commonly have multiple items to which individuals are asked to respond. An important distinction between these types of instruments and qualitative methods for gathering similar information is the use of a limited number of standardized, mutually exclusive options for each question or statement on the survey. A common example is some sort of rating scale. Respondents typically are instructed to select only one response for each item. The advantage of this approach is the ability to statistically evaluate the information gathered using quantitative analytic techniques. In contrast, qualitative approaches intentionally seek the individuals' own words to describe their experiences.

Investigators developing new self-report measures start the process by crafting an initial set of operational definitions or survey items. The focus of these definitions also is considered. Self-report measures with a general focus, referred to as "generic instruments," can be applied to the widest variety of situations or with an assortment of patients or clients. Other measures may focus on specific conditions (e.g., arthritis), body regions (e.g., knee), or satisfaction with particular aspects of the episode of care.[7] Methods used to develop operational definitions may include review of prior literature, consultation with content experts, focus groups of patients, clients and/or caregivers, or elaborations of theory. Once a list of survey items is generated, then testing and refinement with subjects of interest continues through a series of iterations designed to[7]:

- Create the most complete but efficient (parsimonious) set of items for the survey;
- Establish the relationship among multiple items intended to measure one aspect of the phenomenon;
- Establish the stability, interpretability, and meaningfulness of scores with a group of subjects for whom the survey is designed; and
- Establish the relationship between the survey and a previously established instrument (or instruments).

If the research project is well funded and has access to a large number of subjects, then the investigators also may explore the instrument's performance in a second group of individuals with the same diagnosis, clinical problem, or circumstances. In addition, the usefulness of the instrument measuring change over time may be demonstrated. Further studies are required to explore the measurement properties of the instrument using subjects with a related but distinct diagnosis or clinical problem, as well as versions of the survey in different languages.

Salaffi et al. reported on the development and testing of the Recent-Onset Arthritis Disability (ROAD) questionnaire. In the first paper they described a five-step process through which 122 survey items were generated and ultimately reduced to 12 for the final instrument. The process involved both statistical and qualitative components typical of self-report outcomes measure development.[42] The companion paper described the methods used to evaluate the questionnaire's measurement reliability, validity, and ability to detect change.[43] The need for two research publications to convey the development and testing steps is common when any new measures are created. As a result, evidence-based physical therapists must be prepared to search for more than one article to fully answer their clinical questions.

Secondary Analyses

In their most common form, secondary analyses are reports about a collection of previously completed individual studies. The motivation to conduct this type of secondary analysis stems from the reality that one single research study often does not provide a definitive conclusion about the usefulness of a diagnostic test, clinical measure, prognostic factor, intervention, clinical prediction rule, outcome, or self-report outcomes measure. The primary reasons for this limitation in clinical research are the difficulty locating and enrolling a large enough group of individuals in the study, as well as ethical and logistical challenges to testing, manipulating, and controlling patients who may already be vulnerable based on their condition or disorder. Lack of funding of large-scale studies also poses a problem for many investigators. As a result, several smaller studies may exist addressing a specific topic that, cumulatively, may provide stronger evidence to answer a clinical question.

One form of secondary analysis is the narrative review (previously referred to as a "literature review"). A *narrative review* is a paper in which the authors describe prior research on a particular topic without using a systematic search and critical appraisal process. Current patient/client management also may be described in an anecdotal fashion. By definition, these articles are biased representations of a cumulative body of literature because standardized methods for article identification, selection, and review were not implemented.[10] **Table 5-5** lists some narrative reviews relevant to physical therapist practice. The Clinical Summaries feature of the PTNow website also contains reviews created by American Physical Therapy Association members on a variety of topics.[49] Although these narrative reviews are ranked lower on the evidence hierarchy, they may be useful in identifying other individual articles that have a true research design of some kind that is worth reading and evaluating.

DiCenso and colleagues describe other types of "summary" products, such as clinical decision support systems, clinical practice guidelines, and various evidence-based abstractions of the published literature.[14] When developed through a systematic process that emphasizes high-quality research, these products can be reliable and efficient resources for busy physical therapists. Readers are reminded, however, that these resources have features that differentiate them from true research designs.

TABLE 5-5   **Examples of Narrative Reviews Pertinent to Physical Therapy**

- Alon G. Functional electrical stimulation (FES). The science is strong, the clinical practice not yet – a review of the evidence. *Arch Phys Rehabil Med.* 2016;59S:e26-e27.

- Smith AC, et al. A review on locomotor training after spinal cord injury: re-organization of spinal neuronal circuits and recover of motor function. *Neural Plast.* 2016; 2016:1216258.

- Edwards P, et al. Exercise rehabilitation in the non-operative management of rotator cuff tears: a review of the literature. *Int J Sports Ther.* 2016;11(2):279-301.

- Cameron S, et al. Early mobilization in the critical care unit: a review of adult and pediatric literature. *J Crit Care.* 2015;30(4):664-672.

- Taghian NR, et al. Lymphedema following breast cancer treatment and impact on quality of life: a review. *Crit Rev Oncol Hematol.* 2014;92(3):227-234.

Systematic Reviews

As their name implies, systematic reviews are the antithesis of the narrative review and are located at the top of most evidence hierarchies. A *systematic review,* or *synthesis,* is a true research product with the following design elements and controls:

- A specific research question to be addressed;
- Detailed inclusion and exclusion criteria for selection of studies to review;
- Elaborate and thorough search strategies;
- Standardized review protocols that often include trained reviewers other than the primary investigators;
- Standardized abstracting processes for capturing details about each study included in the review; and
- Pre-established quality criteria with which to rate the value of the individual studies, usually applied by masked reviewers.

Systematic reviews look like typical research articles in the sense that they begin with an introduction and purpose statement, follow with methods and results sections, and conclude with a discussion and summary statement about what the cumulative weight of the evidence suggests. The most well-known and prolific source of systematic reviews is the Cochrane Collaboration[50]; however, similar methods for conducting systematic reviews are implemented by investigators independent of this international group.

Richards et al. performed a systematic review of prospective randomized controlled trials evaluating the effectiveness of various physical therapy interventions for the prevention and treatment of back and pelvic pain in pregnant women.[51] Both electronic and paper databases were searched. As is often the case, the review authors identified more studies (26) than they were able to include (4) in their analysis because of the poor quality of many research designs, as well as the lack of other elements specified by the inclusion criteria. The total number of subjects from the studies they reviewed was 566, whereas the number of subjects in the individual studies ranged from 60 to 301. Three of the four studies were judged to have low-to-moderate risk of bias based on pre-established criteria. The variety of treatments assessed and outcomes measured prevented the authors from making a definitive conclusion about the effectiveness of physical therapy for pregnant women with low back or pelvic pain. However, the identification of individual high-quality clinical trials may be a secondary benefit of systematic reviews even when the review itself results in equivocal conclusions.

Meta-Analyses

Whenever feasible, authors conduct additional statistical analyses by pooling data from the individual studies in a systematic review. This approach requires that the interventions and outcomes of interest in individual studies be similar. When these criteria are met, authors can create a much larger sample size than any one study, thereby increasing the statistical *power* of the analysis and the representativeness of the *sample.* This form of a systematic review is referred to as a *meta-analysis.*

Mckoy et al. performed a meta-analysis as part of their systematic review of active cycle of breathing techniques compared to other airway clearance techniques for patients with cystic fibrosis.[52] Five of the 19 studies included in the overall systematic review were used for the meta-analysis (total number of subjects = 192). Once again, many of the individual trials were limited in their design quality. Data pooled from the five studies revealed no statistically significant difference between active cycle of breathing and any other technique used in terms of "participant preference, quality of life, exercise tolerance, lung function, sputum weight, oxygen saturation or number of pulmonary exacerbations". It is important to note that the authors did not conclude that active cycle of breathing was "ineffective";

rather, they stated that there "insufficient evidence to support or reject use" of this technique. In other words, the pooled statistical results did not indicate that one method was more effective than another. This conclusion requires readers to use their clinical expertise and judgment regarding which treatment technique they will use based on this evidence, a common result of systematic reviews and meta-analyses of physical therapy research. Only when the individual studies are consistently high in quality will these types of reviews start to draw more definitive directional conclusions.

Qualitative Studies

Qualitative studies in health care often focus on the perspectives and interactions of patients or clients, family members, caregivers, providers and others engaged in the health care enterprise. The investigations are intended to capture in the subjects' own words and/or through the researchers' direct observations the experiences that unfold in their natural context. As noted previously, three qualitative research methodologies are common in physical therapy literature: ethnographic, grounded theory and phenomenologic. The following examples illustrate each format:

- Ethnographic (observations): Hoffman used a nonparticipant observation approach to explore how physical therapists taught individuals to manage their bodies and their prostheses following lower limb amputation. The author documented physical therapy sessions at one rehabilitation hospital in Israel using audiotape and field notes. Four themes he labeled "prosthetics only", "compensatory skills", "enduring pain", and "talking prosthetics" were identified as oriented toward recovery of socially acceptable body habits and movements (i.e., body techniques). The findings suggest additional avenues for investigation related to the perceptions that individuals with lower limb amputations have regarding the methods physical therapists use to facilitate their functional recovery.[53]
- Grounded theory (empirically driven theory): McCay et al. used a grounded theory methodology to explore perceptions of the impact of knee pain and dysfunction on individuals between 35–65 years old. Written and audio-recorded data from 41 participants were collected via focus groups and from an additional 10 individuals via personal semi-structured interview. An iterative, concurrent analytic process involving all study authors was used to identify two themes: 1) disruption of the individual's physical, social and emotional life, and 2) an altered view of one's body and overall self. The authors used these findings to argue for a paradigm shift toward early intervention for younger people with mild knee pain and dysfunction to help keep them physically active and engaged in their personal context.[54]
- Phenomenologic (interviews): Waterfield et al. queried 21 physical therapists via focus group or semi-structured telephone interview about their subjective experiences and perceptions of the role of acupuncture in pregnant women with low back pain. The interviews were recorded and transcribed so that themes could be identified. Accumulated responses were validated with the study participants. Thematic findings included reluctance to apply acupuncture to pregnant women due to perceived safety concerns, mistrust of the available evidence and fear of litigation. The results of this study were used to prepare other physical therapists for participation in a randomized controlled trial examining the effectiveness of acupuncture in pregnant women with low back pain.[55]

Summary

Research designs describe the approach investigators will use (or have used) to answer their questions. They also reflect the investigators' philosophical perspective regarding the inherent objectivity or subjectivity of the phenomenon of interest. Research designs provide details about the manner in which subjects will be selected and managed, how variables will be measured and/or manipulated, the timing of subject and investigator activities, the time frame of the study, and the means by which unwanted influences will be minimized or avoided. Each design has inherent strengths and weaknesses with which investigators must contend in order to have confidence in a study's findings.

Different research questions are answered best by specific research designs. The randomized clinical (controlled) trial is the most effective approach with regard to controlling unwanted influences and demonstrating cause-and-effect relationships between variables. As a result, this design is most appropriate for questions pertaining to interventions. Other designs that do not include randomization to groups are more useful when examining questions about diagnostic factors, clinical measures, prognostic indicators, clinical prediction rules, and patient or client outcomes. However, researchers must find additional means to control for extraneous factors that may interfere with these studies' results. Qualitative research designs are well suited to capturing, in their own words, the perceptions and experiences of participants in the health care encounter. These designs often inform the therapeutic relationship by providing insight into patients' or clients' (and families'/caregivers') points of view. Evidence-based physical therapists must be able to identify and evaluate the strength of a study's research design to determine whether the results provide important and useful information that should be considered during the patient/client management process.

Exercises

1. Differentiate between the quantitative and qualitative research paradigms and provide an example of a research question relevant to physical therapist practice that might be answered in each approach.
2. Describe the general features of experimental research designs. Include important strengths and weaknesses. Provide an example relevant to physical therapist practice of the type of question that is best answered by this approach.
3. How is an experimental research design different from a quasi-experimental design? What additional challenges occur as a result of using the quasi-experimental approach? Provide an example relevant to physical therapist practice to illustrate your points.
4. Describe the general features of nonexperimental research designs. Include important strengths and weaknesses. Provide an example relevant to physical therapist practice of the types of questions that are best answered by this approach.
5. Discuss the primary methods of control for extraneous (unwanted) influences in experimental, quasi-experimental, and nonexperimental research designs. Provide examples relevant to physical therapist practice to illustrate your points.
6. Differentiate between an impairment measure and a self-report outcomes measure that reflects the patient or client's perspective. Provide examples relevant to physical therapist practice to illustrate your points.
7. Differentiate between narrative reviews and systematic reviews. Why are systematic reviews the preferred approach to answering questions about the cumulative weight of the evidence?
8. Describe the general approaches to qualitative research and the questions they answer. Provide examples relevant to physical therapist practice to illustrate your points.

References

1. Carter RE, Lubinsky J, Domholdt E. *Rehabilitation Research: Principles and Applications.* 4th ed. St. Louis, MO: Elsevier Saunders; 2011.

2. Helewa A, Walker JM. *Critical Evaluation of Research in Physical Rehabilitation: Towards Evidence-Based Practice.* Philadelphia, PA: W.B. Saunders; 2000.

3. Guyatt G, Rennie D. *Users' Guides to the Medical Literature: A Manual for Evidence-Based Clinical Practice.* 3rd ed. Chicago, IL: AMA Press; 2014.

4. McEwen I. *Writing Case Reports: A How to Manual for Clinicians.* 3rd ed. Alexandria, VA: American Physical Therapy Association; 2009.

5. Information for Authors: "Full" Traditional Case Reports. Available at: http://ptjournal.apta.org/content /information-authors-full-traditional-case-reports. Accessed July 31, 2016.

6. Batavia M. *Clinical Research for Health Professionals: A User-Friendly Guide.* Boston, MA: Butterworth-Heinemann; 2001.

7. Portney LG, Watkins MP. *Foundations of Clinical Research: Applications to Practice.* 3rd ed. Upper Saddle River, NJ: Prentice Hall Health; 2009.

8. Straus SE, Richardson WS, Glaziou P, Haynes RB. *Evidence-Based Medicine: How to Practice and Teach EBM.* 3rd ed. Edinburgh, Scotland: Elsevier Churchill Livingstone; 2005.

9. Campbell DT, Stanley JC. *Experimental and Quasi-Experimental Designs for Research.* Boston, MA: Houghton Mifflin; 1963.

10. Herbert R, Jamtvedt G, Hagen KB, Mead J. *Practical Evidence-Based Physiotherapy.* 2nd. Edinburgh, Scotland: Elsevier Butterworth-Heinemann; 2011.

11. Greiner AC, Knebel E, eds. Health Professions Education: A Bridge to Quality. Institute of Medicine Website. Available at: https://www.nap.edu/read/10681/chapter/1. Accessed July 16, 2016.

12. Green J, Thorogood N. *Qualitative Methods for Health Research.* 2nd ed. London, England: Sage; 2009.

13. Cook TD, Campbell DT. *Quasi-experimentation: Design and Analysis Issues for Field Settings.* Boston, MA: Houghton Mifflin Company; 1979.

14. DiCenso A, Bayley L, Haynes RB. Accessing pre-appraised evidence: fine-tuning the 5S model into a 6S model. *Evid Based Nurs.* 2009;12(4):99–101.

15. Hesse-Biber SN, Leavy P. *The Practice of Qualitative Research.* 3rd ed. Thousand Oaks, CA: Sage; 2016.

16. Denizen NK, Lincoln Y (eds). *The SAGE Handbook of Qualitative Research.* 4th ed. Thousand Oaks, CA: Sage; 2011.

17. Sackett DL, Wennberg JE. Choosing the best research design for each question. *BMJ.* 1997;315(7123):1636.

18. Cook C, Beatty S, Kissenberth MJ et al. Diagnostic accuracy of five orthopedic clinical tests of superior labrum anterior posterior (SLAP) lesions. *J Shoulder Elbow Surg.* 2012;21(1):13–22.

19. Reese NB, Bandy WD. Use of an inclinometer to measure flexibility of the iliotibial band using the Ober test and the modified Ober test: differences in magnitude and reliability of measurements. *J Orthop Sports Phys Ther.* 2003;33(6):326–330.

20. Irwin CB, Sesto ME. Reliability and validity of the multi-axis profile dynamometer with younger and older participants. *J Hand Ther.* 2010;23(3):281–289.

21. Wang CH, Hsueh IP, Sheu CF, et al. Psychometric properties of 2 simplified 3-level balance scales used for patients with stroke. *Phys Ther.* 2004;84(5):430–438.

22. Grimes DA, Schulz KF. Bias and causal associations in observational research. *Lancet.* 2002;359(9302):248–252.

23. Alemdaroglu E, Uçan H, Topçuoglu AM, Sivas F. In-hospital predictors of falls in community-dwelling individuals after stroke in the first 6 months after a baseline evaluation: a prospective cohort study. *Arch Phys Med Rehabil.* 2012;93(12):2244–2250.

24. Bland MD, Sturmoski A, Whitson M, et al. Prediction of discharge walking ability from initial assessment in a stroke inpatient rehabilitation facility population. *Arch Phys Med Rehabil.* 2012;93(8):1441–1447.

25. Sasco AJ, Secretan MB, Straif K. Tobacco smoking and cancer: a brief review of recent epidemiological evidence. *Lung Cancer.* 2004;45(2):S3–S9.

26. Wang K, Ho V, Hunter-Smith DJ et al. Risk factors in idiopathic adhesive capsulitis: a case control study. *J Shoulder Elbow Surg.* 2013:22(7)e24–e29.

27. Cotchett MP, Munteanu SE, Landorf KB. Effectiveness of trigger point dry needling for plantar heel pain: a randomized controlled trial. *Phys Ther.* 2014;94(8):1083–1094.

28. Bhambhani Y, Rowland G, Farag M. Effects of circuit training on body composition and peak cardiorespiratory responses in patients with moderate to severe traumatic brain injury. *Arch Phys Med Rehabil.* 2005;86(2):268–276.

29. Robitaille Y, Laforest S, Fournier M, et al. Moving forward in fall prevention: an intervention to improve balance among older adults in real-world settings. *Am J Public Health.* 2005;95(11):2049–2056.

30. Carr S, Fairleigh A, Backman C. Use of continuous passive motion to increase hand range of motion in a woman with scleroderma: a single-subject study. *Physiother Can.* 1997;49(4):292–296.

31. Wainner RS, Fritz JM, Irrgang JJ, et al. Development of a clinical prediction rule for the diagnosis of carpal tunnel syndrome. *Arch Phys Med Rehabil.* 2005;86(4):609–618.

32. Gravel J, Hedrei P, Grimard G, Gouin S. Prospective validation and head-to-head comparison of 3 ankle rules in a pediatric population. *Ann Emerg Med.* 2009;54(4):534–540.

33. Stiell IG, Greenberg GH, McKnight RD, et al. Decision rules for the use of radiography in acute ankle injuries. Refinement and prospective validation. *JAMA.* 1993;269(9):1127–1132.

34. Matchar DB, Rudd AG. Health policy and outcomes research 2004. *Stroke.* 2005;36(2):225–227.

35. Outcomes Research Fact Sheet. Agency for Healthcare Research and Quality Website. Available at: https://archive.ahrq.gov/research/findings/factsheets/outcomes/outfact/outcomes-and-research.html. Accessed September 1, 2016.

36. Iezzoni LI. Using administrative data to study persons with disabilities. *Millbank Q.* 2002;80(2):347–379.

37. National Quality Forum. National Quality Forum Website. Available at: www.qualityforum.org. Accessed September 1, 2016.

38. Jette AM. Outcomes research: shifting the dominant research paradigm in physical therapy. *Phys Ther.* 1995;75:965–970.

39. Focus on Therapeutic Outcomes, Inc. Website. Available at: www.fotoinc.com. Accessed September 1, 2016.

40. Jewell DV, Riddle DL. Interventions associated with an increased or decreased likelihood of pain reduction and improved function in patients with adhesive capsulitis: a retrospective cohort study. *Phys Ther.* 2009;89(5):419–429.

41. American Physical Therapy Association. *Guide to Physical Therapist Practice 3.0.* Available at: http://guidetoptpractice.apta.org. Accessed July 16, 2016.

42. Salaffi F, Bazzichi L, Stancati A, et al. Measuring functional disability in early rheumatoid arthritis: the validity, reliability and responsiveness of the Recent-Onset Arthritis Disability (ROAD) index. *Clin Exp Rheumatol.* 2005;23(5):628–636.

43. Salaffi F, Stancati A, Neri R, et al. Development of a functional disability measurement tool to assess early arthritis: The Recent-Onset Arthritis Disability (ROAD) questionnaire. *Clin Exp Rheumatol.* 2005;23(5 suppl):S31–S42.

44. Patel AS, Siegert RJ, Creamer D, et al. The development and validation of the King's Sarcoidosis Questionnaire for the assessment of health status. *Thorax.* 2013;68(1):57–65.

45. Thompson DR, Jenkinson C, Roebuck A, et al. Development and validation of a short measure of health status for individuals with acute myocardial infarction: The myocardial infarction dimensional assessment scale (MIDAS). *Qual Life Res.* 2002;11(6):535–543.

46. Beattie PF, Pinto MB, Nelson MK, Nelson R. Patient satisfaction with outpatient physical therapy: instrument validation. *Phys Ther.* 2002;82(8):557–565.

47. Beattie P, Turner C, Dowda M, et al. The MedRisk Instrument for Measuring Satisfaction with Physical Therapy Care: a psychometric analysis. *J Orthop Sports Phys Ther.* 2005;35(1):24–32.

48. Price P, Harding K. Cardiff Wound Impact Schedule: the development of a condition-specific questionnaire to assess health-related quality of life in patients with chronic wounds of the lower limb. *Int Wound J.* 2004;1(1):10–17.

49. PTNow. Available at: http://www.ptnow.org/Default.aspx. Accessed September 1, 2016.

50. The Cochrane Library. The Cochrane Collaboration. Available via Wiley Interscience website at: http://www.cochranelibrary.com. Accessed September 1, 2016.

51. Richards E, van Kessel G, Virgara R, Harris P. Does antenatal physical therapy for pregnant women with low back pain or pelvic pain improve functional outcomes? A systematic review. *Acta Obstet Gynecol Scand*. 2012;91(9):1038–1045.

52. Mckoy NA, Wilson LM, Saldanha IJ, Odelola OA, Robinson KA. Active cycle of breathing techniques for cystic fibrosis. *Cochrane Database Syst Rev*. 2016, Issue 7.

53. Hoffman M. Bodies completed: on the physical rehabilitation of lower limb amputees. Health. 2012;17(3):229–245.

54. McCay C, Jaglal SB, Sale J, Badley EM, Davis AM. A qualitative study of the consequences of knee symptoms: "It's like you're an athlete and you go to a couch potato." *BMJ Open*. 2014;4e006006.

55. Waterfield J, Bartlam B, Bishop A, et al. Physical therapists' views and experiences of pregnancy-related low back pain and the role of acupuncture: qualitative exploration. *Phys Ther*. 2015;95(9):1234–1243.

CHAPTER 6

RESEARCH SUBJECTS

OBJECTIVES

Upon completion of this chapter, the student/practitioner will be able to do the following:

1. Differentiate between a study population and sample.

2. Discuss the purpose and characteristics of inclusion and exclusion criteria used to identify potential subjects.

3. Describe probabilistic subject selection methods and discuss their strengths and limitations.

4. Describe nonprobabilistic subject selection methods and discuss their strengths and limitations.

5. Describe methods for assigning subjects to groups within a study and discuss their strengths and limitations.

6. Discuss methods for controlling extraneous influences related to subject participation in a study.

7. Discuss the role of sample size in the statistical analysis of a study's results.

TERMS IN THIS CHAPTER

Accessible population: The pool of potential research subjects available for researchers to study.[1]

Assignment (also referred to as *allocation*): The process by which subjects are placed into two or more groups in a study.

Block assignment: An assignment method in which the number of individuals in each group is predetermined; investigators randomly assign subjects to one group at a time until each quota is met.

Cluster sampling: A probabilistic sampling method in which subjects are randomly selected from naturally occurring pockets of the population of interest that are geographically dispersed.

Convenience sampling: A nonprobabilistic sampling method in which investigators select subjects who are readily available (such as students).

Exclusion criteria: A list of characteristics that may influence, or "confound," the outcomes of a study; researchers use these criteria to eliminate individuals (or units of analysis such as organizations) with these characteristics as subjects in a study.

Extraneous variables: Individual, organizational, or environmental characteristics other than the factor of interest (i.e., test, predictor, intervention) that may influence the outcome of a study.

Inclusion criteria: A list of specific attributes that will make an individual (or a unit of analysis such as an organization) eligible for participation in a specific study.

Masked (also referred to as *blinded*): (1) In diagnostic test and clinical measure papers, the lack of knowledge about previous test/measure results; (2) in prognostic factor papers, the lack of knowledge about whether a subject has the predictive factor of interest; and (3) in intervention papers, the lack of knowledge about to which group a subject has been assigned.

Matched assignment: An assignment method in which subjects are first divided into subgroups based on a specific characteristic such as age, gender, and so forth; members of each subgroup are then randomly assigned to each group in the study to balance the characteristics across the groups.

Nonprobabilistic sampling: Methods for choosing subjects that do not use a random selection process; as a result, the sample may not represent accurately the population from which it is drawn.

Power: The probability that a statistical test will detect, if present, a relationship between two or more variables or a difference between two or more groups.[1,2]

Primary data: Data collected in real time from subjects in a study; used in prospective research designs.

Probabilistic sampling: Methods for choosing subjects that use a random selection process to increase the chance of obtaining a sample that accurately represents the population from which it is drawn.

Purposive sampling: A nonprobabilistic sampling method in which investigators hand select specific individuals to participate based on characteristics important to the researchers.

Random assignment by individual: An assignment method in which each subject is randomly allocated to a group based on which side of a coin lands upright or which number is pulled from a hat.

Sample: A collection of individuals (or units of analysis such as organizations) taken from a population of interest for the purposes of a research study.

Sampling error: Occurs when a sample has characteristics that are different from other samples and from the population from which the samples are drawn.

Sampling frame: A list of potential subjects obtained from various public or private sources.

Secondary data: Data that have been collected previously by others for nonresearch purposes that are used by investigators to answer a research question; used in retrospective research designs.

Selection (also referred to as *sampling*): The process by which subjects are chosen from a potential candidate pool.

Simple random sample: A probabilistic sampling method in which each potential subject has an equal chance of being selected.

Snowball sampling: A nonprobabilistic sampling method in which the initial subjects in a study recruit additional participants via word-of-mouth communication.

Stratified random sampling: A probabilistic sampling method in which subgroups of a population are identified and randomly selected to ensure their inclusion in a study.

Subjects: Individuals, organizations, or other units of analysis about whom information will be gathered for the purposes of a research study.

Systematic assignment: An assignment method in which subjects count off the group numbers until everyone is placed in a group.

Systematic sampling: A probabilistic sampling method in which the first subject is randomly selected from a group organized according to a known identifier (such as a birth date) and then all remaining subjects are chosen based on their numerical distance from the first individual.

Target population: The total aggregate of individuals to whom investigators wish to apply their research findings.[1]

Type II error: A result from a statistical test that indicates no significant relationship or difference is present when in fact one exists (i.e., a false negative).[2]

CLINICAL SCENARIO

Do These Studies Apply to Me?

© Photographee.eu/Shutterstock

One of the research articles Anne found online was about risk factors for elbow pain. She indicated that participants in the study were volunteers from a large general medical practice in a European country. Seventy-eight percent of the subjects were men with an average age of 52 years. In addition, 42% of the participants were current smokers, 23% were overweight or obese, and only 18% engaged in regular physical activity or exercise. She read on a medical website that men and women were equally affected by this problem; so she wondered why the subjects in this study were so different.

How will you help her understand the challenges of recruiting individuals for study enrollment?

Introduction

Clinical research related to patient/client management requires data obtained from people. The research question or purpose identifies the general group of people from whom that information is needed. In technical terms, this general group is referred to as the study's target population. The *target population* is the total aggregate of individuals to whom researchers wish to apply their study's findings.[1] All athletes who undergo anterior cruciate ligament reconstruction or all children with asthma are examples of target populations that may be of interest to physical therapist researchers. Every member of these target populations may not be accessible to investigators because of the large population and their geographic distribution. In addition, some members of these populations may not be identifiable. As a result, researchers define the *accessible population* of individuals who are potential participants in their study. Athletes undergoing ligament surgery in hospitals in a large metropolitan area or children with asthma who are managed through community health centers in one state are examples of accessible populations.

Even though the accessible population is a smaller subset of the target population, it is often too large to study in its entirety; therefore, investigators must choose a smaller number of individual representatives.[2] The research design specifies the methods by which these individuals, referred to as *subjects*, will be selected from the accessible population, as well as in which activities they will participate during the study. A collection of subjects for a study is called a *sample*. Depending on the study's design, the sample may be composed of people from whom data will be collected in real time during the project (*primary data*) or it may be made up of people from whom data were previously collected as part of routine health care delivery or during participation in a prior research activity (*secondary data*).

Evidence-based physical therapists must evaluate a study's design to determine if the results answer the research question in a useful and believable fashion. Three design steps pertaining to a study's subjects are essential ingredients of a successful project:

1. Identification of potential candidates for study;
2. Selection of an appropriate number of individuals from the candidate pool; and
3. Management of the subjects' roles and activities during the study.

Appropriate subject identification, selection, and management enhance a study's usefulness and believability, as well as the relevance of its results for similar individuals who were not study participants. In addition to these design considerations, a sufficient number of appropriate subjects are needed to increase the probability that a statistically significant result will be found if it exists. This chapter discusses commonly used methods by which subjects may be identified, chosen, and handled during their participation in clinical research, as well as issues related to sample size.

Subject Identification

The research question or purpose indicates in general terms the population of interest for a study. For example, in the studies itemized in **Table 6-1**, the populations of interest included "people with spinal cord injury,"[3] "people with Parkinson's disease,"[4] "older adults,"[5] and "participants . . . with a diagnosis of stroke of any type."[6] Ideally, individuals who are candidates for each of these studies should have characteristics that are consistent with each population's description while also being free of other attributes that may influence, or "confound," the results of the project. The characteristics of interest are referred to collectively as *inclusion criteria*, and the undesirable attributes are referred to as *exclusion criteria*.

Inclusion criteria define in more detail the characteristics that individuals from the population of interest must possess to be eligible for the study. These characteristics often are demographic, clinical, and/or geographic.[1] For example, potential subjects in Ho et al.'s study had to be individuals with a spinal cord injury who were at least 18 years old and who had stage III or IV pressure ulcers with "clinically clean" wound beds.[3] Similarly, potential candidates for Bhatt et al.'s study had to be people with Parkinson's disease who were managed at a "movement disorder clinic" in Hong Kong, were stable on their medical regimen, and were able to rise to standing independently.[4]

TABLE 6-1	Studies Relevant to Physical Therapy

Randomized Clinical Trial

Ho CH, et al. Pulsatile lavage for the enhancement of pressure ulcer healing: a randomized controlled trial. *Phys Ther.* 2012;92(1):38-48.

Quasi-Experimental Study

Bhatt T, et al. Effect of externally cued training on dynamic stability control during the sit-to-stand task in people with Parkinson's disease. *Phys Ther.* 2013;93(4):492-503.

Observational Study

Farlie MK, et al. Clinical markers of the intensity of balance challenge: observational study of older adult responses to balance tasks. *Phys Ther.* 2016;96(3):313-323.

Summary

Yamato TP, et al. Virtual reality for stroke rehabilitation. *Phys Ther.* 2016;96(10):1508-1513.

Inclusion criteria must be broad enough to capture all potentially eligible individuals without admitting too many extraneous variables. For example, Ho et al. were interested in the effectiveness of two treatment techniques with respect to the healing rate of moderate to severe pressure ulcers that did not require mechanical debridement.[3] Specifying which clinical signs will identify individuals with "clinically clean wound areas" is necessary to avoid also enrolling subjects with different problems, such as the presence of necrosis or eschar, for whom the treatment effects may be different. However, had the authors made the inclusion criteria too narrow and enrolled only individuals with clean stage I and II pressure ulcers, they may have biased the study in favor of a positive treatment effect because these subjects may have recovered on their own even if the treatment did not work. In addition, the study's results would not be applicable to patients with more severe forms of the disorder. Support for selected inclusion criteria often is provided in the literature reviewed for the current study. Nevertheless, evidence-based physical therapists should judge for themselves whether the inclusion criteria are sufficient to make the study credible given the research question or purpose.

Exclusion criteria define in more detail the characteristics that will make individuals ineligible for consideration as subjects. These criteria reflect extraneous variables that potentially will interfere with the study's outcome.[2] Exclusionary factors also may be demographic, clinical, or geographic. Ho et al. listed five exclusion criteria: two related to the status of the wounds, one described indications of other wound etiologies, one referred to other systemic diseases, and one referred to medical management of the ulcers.[3] Bhatt et al. also excluded individuals who could not follow instructions.[4] The inability of potential study candidates to understand and respond consistently to directions provided or to answer questions consistently in oral or written form are common exclusion criteria because of the likelihood of unstable subject performance and inaccurate or incomplete data. As with inclusion criteria, justification for exclusion criteria may be found in the background literature reviewed at the outset of the project. Evidence-based physical therapists must still determine for themselves whether extraneous variables were introduced because certain relevant exclusion criteria were not implemented in a study.

Once the inclusion and exclusion criteria are established, researchers must determine how they will locate potential subjects. Individuals who already belong to a specific group may be identified through records maintained by private or public organizations. For example, lists of potential subjects may be available from hospital medical records, insurance company beneficiary files, health care professional licensing boards, professional association membership rosters, or university registrars, to name just a few options. When such a list exists, it is referred to as a *sampling frame*. The advantage of a sampling frame is that potential candidates are identified all at once, thereby expediting the selection process. If the investigators are interested in individuals at the time of their admission to a group, such as newly evaluated or diagnosed patients, then they will have to wait for these individuals to present themselves to participating clinicians because there will not be a preexisting sampling frame with which to identify them. The nature of the research question and the availability of records for use determine whether the use of a sampling frame is appropriate and feasible.

Additional methods for locating potential subjects include advertising in local media, direct solicitation or personal invitation, recruitment through clinical facilities, or recruitment through other organizations such as schools, churches, civic associations, colleges, and universities. The extent of the recruitment effort depends on the definition of the accessible population, as well as practical issues related to cost (e.g., the price of an advertisement) and logistics (e.g., number of research assistants, ability to access enrollment locations, etc.).

Subject Selection

After potential candidates are identified, investigators must use a method for selecting individuals to participate in the study. Ideally, subjects will represent the population from which they are drawn so that any conclusions may be extrapolated to the larger group of people. The two general approaches to subject *selection* are probabilistic sampling methods and nonprobabilistic sampling methods. Which approach is used often depends on a number of logistical factors, including the likelihood that a sufficient number of potential subjects exists and is available for study, the ability of subjects to get to researchers or vice versa, and the time frame in which the study is to be completed. The availability of sufficient funds often is a deciding factor.[2] Exploratory or pilot studies, as well as those that are self-funded, often use less involved sampling methods.

Probabilistic Sampling Methods

Probabilistic sampling refers to the use of a method for randomly selecting subjects for participation in studies that implement a quantitative research paradigm. Random selection is the approach most likely (although not guaranteed) to capture a representative group of eligible subjects because the rules of probability suggest that repeated sampling will produce collections of similar individuals.[1] This potential similarity among samples is important because investigators want to attribute their study findings to the larger population from which subjects were selected. To do that, investigators either must demonstrate, or assume, that their study findings are reproducible every time they draw a sample from the target population. Samples from the same population that differ from one another, or from the population itself, reflect a problem referred to as *sampling error*. In addition to minimizing sampling error, a random selection process minimizes the opportunity for investigators to introduce bias into the study by using their own judgment or preferences to decide which individuals should serve as subjects.

The most basic probabilistic sampling method is referred to as the *simple random sample*. A simple random sample minimizes sampling error because each potential subject has an equal chance of being selected. In this method, every subject that meets the inclusion criteria is assigned a number. Which individuals are selected is determined by identification of their numbers through methods as crude as drawing a piece of paper out of a hat or as sophisticated as using a random number generator. Long et al. surveyed a random sample of 1,000 physical therapists self-identified as pediatric service providers generated from a sampling frame of members of the Pediatric Section of the American Physical Therapy Association.[7] The sample represented 20% of the overall accessible population, a result that was logistically feasible through an automated selection process. An alternative method in this case is a *systematic sampling* approach in which potential subjects are organized according to an identifier such as a birth date, Social Security number, or patient account number. Only the first subject is selected randomly from this group, and then all remaining subjects are chosen based on their numerical distance (e.g., every 10th person) from the first individual.

Stratified random sampling is a more complex probabilistic selection method used when investigators have an interest in capturing subgroups within the population. Subgroups often are based on naturally occurring differences in the proportion of a particular subject characteristic such as gender, race, age, disease severity, or functional level within a population. For example, imagine a study in which the researchers want to know whether risk factors for a disease differ depending on the age of the individual. In this hypothetical study, the individuals in the population range in age from 18 to 65 years. Twenty percent of these individuals are 18 to 25 years old, 35% are 26 to 40 years old, and 45% are 41 to 65 years old. To answer their question, the investigators in this study might select a simple random sample from the entire population; however, doing so may result in such a small number of representatives from a particular age group that analyzing the differences in risk becomes difficult statistically. If the investigators wish to preserve the natural proportions of subjects' ages in their sample, then they will use the stratified sampling method. **Table 6-2** provides a comparison of hypothetical samples (500 subjects each) from this population of 2,500 individuals selected using the simple random sample and stratified random sampling techniques.

Researchers also may use stratified random sampling to ensure that certain members of the population are included in the study regardless of their proportion in the overall population. For example, Peel et al. oversampled subjects based on race, gender, and geographic location to ensure adequate representation of these characteristics in their study of a mobility assessment method in older community-dwelling residents.[8]

TABLE 6-2	Percentage of Hypothetical Subjects Selected from Different Age Groups Using Different Sampling Techniques*		
		Sampling Technique	
	Accessible Population	**Simple Random Sample**	**Stratified Random Sample**
Age Group	**Number of Individuals (% of total population)**	**Number of Subjects (% of total sample)**	**Number of Subjects (% of total sample)**
18–25 years old	500 (20%)	165 (33%)	100 (20%)
26–40 years old	875 (35%)	195 (39%)	175 (35%)
41–65 years old	1,125 (45%)	140 (28%)	225 (45%)
*Total number of subjects = 500.			

Cluster sampling is a probabilistic selection method used when naturally occurring pockets of the population of interest are geographically dispersed. For example, imagine a prospective study in which investigators want to determine the effect of a new body mechanics education program for patients with low back pain in the state of Virginia. The naturally occurring clusters in this study might be major cities within the state and outpatient physical therapy clinics within these cities. **Figure 6-1**

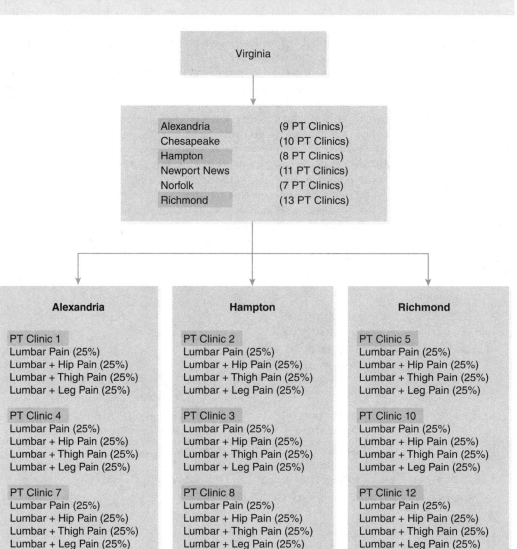

FIGURE 6-1 Cluster sampling plan in a hypothetical study of physical therapy visits in major cities in Virginia.

illustrates this sampling technique using metropolitan areas with a population between 100,000 and 300,000 residents.[9] The highlighted cities are randomly selected in the first step. Each city has a fictitious number of physical therapy clinics in which at least 50% of the patients served have low back pain. Three clinics in each city are randomly selected in the second step of the sampling process. Finally, each clinic has patients with low back pain who fall into one of four back pain categories. In the last step of the sampling process, the investigators randomly select 25% of the patients from each back pain category within each clinic. The primary benefit of cluster sampling is an improved ability to identify potential subjects when a sampling frame is not available. In addition, costs may be reduced if travel is required because only nine clinics among three cities are involved rather than every physical therapy clinic in every major metropolitan area in Virginia.

As noted previously, probabilistic selection methods are preferred because of the enhanced likelihood that the subjects in a study will represent the target population to which the findings will be applied. Unfortunately, researchers often have challenges implementing these approaches. A query of the full-text archive of the journal *Physical Therapy* using the term "random sample" in the "full text, abstract, or title" search field returned only 214 citations out of thousands dating back to 1980. The overwhelming majority of published studies relied on nonprobabilistic selection techniques.

Nonprobabilistic Sampling Methods

Nonprobabilistic sampling refers to methods for choosing subjects that do not involve a random selection process. These methods commonly are used in clinical research because they are easier to implement and cost less.[2] In addition, nonprobabilistic approaches may be needed when the length of time required to generate a large enough subject candidate pool will prevent the study's completion or when a potential sample size is already small (as in the case of a rare disorder).[10] These last two scenarios are common occurrences in clinical research, especially in those studies in which subject enrollment depends on new patients being identified and willing to participate. The absence of a random selection process means that the rules of probability are not in effect; therefore, nonprobabilistic sampling methods increase the opportunity for sampling error. As a result, the sample drawn likely will not be representative of the population and may even be so different as to result in outcomes that cannot be reproduced with repeated study. In spite of this important limitation, nonprobabilistic selection methods are the most frequently used approaches in quantitative clinical research.

The most basic nonprobabilistic method is referred to as *convenience sampling*. In this approach, the investigators recruit easily available individuals who meet the criteria for the study. Common strategies for locating potential subjects include personal requests for volunteers to known assemblies of people (such as students) or direct invitation to passersby on a street or in a mall.[10] Ho et al. and Bhatt et al. recruited subjects from medical facilities.[3,4] In effect, these individuals are "convenient" because of the ease of locating and contacting them. Often subjects are chosen consecutively as they become available or make themselves known. A challenge when using convenience sampling is the effect on study outcomes of potential dissimilarities between the individuals who volunteer and those who do not. For example, elderly residents of an assisted living community who sign up for a project about the effects of exercise on balance and falls may be more concerned about their safety than those who do not respond to the recruitment request. In this scenario, it is possible that these concerns will motivate the study participants to exercise more aggressively or more consistently than those who are not worried about their own safety. This differential in performance may result in a statistically significant improvement in balance and falls for participants in the experimental exercise program that cannot be reproduced in subjects whose lack of concern about their safety translates into minimal effort with exercise.

Snowball sampling is a nonprobabilistic technique in which the investigators start with a few subjects and then recruit more individuals via word of mouth from the original participants. This approach is particularly useful when it is difficult to locate potential study candidates because their identity is unknown or purposefully concealed from public knowledge. For example, investigators interested in identifying risk factors for skin breakdown in homeless veterans may ask individuals who received wound care at a local Veterans Affairs clinic to help recruit other members of the street population who served in the military. Similarly, researchers examining the effectiveness of a treatment for repetitive motion injuries in undocumented farm workers might use a snowball sampling approach because potential subjects may hide their immigration status for fear of criminal penalty or deportation.

The haphazardness (i.e., "randomness") of convenience and snowball sampling techniques should not be confused with actual random sampling methods. Although it is true that the investigators do not have control over who responds to their invitations or who will be contacted via word of mouth, these processes lack the ability to give every individual within range an equal opportunity for selection. In the absence of an equal opportunity, the rules of chance inherent in a randomized selection process cannot be applied. As a result, future samples from the same population are likely to be dissimilar.

Finally, *purposive sampling* is an approach in which the investigators make specific choices about who will serve as subjects in their study. This method is different from convenience sampling because the researchers do not rely simply on the spontaneous availability of the potential subjects. Rather, the investigators make judgments about which individuals are appropriate to participate and enroll them. This approach is commonly used in qualitative studies in which representatives with content knowledge or expertise from known groups are desired to ensure that a variety of perspectives are obtained. For example, investigators studying the perceived value of a case management system with respect to the rehabilitation and return-to-work of injured shipyard employees might interview subjects specifically selected from the shipyard executive staff, the shipyard human resources staff, employees with work-related injuries, case managers, physicians, and rehabilitation staff. These groups all have an interest in the outcomes of the injured workers' rehabilitation; therefore, their inclusion in the study is necessary to ensure that all perceptions of the usefulness of case management are considered. Unlike convenience and snowball sampling, purposive sampling may result in a reasonably representative sample as long as the researchers carefully consider all of the relevant characteristics before selecting their subjects.[2]

Subject Management Within the Study

Subjects are enrolled in a study to collect data about them as they proceed through specified activities relevant to the research question. Which activities an individual subject will participate in is governed by the research design. If the design is an experiment that requires group comparisons to evaluate the effectiveness of an intervention, then the first issue to be determined is the group assignment for each subject. Ideally, the *assignment* process will lead to groups of equal size across which subject characteristics are evenly distributed. Balanced groups are important to isolate the effect, if any, of the experimental intervention on the study's outcome. If the groups are different at the outset of the study, then the outcome may be a result of these initial differences. As might be expected, a randomization process for subject assignment increases the likelihood of achieving group equality through the rules of chance.

Random Assignment Methods

The simplest approach among these methods is *random assignment by individual*. In this scenario each subject is assigned, or allocated, to a group according to which group number is randomly pulled from a hat or which side of a coin lands upright. The problem with this approach is that groups may be unequal in both number and distribution of characteristics, especially if the overall sample size is small.[2] An alternative strategy is to use *block assignment* in which the size of the groups is predetermined to ensure equal numbers. The investigators then randomly assign the identified number of subjects to the first group, then the second group, and so forth. Ho et al. and Bhatt et al. implemented this approach to achieve two groups of equal size at the start of their studies.[3,4] Investigators implementing a third option, *systematic assignment*, use a list of the subjects and repeatedly count off the group numbers until everyone is assigned. **Table 6-3** illustrates this method for a hypothetical study with four groups. Based on the list in the table, Group 1 will contain subjects A, E, and I; Group 2 will contain subjects B, F, and J, and so on.

Finally, *matched assignment* is used when investigators want all groups to have equal numbers of subjects with a specific characteristic. Subjects first are arranged into subgroups according to attributes such as gender, age, or initial functional status. Then each member of the subgroup is randomly assigned to the study groups. Matching is a method of controlling for the potential effects of these specific characteristics on the outcome. Unfortunately, this approach can be both time intensive and expensive because investigators need to identify enough potential subjects with whom matching can be performed.[2] Nevertheless, some physical therapist researchers have implemented this technique. Gerber et al. randomly assigned patients status post anterior cruciate ligament reconstruction into two groups representing different rehabilitation protocols. They matched subjects based on graft type, sex, and age because of the potential influence of these factors on subsequent muscle volume, ligament laxity, and function.[11]

Each of these assignment methods presupposes that all of the subjects have been identified and can be distributed to groups at the same time. However, clinical research often deals with patients who are identified one at a time as they present with the relevant diagnosis or problem. This method of obtaining subjects may take months or years to complete depending on disease or problem prevalence. If researchers waited until all subjects were assembled to perform the assignment process, the study would be delayed unnecessarily. To avoid this problem, investigators identify subjects based on their order of admission to the study—that is, the first subject enrolled, the second subject enrolled, and so on. If 50 subjects are needed for a study, then 50 consecutive enrollment numbers are randomly assigned to the study groups in advance of actual subject identification. As each subject is enrolled, his or her group assignment already has been determined, and the study can proceed without disruption.

TABLE 6-3   Systematic Assignment of Subjects to Four Groups in a Hypothetical Study

Subject Identification	Group Number
Subject A	Group 1
Subject B	Group 2
Subject C	Group 3
Subject D	Group 4
Subject E	Group 1
Subject F	Group 2
Subject G	Group 3
Subject H	Group 4
Subject I	Group 1
Subject J	Group 2
Subject K	Group 3
Subject L	Group 4

Nonrandom Assignment Methods

Nonrandom assignment to groups occurs when subjects are members of naturally occurring groups in which the investigators have an interest or when investigators make their own decisions about which subjects go in which groups. Nonrandom groups commonly are used in retrospective studies about prognostic factors. Begnoche et al. compared two groups of children with cerebral palsy based on their Gross Motor Function Classification System score in an effort to identify factors that may predict independent walking ability 1 year after initial data were collected.[12] The authors of this study did not "assign" the subjects to these groups. Rather, they used specific identifying criteria to determine the preexisting group membership of each child. Nonrandom assignment also may be used in studies of interventions. For example, a hypothetical study about the effectiveness of rigid removable dressings following below knee amputations might compare limb girth and wound-healing time in a group of patients whose surgeon requires the dressings postoperatively to a group of patients whose surgeon does not believe in or use them. In both of these examples, the lack of randomization reduces the likelihood that groups will be equal in size or in distribution of potentially confounding characteristics. As a result, the investigators may require statistical methods to adjust for extraneous influences introduced into the study.

Other Subject Management Issues

Assignment to groups is one of many methods investigators use to manage subjects in a study. All of these tactics are intended to minimize the chance that an unwanted factor or factors (i.e., *extraneous variables*) will influence the outcome of the study. For example, investigators may follow pre-established protocols for dealing with subjects to reduce the possibility that variations in researcher behavior will result in changes in subject performance. Protocols may be written as scripts for instructions or as a specific sequence to follow for testing or providing the study interventions. Similarly, every subject is provided with the information necessary for appropriate participation in relevant study activities.[1] Training and practice sessions may be scheduled to ensure that individuals understand what is expected of them, can perform the tasks appropriately, and have time to overcome any learning curves that may result in an inconsistent performance.

Participation in a study usually means that subjects must avoid a change in their daily routine until the project is concluded. For example, subjects in an aerobic exercise effectiveness study may be instructed to maintain their usual activity levels and to postpone starting a new exercise program until after they have completed the project. This restriction is implemented to isolate the effect, if any, of the experimental aerobic exercise technique. A change in subjects' routines could influence their performance on the outcome measures and perhaps produce an inaccurate representation of the impact of the aerobics program.

Finally, subjects in studies with two or more groups may not be informed of their assignment to minimize changes in their behavior as a result of this knowledge. This strategy of keeping subjects in the dark about their group assignment is referred to as *masking* or *blinding*. Investigators also may ask subjects not to discuss the study's activities with other people during their participation. Conversations with individuals from other groups might result in subjects learning about their assignment and changing their behavior in response to this knowledge. Similarly, study personnel providing the treatment regimens or collecting outcome measures may be masked so that they do not change their behavior upon learning to which group a subject has been assigned. Unfortunately, in physical therapy research it is often difficult to mask subjects or investigators to group assignment because of the movement-based nature of most interventions.

Sample Size

Researchers are required to report the number of subjects who ultimately participated in the study. This number represents the sample size, the standard notation for which is "$n =$," where the letter "n" stands for the word "number." An essential consideration is the minimum number of subjects that will be required to ensure that important relationships between (or among) variables or differences between (or among) groups can be detected statistically if they are present. The probability that a statistical test will identify a relationship or difference if it is present is referred to as the *power* of the test.[1,2] The concern is that an insufficient number of subjects will produce a result that incorrectly indicates that no significant relationship or difference exists. This false-negative finding—failure to detect a relationship or difference when it is present—is called a *type II error*.[2] Because of the many challenges in clinical subject recruitment and enrollment, investigators must be persistent in their efforts to achieve an adequate sample size. Fortunately, software programs are available that can be used to calculate the minimum number of subjects needed for adequate statistical power prior to the start of the study.

Summary

Clinical studies require human subjects from whom to collect data to answer the research questions. Identification of potential subjects starts with the establishment of specific inclusion and exclusion criteria. Once a candidate pool is determined, random selection of subjects is preferred because of the increased likelihood of drawing a representative sample from the target population. Unfortunately, random selection methods often are difficult to use when attempting to study patients who may be limited in number and availability. Nonrandom selection methods are used most commonly in clinical research, but they may result in biased samples whose outcomes may not be reproducible.

Once subjects are selected, they must be managed throughout the study to minimize any changes in their behavior that may affect the outcome. Studies that evaluate the effectiveness of interventions among two or more groups require a method for subject assignment to the groups. Random assignment methods are preferred because of the likelihood that they will distribute equally the subject characteristics that may influence the outcome. Finally, the statistical power of a study to detect relationships or differences when they exist depends in part on an adequate sample size, an estimate of which can be calculated prior to the start of a research project.

Exercises

1. Create a hypothetical research question you might pursue as a physical therapist researcher. From this scenario
   a. Identify the target population of interest and explain why it might be difficult to study in its entirety.
   b. Identify an accessible population for study and explain why this group of individuals is easier to study.
   c. Identify three inclusion criteria and three exclusion criteria you will use to identify eligible subjects. Provide a rationale for each criterion.
2. Discuss the general strengths and weaknesses of probabilistic and nonprobabilistic sampling methods. Pick one method from each sampling approach and explain how it would be used in your study from the scenario in question 1.
3. Discuss the benefits of random assignment of subjects to groups in studies evaluating the effectiveness of interventions. Why do these benefits enhance the study's credibility? Provide an example relevant to physical therapist practice to support your answer.
4. Provide three examples of subject management during a study relevant to physical therapist practice. Why is the control over subject and researcher behavior so important?
5. Explain the concept of statistical power. Why is a type II error a concern in research? Provide an example relevant to physical therapist practice to support your answer.

References

1. Portney LG, Watkins MP. *Foundations of Clinical Research: Applications to Practice.* 3rd ed. Upper Saddle River, NJ: Prentice Hall Health; 2009.

2. Carter RE, Lubinsky J, Domholdt E. *Rehabilitation Research: Principles and Applications.* 4th ed. St. Louis, MO: Elsevier Saunders; 2011.

3. Ho CH, Bensitel T, Wang X, Bogie KM. Pulsatile lavage for the enhancement of pressure ulcer healing: a randomized controlled trial. *Phys Ther.* 2012;92(1):38–48.

4. Bhatt T, Yang F, Mak MKY, et al. Effect of externally cued training on dynamic stability control during the sit-to-stand task in people with Parkinson's disease. *Phys Ther.* 2013;93(4):492–503.

5. Farlie MK, Molloy E, Keating JL, Haines TP. Clinical markers of the intensity of balance challenge: observational study of older adult responses to balance tasks. *Phys Ther.* 2016;96(3):313–323.

6. Yamato TP, Pompeu JE, Pompeu SMAA, Hassett L. Virtual reality for stroke rehabilitation. *Phys Ther.* 2016;96(10):1508–1513.

7. Long TM, Perry DF. Pediatric physical therapists' perceptions of their training in assistive technology. *Phys Ther.* 2008;88(5):629–639.

8. Peel C, Sawyer Baker P, Roth DL, et al. Assessing mobility in older adults: the UAB Study of Aging Life-Space Assessment. *Phys Ther.* 2005;85(10):1008–1019.

9. Virginia Population Estimates. Weldon Cooper Center for Public Service website. Available at: http://www.coopercenter.org/demographics/virginia-population-estimates. Accessed September 1, 2016.

10. Batavia M. *Clinical Research for Health Professionals: A User-Friendly Guide.* Boston, MA: Butterworth-Heinemann; 2001.

11. Gerber JP, Marcus RL, Dibble LE, et al. Effects of early progressive eccentric exercise on muscle size and function after anterior cruciate ligament reconstruction: a 1-year follow-up study of a randomized clinical trial. *Phys Ther.* 2009;89(1):51–59.

12. Begnoche DM, Chiarello LA, Palisano, RJ et al. Predictors of independent walking in young children with cerebral palsy *Phys Ther.* 2016;96(2):232–240.

CHAPTER 7

VARIABLES AND THEIR MEASUREMENT

OBJECTIVES

Upon completion of this chapter, the student/practitioner will be able to do the following:

1. Differentiate among and discuss the roles of independent, dependent, and extraneous variables.

2. Identify the number of levels of independent variables in a study.

3. Differentiate among and discuss the mathematical properties of nominal, ordinal, interval, and ratio levels of measurement.

4. Differentiate between norm-referenced and criterion-referenced measures.

5. Discuss the concept of measurement error and its implications for research findings.

6. Discuss the following forms of, and factors influencing, measurement reliability, including:

   a. Reproducibility (or test–retest reliability);

   b. Internal consistency;

   c. Parallel forms reliability;

   d. Split-half reliability;

   e. Intrarater reliability; and

   f. Interrater reliability.

7. Discuss the following forms of, and factors influencing, measurement validity, including:

   a. Face validity;

   b. Content validity;

   c. Construct validity;

   d. Convergent validity;

   e. Discriminant validity;

   f. Criterion validity;

   g. Concurrent validity; and

   h. Predictive validity.

8. Discuss the importance of, and potential barriers to, responsiveness to change in measures.

TERMS IN THIS CHAPTER

Ceiling effect: A limitation of a measure in which the instrument does not register a further increase in score for the highest scoring individuals.[1]

Concept: A mental image of an observable phenomenon that is expressed in words.[1]

Concurrent validity: A method of criterion validation that reflects the relationship between a measure of interest and a measure with established validity ("criterion measure"), both of which have been applied within the same time frame.[1]

Construct: A nonobservable abstraction created for a specific research purpose; defined by observable measures such as events or behaviors.[2]

Construct validity: The degree to which a measure matches the operational definition of the concept or construct it is said to represent.[1]

Content validity: The degree to which items in an instrument represent all of the facets of the variable being measured.[3]

Continuous variable: A variable whose values are on a scale with a theoretically infinite number of measurable increments between each major unit.

Convergent validity: A method of construct validation that reflects the degree to which two or more measures of the same phenomenon or characteristic will produce similar scores.[2]

Criterion referenced: Scores from measures that are compared to an absolute standard to judge an individual's performance.[1]

Criterion validity: The degree to which a measure of interest relates to a measure with established validity ("criterion measure").[2]

Dependent variable: The outcome of interest in a study.

Dichotomous variable: A variable for which only two values are possible.

Discrete variable: A variable for which the value is a distinct category.

Discriminant validity: A method of construct validation that reflects the degree to which an instrument can distinguish between or among different phenomena or characteristics.[2]

Experimental design: A research design in which the behavior of randomly assigned groups of subjects is measured following the purposeful manipulation of an independent variable(s) in at least one of the groups; used to examine cause-and-effect relationships between an independent variable(s) and an outcome(s).[1,4]

Extraneous variable: Individual, organizational, or environmental characteristics other than the factor of interest (i.e., test, predictor, intervention) that may influence the outcome of a study.[1]

Face validity: A subjective assessment of the degree to which an instrument appears to measure what it is designed to measure.[3]

Factorial design: An experimental research design in which the effects of two or more independent variables, and their interactions with one another, are evaluated.[1]

Floor effect: A limitation of a measure in which the instrument does not register a further decrease in score for the lowest scoring individuals.[1]

Independent variable: Traditionally defined as the variable that is purposefully manipulated by investigators in an effort to produce a change in outcome.

Internal consistency: The degree to which subsections of an instrument measure the same concept or construct.[2]

Interrater reliability: The stability of repeated measures obtained by two or more examiners.

Interval level of measurement: A measure that classifies objects or characteristics in rank order with a known equal distance between categories but that lacks a known empirical zero point.

Intrarater reliability: The stability of repeated measures obtained by the same examiner.

Measurement: The process by which values are assigned to variables.

Measurement error: "The difference between the true value and the observed value."[3(p.62)]

Measurement reliability: The extent to which repeated measurements agree with one another. Also referred to as "stability," "consistency," and "reproducibility."[3]

Measurement validity: The degree to which a measure captures what it is intended to measure.[3]

Minimal detectable change (MDC): The amount of change that just exceeds the standard error of measurement of an instrument.[3]

Nominal level of measurement: A measure that classifies objects or characteristics but lacks rank order and a known equal distance between categories.

Nonexperimental design (also referred to as an *observational study*): A study in which controlled manipulation of the subjects is lacking[1]; in addition, if groups are present, assignment is predetermined based on naturally occurring subject characteristics or activities.[5]

Norm referenced: Measures the scores of which are compared to the group's performance to judge an individual's performance.[1]

Ordinal level of measurement: A measure that classifies objects or characteristics in rank order but lacks the mathematical properties of a known equal distance between categories; may or may not have a natural zero point.

Parallel forms reliability: Reliability of a self-report instrument established by testing two versions of the tool that measure the same concepts or constructs.

Predictive validity: A method of criterion validation that reflects the degree to which the score on a measure predicts a future criterion score.[2]

Quasi-experimental design: A research design in which there is only one subject group or in which randomization to more than one subject group is lacking; controlled manipulation of the subjects is preserved.[6]

Ratio level of measurement: A measure that classifies objects or characteristics in rank order with a known equal distance between catego0ries and a known empirical zero point.

Reproducibility (also referred to as *test–retest reliability*): The stability of a measure as it is repeated over time.[1]

Responsiveness: The ability of a measure to detect change in the phenomenon of interest.

Split-half reliability: Reliability of a self-report instrument established by testing two versions of the tool that are combined into one survey administered at one time; investigators separate the items and compare results for the two forms after subjects complete the instrument.

Standard error of measurement: The extent to which observed scores are disbursed around the true score; "the standard deviation of measurement errors" obtained from repeated measures.[1(p.482)]

Variable: A characteristic of an individual, object, or environmental condition that may take on different values.

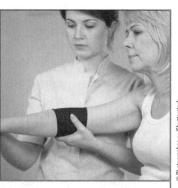

© Photographee.eu/Shutterstock

CLINICAL SCENARIO

Are These Pain Scales Accurate?

Anne's primary complaint was the extent to which her elbow pain interfered with her work activities and physical fitness routines. As she searched for information about symptom management, she noticed the following different methods for measuring pain displayed on various medically oriented websites:

- A simple "yes/no" question
- A list of numbers from 0–10
- A sequence of cartoon faces with words indicating less to more severe levels
- A 100-millimeter line

How will you explain the different approaches to pain measurement each of these scales represents and the methods for verifying their accuracy?

Introduction

Investigators require information to answer their research questions. The nature of the information is indicated by the question or purpose statement itself as well as by the research paradigm from which the investigator is operating. For example, qualitative studies that explore patients' perspectives about their health care experiences need to collect each subject's thoughts and observations. The data obtained are the participants' and/or the researchers' words from which cohesive themes are discerned. There is structure to the information-gathering process itself but investigators do not presuppose what the responses will be or attempt to impose artificial limits on their form. Respect for the natural context in which the information was generated is paramount to generating meaning in relation to the research question posed.

Quantitative studies about aspects of physical therapist patient/client management, on the other hand, focus on information that is collected under controlled conditions after operational definitions for the measurement of each data element have been established. For example, investigations comparing the accuracy of a new diagnostic test to a previously established approach require details about the types of tests applied and the rules used to classify the results. Similarly, studies about interventions require details about the treatments provided and the type and magnitude of their effects. In the quantitative research paradigm, the tests, diagnoses, treatments, and effects are referred to generically as "variables." Quantitative study designs should specify what variables will be included and how they will be measured. Ideally, the measurement instruments or techniques used will have established performance records that indicate their consistency and appropriateness for use in the study. This chapter discusses different types of variables, as well as the characteristics of measures, used in quantitative research.

Variables

Variables are characteristics of individuals, objects, or environmental conditions that may have more than one value. Attributes of individuals commonly used in clinical research on individuals include, but are not limited to, age, gender, race/ethnicity, type of pathology, and the degree of impairment in body functions and structures, activity limitations, and participation restrictions. Performance characteristics, such as strength, flexibility, endurance, balance, and task-specific skill level, are analogous attributes that may be used in research on individuals who are healthy or who have stable chronic disease. Characteristics of objects often refer to the nature of diagnostic tests and interventions, whereas characteristics of environmental conditions describe the study's context. In *nonexperimental designs*, investigators acquire information about variables of interest without purposefully trying to influence their behavior or expression. *Experimental* and *quasi-experimental designs*, however, are defined by the intentional manipulation of some of the variables in the study. Different study designs, therefore, require different types of variables.

Independent Variables

An *independent variable* traditionally is defined as the variable that is purposefully manipulated by investigators in an effort to produce a change in an outcome. In clinical research, independent variables are the interventions that are evaluated through the use of experimental and quasi-experimental designs. For example, Seynnes et al. examined the impact of an exercise program on strength and function in frail elders.[7] The independent variable was a resistance training program that was implemented by the investigators according to a specific protocol under controlled conditions. Purposeful manipulation of the variable was achieved through the creation of a high-intensity exercise group, a low-moderate intensity exercise group, and a placebo group. These three groups reflect three "levels" of the independent variable. Investigators define levels when they determine what forms the independent variable will take in a study.

Intervention studies may have one or more independent variables, a situation that increases the complexity of the research design because of the potential interaction between the independent variables at their different levels. Studies in which this interaction is anticipated are referred to as *factorial designs*. For example, Bower et al. used a 2 × 2 factorial design in their study of the effects of physiotherapy in children with cerebral palsy.[8] The designation "2 × 2" refers to the number of independent variables—"objective setting" and "physiotherapy"—and the number of levels within each (objective setting = aims, goals; physiotherapy = routine, intense). **Table 7-1** illustrates the interaction among the levels of each variable that results in the creation of four groups for study

TABLE 7-1   Factorial Design with Two Independent Variables

		Physiotherapies	
		Routine (R)	**Intense (I)**
Objective Setting	**Aims (A)**	AR	AI
	Goals (G)	GR	GI

Reprinted from *Developmental Medicine and Child Neurology*, Randomized controlled trial of physiotherapy in 56 children with cerebral palsy followed for 18 months, Bower E, Michell D, Burnett M, Campbell MJ, McLellan DL, pp. 4–15. Copyright © 2001, with permission from Wiley.

(1) aims × routine physiotherapy (AR), (2) aims × intense physiotherapy (AI), (3) goals × routine physiotherapy (GR), and (4) goals × intense physiotherapy (GI). Evidence-based physical therapists must be attentive to the number and definition of independent variables in a study to understand the potential cause(s) of change in the outcome of interest.

Investigators also may refer to the use of independent variables in studies of prognostic factors. The usefulness of independent variables (also referred to as "factors" or "predictors") in these studies is determined based on their ability to predict the outcome of interest. Although they are not purposefully manipulated like interventions, they are variables that may assume different values that the investigators can measure. For example, Hulzebos et al. evaluated the role of 12 factors, including patient age, presence of diabetes, smoking history, and pulmonary function, in predicting the development of pulmonary complications after elective coronary artery bypass surgery.[9] Independent variables in studies of prognostic factors cannot be said to "cause" a change in the outcome; rather, they may be "related to" it depending on the results obtained.

Some authors also may refer to interventions as independent variables when they are part of observational studies collectively referred to as outcomes research. This designation is tricky, however, because clinicians apply these interventions beyond the control of the researchers. In other words, purposeful manipulation according to specific study protocols does not occur. Unless the clinicians already implement treatments in a standardized fashion, the application of the term *independent variable* is confusing rather than helpful. Nevertheless, a statistical analysis of observed data in a before treatment–after treatment format implies the application of an independent variable in these studies.

The term *independent variable* does not apply to purely descriptive studies or to studies in which relationships between variables are evaluated in the absence of a predictive model. A hypothetical study characterizing the signs and symptoms of different forms of multiple sclerosis is an example of the first scenario. The investigator conducting this study does not manipulate anything nor is there an outcome of interest for which an independent variable might be responsible. Therefore, use of the term is irrelevant in this case. A hypothetical study that investigates the possible relationship between geographic place of residence and the form of multiple sclerosis is an example of the second scenario. In this case, both factors may be classified generally as variables. However, the goal of the study is to determine simply the degree to which the value of one is aligned with the value of the other. In the absence of a predictive model, identification of either residence or type of multiple sclerosis as the independent variable is arbitrary.

Dependent Variables

A *dependent variable* is the outcome of interest in a study. Studies about interventions investigate the causal link between an independent variable and change in the dependent variable. Seynnes et al. evaluated the change in the dependent variables "strength," "function," and "self-reported disability," that may be caused by different intensities of the independent variable "resistance training."[7] Similarly, Bower et al. examined what effects, if any, the independent variables "goal setting" and "physiotherapy" produced on the dependent variables "motor function" and "motor performance."[8] In studies about prognostic factors, in contrast, investigators presume that the value of the dependent variable is predicted by, rather than caused by, the independent variable. This distinction is consistent with studies that examine differences versus studies that examine relationships. Note that individual studies of relationships cannot establish a causal connection between an independent and dependent variable. As a result, Hulzebos et al. could identify factors such as age and smoking history that increased the risk of postoperative pulmonary complications (the dependent variable), but they could not conclude that either of these independent variables caused the adverse outcomes.[9]

Extraneous Variables

An *extraneous variable* is a factor other than the independent variable that is said to influence, or confound, the dependent variable.[1] The potential for extraneous variables is the principal reason why controls through study design and statistical adjustment are attempted in quantitative research. Subjects, investigators, equipment, and environmental conditions are just some of the sources of confounding influences in a study. For example, subject performance may wax and wane over the course of time due to fatigue or alertness levels. Investigators may have varying levels of experience with the outcome measure used. Equipment may lose accuracy with repeated use. Room temperature and lighting may impede a subject's ability to execute a task. Any of these problems may influence the outcome of the study resulting in misleading conclusions about the impact of, or relationship to, the independent variables. Researchers must anticipate which of the many potential extraneous variables are most likely to be a threat to their study and try to control or adjust for them. Evidence-based physical therapists must determine the success with which this control or adjustment was performed, as well as whether any important factors were ignored or overlooked.

Table 7-2 itemizes different types of variables in the Seynnes et al. and the Hulzebos et al. studies.[7,9] Note that the extraneous variables are defined as "potential" because these were identified, but not controlled for, in these studies.

Other Terminology Related to Variables

In addition to the labels *independent*, *dependent*, and *extraneous*, variables may be characterized by the general methods by which they are measured. Variables whose possible values are distinct categories are referred to as *discrete variables*. Weight-bearing status characterized as "none," "toe-touch," "foot-flat," "as tolerated," and "full" is an example of a discrete variable. When only two values are possible—such as "male–female" or "disease present–disease absent"—then the discrete variable is further described as *dichotomous*. Investigators also may operationally define a quantitative variable in discrete terms, such as "<5 hospitals in a region" and "≥6 hospitals in a region." In contrast, values of variables that are on a scale with a theoretically infinite number of measurable increments between each major unit are referred to as continuous. Distance walked characterized in feet or meters is an example of a *continuous variable*.

Measurement

If investigators wish to gain an understanding of the role and behavior of variables in a study, then they must determine a method by which to assign values to them. Values may be descriptive or numeric in nature; in both cases their assignment should be guided by clearly defined rules that are consistently applied in a study.[1,3] The process of value assignment is referred to as *measurement*. Measurement of variables is a necessary step to perform descriptive or inferential statistical analysis of the information obtained by quantitative research.

Levels of Measurement

Four levels of measurement create a continuum from descriptive to numeric value assignment: nominal, ordinal, interval, and ratio. A *nominal level of measurement* is one in which values are named categories without the mathematical properties of rank and a known equal distance between them. Hair color (i.e., blond, brunette, auburn) and sex (i.e., male, female), as well as survey questions that have "yes–no" response options, are examples of variables captured with nominal measures. That is, the categories used for each variable are assumed to be equal—one is not greater

TABLE 7-2   Types of Variables in Selected Intervention and Prognosis Studies

Intervention Study: Seynnes et al.[7]		
Independent Variable	**Dependent Variables**	**Potential Extraneous Variables**
Training Intensity (three levels)	Muscle strength	Overall subject health status
• Sham (placebo)	Muscle endurance	Subject psychological status
• Low to moderate	Functional limitation 1	Subject emotional status
• High	Functional limitation 2	Environmental conditions during training
	Functional limitation 3	
	Disability	

Prognosis Study: Hulzebos et al.[9]		
Independent Variables	**Dependent Variable**	**Potential Extraneous Variables**
Gender	Postoperative pulmonary complications (four grades)	Physician documentation
Body mass index		Operation time
Age		Medications for cardiac conditions
History of cigarette smoking		Prior cardiac surgery
Coughing		Evidence of heart failure
Forced expiratory volume in 1 second		Previous myocardial infarction
Inspiratory vital capacity		Electrocardiographic changes
Maximal expiratory pressure		Anesthesiology classification
Maximal inspiratory pressure		
History of COPD		
Diabetes mellitus		
Specific Activity Scale Score		

than or less than the other in value (rank). As a result, any statistical analysis must be performed using the frequencies (i.e., numbers or percentages) with which these characteristics occur in the subjects in the study.

An *ordinal level of measurement* also classifies characteristics without a known equal distance between them; however, categories have a rank order relative to one another. Ordinal measures are frequently used in questionnaires in which subject opinion or perception is solicited. A common clinical example is a survey of patient satisfaction in which the response options are displayed with both word and numerical anchors (**Figure 7-1**). In this case, the numerals are symbols, not quantities. The variable "weight-bearing status" progresses in value from "none" to "full" with categories

FIGURE 7-1	An ordinal scale used for responses in a hypothetical patient satisfaction survey.

Completely Dissatisfied	Somewhat Dissatisfied	Neutral	Somewhat Satisfied	Completely Satisfied
1	2	3	4	5

in between reflecting increases in the amount of weight bearing allowed. These increases are not measured with numbers but are indicated with modifying words. Traditionally, the absence of a known distance between each level of these scales means that mathematical functions cannot be performed directly with the measure. As a result, quantities in ordinal levels of measurement are determined based on the number or percentage of each response or category selected.

An *interval level of measurement* is a scale that assigns numeric, rather than descriptive, values to variables. These values are numbers that have rank and a known equal distance between them but do not have a known zero point. In other words, the value "0" does not reflect the absence of the characteristic. The classic example of an interval scale is the measurement of temperature in Fahrenheit or Celsius. Zero degrees on either scale represents an actual temperature, not the lack of temperature. Theoretically, the possible values extend to infinity on either side of both scales. The lack of a known empirical zero point means that the quantities identified with an interval scale may have positive and negative values. In addition, they may be added and subtracted from one another, but they are not appropriate for multiplication or division.

A *ratio level of measurement* has all of the necessary mathematical properties for manipulation with addition, subtraction, multiplication, and division. These quantities have rank order, a known equal distance between them, and a known empirical zero point. The presence of an empirical zero point means that these scales cannot have negative values. Height, weight, blood pressure, speed, and distance are just a few of the many clinical examples of ratio level measures.

Table 7-3 summarizes the four levels of measurement along with relevant clinical examples. **Table 7-4** illustrates the application of these concepts using the dependent variables from Seynnes et al.[7]

Note that classifying a measure is not always a straightforward exercise. Consider the example "assistive device" in which the values are "cane," "walker," and "wheelchair." On the surface this would appear to be a nominal measure—classification without rank. Inherently, a cane has no more or less value than a walker or wheelchair. This would be an appropriate designation if the investigators were interested only in the type of device for its own sake. But if the researchers were interested in using "assistive device" as an indication of the level of assistance a subject requires for mobility, then the measure becomes ordinal based on the singular property of each device to provide more (or less) support. The point is that a level of measurement may be defined both by the qualities of the instrument itself *and* by the investigators' intention for its use. Evidence-based physical therapists must discern both of these issues about a study to determine whether the measure is defined and used appropriately.

TABLE 7-3   Levels of Measurement

Level	Clinical Examples
Nominal	Sex (male, female)
	Race/ethnicity (Caucasian, African American, Asian, etc.)
	Religious affiliation (Catholic, Jewish, Muslim, Hindu, etc.)
Ordinal	Weight-bearing status (non-weight-bearing, toe touch, weight bearing as tolerated, etc.)
	Level of assistance required (minimum assist, moderate assist, maximum assist, etc.)
	Manual muscle test grades (trace, poor, fair, good, etc.)
	Patient satisfaction (very dissatisfied, somewhat dissatisfied, neutral, somewhat satisfied, very satisfied)
Interval	Temperature (Celsius, Fahrenheit)
	Calendar year (2000, 2001, 2002, 2003, 2004, 2005, etc.)
Ratio	Height (inches)
	Weight (pounds)
	Circumference (centimeters)
	Blood pressure (millimeters of mercury)
	Speed (meters per second)
	Distance (feet)

TABLE 7-4   Dependent Variables and Their Measures in Seynnes et al.[7]

Dependent Variable	Measure	Type of Measure
Muscle strength	Maximal weight lifted one time (in kilograms)	Ratio
Muscle endurance	Number of repetitions lifting 90% of the maximal amount lifted 1 time (1 rep max)	Ratio
Functional limitation 1	Time required to rise from a chair (in seconds)	Ratio
Functional limitation 2	Stair-climbing power (in watts)	Ratio
Functional limitation 3	Distance walked in 6 minutes (in meters)	Ratio
Disability	Self-report on 0–3 scale (without difficulty, with some difficulty, with much difficulty, unable to do)	Ordinal

Reference Standards in Measurement

A measurement may be characterized not only by its level but also by the standard against which its scores are evaluated. Investigators often wish to compare outcomes scores for individuals or groups with a previously established performance level. When this performance standard is derived from the scores of previously tested individuals, then the measurement is said to be *norm referenced*. Growth curves for children are examples of clinical measurements that are norm referenced. The values for the norms were gathered from a representative sample of healthy individuals characterized by different ages, heights, weights, and genders.[10] **Figure 7-2** is the growth chart for boys from birth to 36 months. Investigators studying infant boys may use this chart to compare the growth of their subjects against these standards.

An alternative to norm-referencing a measurement is to compare the value obtained to a previously established absolute standard. Measures evaluated in this manner are said to be *criterion referenced*. Discharge criteria such as "transfers independently" or "ambulates 300 feet" are examples of clinical situations in which patient performance is judged against an absolute standard. Standardized license and specialist certification exams in physical therapy also use criterion referencing to determine the threshold for passing the test.

Measurement Reliability

If measures were perfect, then every score obtained would be "true," or a precise reflection of the phenomenon of interest. Unfortunately, measures are not perfect, which means that a portion of the value obtained is bound to be the result of variability, or error, that is unrelated to the "true" score. If the error is large enough, then the results of the study may be questioned. For example, it will be difficult to attribute a change in functional balance in elderly subjects (i.e., the outcome) to a new exercise program (i.e., the experimental intervention) if the balance test scores are likely to be different simply because of measurement error. Investigators attempt to minimize *measurement error* through their choice of instruments and the methods for using them. Instruments with an established performance record are preferred but not always available. Collection of measures usually is directed by protocols that are designed to minimize:

- The variability in investigator application of the device or technique;
- The variability in subject performance; and/or
- The potential contribution of device malfunction or failure.

If these choices are appropriate, then researchers and users of evidence should find that scores of the same phenomenon are stable with repeated measurement—that is, the measurement is reliable. Several forms of *measurement reliability* may be evaluated to determine the potential usefulness of scores obtained in a study. Some of these forms pertain to the instrument; others pertain to the person or persons taking the measurements. Investigators may perform these reliability assessments as part of their study or they may refer to previous studies that have evaluated this feature of the instrument. This section discusses forms of reliability.

Instrument Reliability: Reproducibility (or Test–Retest Reliability)

Reproducibility, or *test–retest reliability*, may be established when an instrument is used on two separate occasions with the same subject(s). The challenge with this process is to determine how much time should pass between the two measurements. On the one hand, if the interval is too short, then subject performance may vary due to fatigue, change in motivation, or increased skill with practice—none

FIGURE 7-2 Boys birth to 36 months: length-for-age and weight-for age percentiles.

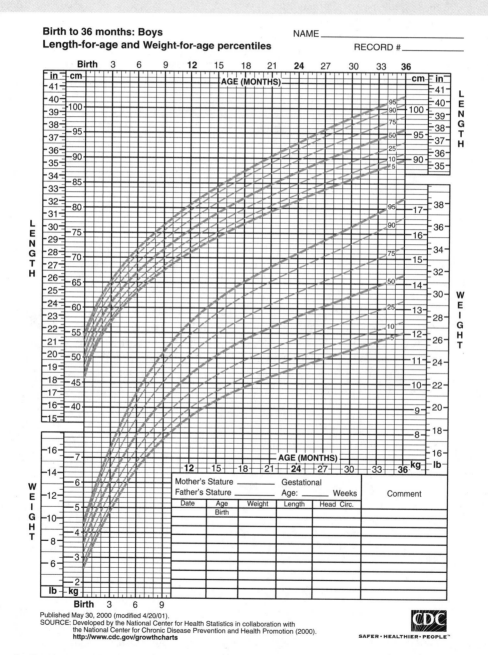

Centers for Disease Control and Prevention. http://www.cdc.gov/nchs/data/nhanes/growthcharts/set1clinical/cj41l017.pdf

of which are related to their "true" score. On the other hand, too long an interval may result in a real change in the variable being measured, in which case the second score will (and should be) different.

Instrument Reliability: Internal Consistency

Internal consistency is a form of reliability that is relevant to self-report instruments, such as health-related quality of life questionnaires. These surveys usually have several items or questions, groups of which are designed to measure different *concepts* or *constructs* within the instrument. For example, the Burden of Stroke Scale (BOSS) is a self-report instrument that assesses the consequences of stroke in terms of three constructs: "physical activity limitations," "cognitive activity limitations," and "psychological distress."[11] Each domain of the BOSS is measured by a number of subscales, each of which is composed of several items (**Figure 7-3**). If the subscales are going to capture different aspects of each domain, then items must relate to one subscale and not to others. Similarly, the subscales should relate to one construct and not to the others. In other words, the instrument should demonstrate internal consistency for each construct.

Instrument Reliability: Parallel Forms

Parallel forms reliability also is relevant to self-report instruments. As the term implies, parallel forms reliability can be established only in cases where two versions of the instrument exist, both of which measure the same constructs or concepts. Each form of the survey is administered on one occasion, and the responses are compared to determine the degree to which they produce the same scores for the same items or concepts.

Instrument Reliability: Split-Half

Split-half reliability eliminates the need for two test administrations by combining the two forms of a survey instrument into one longer version. Subjects complete the entire instrument, and then investigators separate the items for comparison to determine the degree to which scores agree for the same items or concepts.

Rater Reliability

Up to this point, the forms of reliability discussed have pertained to the instrument; however, the stability of a measure also depends on the person or persons collecting it. The consistency of repeated measures performed by one individual is referred to as *intrarater reliability*. For example, a physical therapist responsible for measuring joint range of motion following an experimental stretching technique should be able to obtain nearly the same score for the same position each time the measure is taken within the same time period. However, if several physical therapists from the same clinic take turns collecting data for this study, then the consistency of scores between raters—or *interrater reliability*—must be established.

Measurement Validity

Another essential property of measurement is validity—the ability of a measure to capture what it is intended to capture.[3] In simple terms, a goniometer that measures joint position in degrees is a valid instrument for range of motion, whereas a thermometer is not. Researchers usually are not choosing between two such nonsensical options; rather, they are making a decision between or among multiple instruments that purport to measure the same thing. As is the case with reliability, the selection of an instrument with previously established validity is preferable. Several forms of *measurement validity* may be evaluated to determine the potential usefulness of scores obtained in a study. This section discusses the forms of validity.

FIGURE 7-3   Conceptual model of the Burden of Stroke Scale (BOSS).

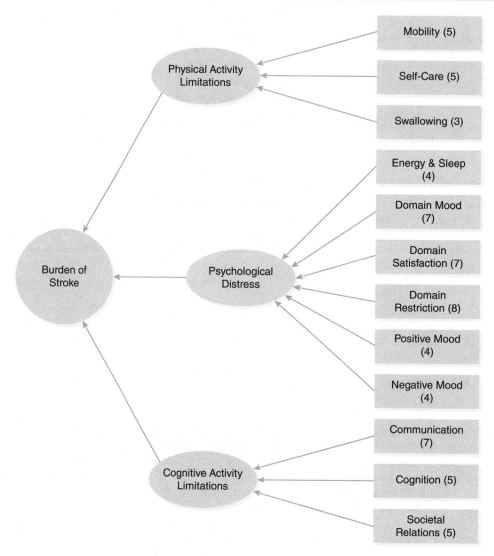

Reprinted from *Journal of Clinical Epidemiology*, *57*(10), Doyle PJ, McNeil MR, Mikolic JM, Prieto L, Hula WD, et al., The Burden of Stroke Scale (BOSS) provides valid and reliable score estimates of functioning and well-being in stroke survivors with and without communication disorders, pp. 997–1007, Copyright © 2004, with permission from Elsevier.

Face Validity

Face validity is both the simplest and most subjective form of measurement validity. Essentially, face validity is tested with the question, "Does this instrument appear to be the appropriate choice to measure this variable?" This is a "yes–no" question without a particular reference standard against which to make the judgment. As a result, investigators should look for instruments for which other forms of validity have been evaluated. However, keep in mind that an instrument that lacks face validity in the eyes of the investigators or subjects likely will not provide the desired information.

Ordinal measures such as surveys, self-report instruments, and qualitative rating scales are most susceptible to this problem because of inadequate operational definition. Consider an employee performance rating system that does not define the labels "does not meet expectations," "meets expectations," and "exceeds expectations." Supervisors may apply these ratings inconsistently because they do not see the relevance of the labels to specific employee behavior. Similarly, employees may not feel compelled to change their behavior to achieve a higher rating because they do not believe the system adequately captures their performance. Despite the subjective nature of face validity, the lack of it may serve as a red flag regarding the potential usefulness of an instrument.

Content Validity

An instrument is said to have *content validity* when it represents all of the relevant facets of the variable it is intended to measure.[3] In addition, the instrument should not contain elements that capture unrelated information. For example, a comprehensive balance test should include activities that challenge an individual's ability to maintain an upright position while sitting and/or standing, but it should not include activities that require the subject to maintain a recumbent position. Similarly, a self-report instrument about the impact of a disease or disorder on lower extremity function should contain items that address the performance of the entire leg (not just the ankle), but it should not include questions about upper extremity function.

Content validity is challenging to determine because there is no external standard or statistical criterion against which an instrument can be judged. The usual method for establishing content validity is to assemble a group of experts whose knowledge is deemed to be extensive enough to identify all of the types of activities or items an instrument should represent. "Experts" may be: (1) health care professionals who specialize in management of the condition of interest addressed by the instrument, (2) individuals who have the condition of interest addressed by the instrument, or (3) a combination of representatives from both groups. This exercise becomes more challenging when the instrument is trying to measure multiple concepts or constructs, as is often the case with measures of health status and disability. A more complex instrument requires greater effort to ensure that all of the relevant facets of a variable are represented appropriately.

Construct Validity

The *construct validity* of an instrument is determined based on the degree to which the measure reflects the operational definition of the concept or construct it is said to represent.[1] Construct validity differs from content validity in that the emphasis is on the definition itself, rather than on the universe of characteristics or items that may compose the definition. For example, "strength," "balance," and "level of dependence" are concepts that physical therapists measure routinely in clinical practice, each of which has more than one definition. "Strength" may be defined as an ability to lift a certain amount of weight a given number of times or an ability to move in relation to gravity. "Balance" may be defined as remaining upright while holding a position in space (static) or while moving (dynamic). "Level of dependence" may be defined in relation to the amount of effort required of the patient or the amount of effort required of the therapist. To assess the construct validity of a measure of each of these concepts, the definition must be specified.

"Patient satisfaction" is an example of a construct that is a challenge to define. If the patient survey only asks questions about the clinical environment—such as how clean it is, how well privacy is protected, and how well the equipment is maintained—then the instrument reflects only satisfaction with the context of care, not the care itself. This definition may be sufficient depending on what clinicians or administrators want to know. However, if the survey also asks questions about the behaviors and competence of the clinical and support staff, then the instrument reflects a broader definition of the construct "patient satisfaction." This holistic representation presumably increases the usefulness of the instrument in a wider variety of scenarios.

The BOSS illustrated in Figure 7-3 is an example of an effort to define a construct—"stroke burden"—in a comprehensive fashion.[11] Construct validity is a moving target because definitions evolve over time through repeated testing that changes people's understanding of the theoretical basis underlying the concept or construct of interest. This is particularly true for newer instruments, such as the BOSS, that have been evaluated to a limited degree.

Convergent Validity

One method with which to evaluate the construct validity of an instrument is to assess the relationship between scores on the instrument of interest and scores on another instrument that is said to measure the same concepts or constructs. If the scores from both instruments yield similar results, they are demonstrating *convergent validity*. Doyle and colleagues used two previously established instruments against which to verify the convergent validity of the BOSS.[12]

Discriminant Validity

Construct validation also may be performed through the assessment of an instrument's discriminant validity. *Discriminant validity* reflects the degree to which an instrument can distinguish between or among different concepts or constructs. For example, if the patient satisfaction survey is able to differentiate appropriately between environment of care and delivery of care, then it is demonstrating discriminant validity. This form of validity also refers to an instrument's ability to differentiate among individuals with different levels of a characteristic of interest such as disease severity, functional level, or degree of disability. The BOSS was able to distinguish between stroke survivors and individuals without stroke as well as between stroke survivors who had communication impairments and those who did not.[11]

Criterion Validity

The *criterion validity* of an instrument reflects the degree to which its scores are related to scores obtained with a reference standard instrument.[2] If the instrument is a diagnostic test, then the reference standard is a superior test whose validity has been established previously. A common example is a comparison between the results of a clinical examination technique to detect soft tissue damage and a radiographic technique, such as a magnetic resonance imaging (MRI) scan. The MRI is the superior test because of its ability to capture images of the potentially affected tissues. By comparison, clinicians must infer damage based on what they see, hear, and feel from the body's exterior. The clinical examination technique will have high criterion validity if it produces the same results as the MRI.

Criterion validity also applies to clinical prediction rules and self-report outcomes instruments. For example, newly developed health status instruments frequently are compared to the Medical Outcomes Trust Short-Form 36 instrument because the latter has been tested successfully with a wide variety of patient populations in different settings and different countries.[13] Whether the instrument is a diagnostic tool or a paper survey, the challenge in both cases is to have a reference standard available in the first place. The validity of the criterion measure depends on whether it measures the same thing as the instrument of interest and produces reliable results, as well as whether there is minimal evidence of bias.[3]

Concurrent Validity

Concurrent validity is a method of evaluating criterion validity that involves administering the test of interest and reference standard test at nearly the same time. The goal is to capture the same behavior, characteristic, or perception with each instrument because the passage of time may result in natural change that confounds the results.

Concurrent validity is of particular interest when researchers wish to use a test of interest that is believed to be more efficient and/or less risky than the criterion test. For example, the use of a validated noninvasive method for measuring blood pressure may be preferable because it can be implemented in any setting and avoids the need for placement of a catheter in a peripheral artery.[14] Concurrent validity also is relevant to self-report instruments, although there may be logistical challenges to performing this assessment if one or both of the questionnaires are lengthy. Subject responses may be influenced by fatigue or loss of interest if an extensive amount of time is required to complete both instruments.

Predictive Validity

Predictive validity is another method for evaluating criterion validity that reflects the degree to which the results from the test of interest can predict a future outcome, preferably measured by a reference standard. Establishing predictive validity often requires a sufficient amount of time to pass before the outcome develops. For example, Werneke and Hart examined the ability of the Quebec Task Force Classification and Pain Pattern Classification systems to predict pain and disability at intake and discharge from rehabilitation, as well as work status one year following discharge for patients with low back pain.[15] Similar efforts are at work when colleges and universities attempt to predict the academic success of applicants to their programs based on performance on prerequisite standardized test scores.

Responsiveness to Change

Change is a central theme in physical therapist practice. Remediation of impairments in body functions and structure, activity limitations, and participation restrictions depends on change that may reflect natural recovery, response to interventions, or both. Change also is the focus of experimental and quasi-experimental research as investigators watch for any effects produced when they manipulate the independent variable. Therapists and investigators alike need instruments that are reliable and valid but also are able to detect change in the phenomenon of interest. This measurement property is referred to as *responsiveness*.

Responsiveness to change depends on (1) the fit between the instrument and the operational definition of the phenomenon of interest, (2) the number of values on the instrument scale, and (3) the standard error of measurement associated with the instrument.[1]

The first requirement for a responsive instrument is construct validity: the measure should match the operational definition of the phenomenon of interest. For example, if joint position is the construct of interest, then the appropriate instrument would be a goniometer rather than a strain gauge. Similarly, disease-specific health-related quality of life surveys address the nuances of specific conditions that are not otherwise captured by more generic instruments.

Second, the more values on the scale of the instrument, the greater the opportunity to detect change when it occurs. For example, a tape measure marked in millimeters will be more responsive to change in the dimensions of a wound bed than a tape measure marked in quarter fractions of an inch.

Finally, the *standard error of measurement* is the extent to which observed scores are disbursed around the "true" score. It makes sense that an instrument with a large standard error of measurement will be less responsive to change because the "true" values are lost in the inaccuracies produced each time a measure is repeated. Responsiveness commonly is determined by calculating the *minimal detectable change* (MDC). The MDC is the amount of change that just exceeds the standard error of measurement of an instrument.[3] Nine of the 12 subscales in the BOSS survey demonstrated responsiveness to change during the first year of recovery after stroke.[12]

Floor and Ceiling Effects

Responsiveness also depends on the range of the scale used. *Floor* and *ceiling effects* occur when the scale of the measure does not register a further decrease or increase in scores for the lowest or highest scoring individuals, respectively. These problems are only relevant in situations in which the variable of interest has further room for change in the first place. For example, a hypothetical disability index for patients with a progressive neurologic disorder may demonstrate a floor effect if the lowest score on the scale reflected individuals who required limited assistance for mobility despite anticipated further decline in function over time. Similarly, a disability index for patients with a reversible disorder may demonstrate a ceiling effect if the highest score reflected individuals who were not completely recovered. Floor and ceiling effects can be avoided with a thorough operational definition of the phenomenon to be measured and careful construction of the measurement instrument.

Interpreting Change

The ability of an instrument to detect change in a phenomenon is complemented by the assignment of meaning to this new state. An ability to walk an additional 25 feet may be immaterial if the individual is still standing in the middle of the room. However, if that same improvement allows the individual to get to the bathroom or the kitchen table independently, then this change makes an impact! The ability of an instrument to detect meaningful change often is an essential criterion for its selection.[16] Whether meaning is derived from the physical therapist or the patient or client also should be considered.

Summary

Variables are characteristics of individuals, objects, or environmental conditions that investigators use in their quantitative research designs to find answers to their questions. Independent variables are the characteristics that are manipulated in intervention studies and the predictors of interest in studies about prognostic factors. Independent variables in nonexperimental outcomes research represent the interventions of interest that usually are applied out of the control of the researchers. Dependent variables are the outcomes of interest. Extraneous variables represent those factors that may affect a study's outcomes apart from the influence of the independent variable(s).

In addition to identifying relevant variables for study, investigators must identify methods for their measurement. Measurement assigns values that range from purely descriptive to numeric in nature. The most useful measurement instruments are those that produce stable results over repeated measures (reliability) and that capture the phenomenon they are designed to measure (validity). Reliability may be assessed in relation to the performance of the instrument as well as to the person taking the measurement. Validity most frequently is established by the degree to which scores on the instrument of interest are related to scores on other instruments. Finally, a responsive instrument is one that detects change in the phenomenon of interest.

Exercises

1. Use your electronic database searching skills to locate an experimental or quasi-experimental study about a physical therapy intervention.
   a. Identify the independent and dependent variables in the study. Discuss the difference between the two types of variables.
   b. Identify two to three actual or potential extraneous variables in the study. Why are these variables problematic for the study's results?
   c. Identify the number of levels and their definition for each independent variable in the study.
2. Give one clinical example each of a discrete variable and a continuous variable relevant to physical therapist practice.
3. Describe how nominal, ordinal, interval, and ratio levels of measurement differ. Classify the type(s) of measurement(s) used for the outcome variable(s) in the study in question 1.
4. Define *measurement error* and discuss its implications with respect to the usefulness of a study's results. Provide a clinical example relevant to physical therapist practice to illustrate your points.
5. Discuss the difference between intrarater and interrater reliability. What is the potential impact on a study's findings if rater reliability is not demonstrated?
6. Describe one method for establishing the reliability of self-report instruments. Provide a clinical example relevant to physical therapist practice to illustrate your points.
7. Differentiate between the content and construct validity of an instrument. Provide a clinical example relevant to physical therapist practice to illustrate your points.
8. Discuss two reasons why an instrument may not be responsive to change. Provide a potential solution to each barrier identified.

References

1. Carter RE, Lubinsky J, Domholdt E. *Rehabilitation Research: Principles and Applications*. 4th ed. St. Louis, MO: Elsevier Saunders; 2011.
2. Polit DF, Beck CT. *Nursing Research: Principles and Methods*. 7th ed. Philadelphia, PA: Lippincott Williams & Wilkins; 2003.
3. Portney LG, Watkins MP. *Foundations of Clinical Research: Applications to Practice*. 3rd ed. Upper Saddle River, NJ; Prentice Hall Health; 2009.
4. Campbell DT, Stanley JC. *Experimental and Quasi-Experimental Designs for Research*. Boston, MA: Houghton Mifflin; 1963.
5. Straus SE, Richardson WS, Glaziou P, Haynes RB. *Evidence-Based Medicine: How to Practice and Teach EBM*. 3rd ed. Edinburgh, Scotland: Elsevier Churchill Livingstone; 2005.
6. Cook TD, Campbell DT. *Quasi-Experimentation: Design and Analysis Issues for Field Settings*. Boston, MA: Houghton Mifflin; 1979.
7. Seynnes O, Singh MAF, Hue O, et al. Physiological and functional response to low-moderate versus high-intensity progressive resistance training in frail elders. *J Gerontol Biol Sci Med Sci*. 2004;59(5):503–509.

8. Bower E, Michell D, Burnett M, et al. Randomized controlled trial of physiotherapy in 56 children with cerebral palsy followed for 18 months. *Dev Med Child Neurol.* 2001;43(1):4–15.

9. Hulzebos EHJ, van Meeteren NLU, de Bie RA, et al. Prediction of postoperative pulmonary complications on the basis of preoperative risk factors in patients who had undergone coronary artery bypass graft surgery. *Phys Ther.* 2003;83(1):8–16.

10. CDC Growth Charts. Centers for Disease Control and Prevention website. Available at: www.cdc.gov /growthcharts/cdc_charts.htm. Accessed September 1, 2016.

11. Doyle PJ, McNeil MR, Mikolic JM, et al. The Burden of Stroke Scale (BOSS) provides reliable and valid score estimates of functioning and well-being in stroke survivors with and without communication disorders. *J Clin Epidemiol.* 2004;57(10):997–1007.

12. Doyle PJ, McNeil MR, Bost JE, et al. The Burden of Stroke Scale provided reliable, valid and responsive score estimates of functioning and well-being during the first year of recovery from stroke. *Qual Life Res.* 2007;16(8):1389–1398.

13. Short Form 36(v2). Medical Outcomes Trust. Available at: http://www.rand.org/health/surveys_tools/mos /36-item-short-form.html. Accessed September 1, 2016.

14. Brinton TJ, Cotter B, Kailasam MT, et al. Development and validation of a noninvasive method to determine arterial pressure and vascular compliance. *Am J Cardiol.* 1997;80(3):323–330.

15. Werneke MW, Hart DL. Categorizing patients with occupational low back pain by use of the Quebec Task Force Classification system versus pain pattern classification procedures: discriminant and predictive validity. *Phys Ther.* 2004;84(3):243–254.

16. Beaton DE, Bombardier C, Katz JN, Wright JG. A taxonomy for responsiveness. *J Clin Epidemiol.* 2001;54(12):1204–1271.

CHAPTER 8

VALIDITY IN RESEARCH DESIGNS

OBJECTIVES

Upon completion of this chapter, the student/practitioner will be able to do the following:

1. Discuss the concept of research validity of a study.

2. Discuss the general consequences of weak research validity of a study.

3. Recognize and discuss the consequences of the following threats to research validity in quantitative studies about interventions:

   a. Selection;

   b. Assignment;

   c. Attrition;

   d. Maturation;

   e. Compensatory rivalry or resentful demoralization;

   f. Diffusion or imitation of treatment;

   g. Statistical regression to the mean;

   h. Compensatory equalization of treatment;

   i. History;

   j. Instrumentation; and

   k. Testing.

4. Describe potential solutions researchers may apply to minimize threats to research validity in quantitative studies about interventions.

5. Discuss the relevance of threats to research validity for quantitative studies about diagnostic tests, clinical measures, prognostic factors, clinical prediction rules, outcomes, and self-report outcomes measures.

6. Define the term *construct validity* as it relates to research designs and discuss its relevance and implications for quantitative studies.

7. Recognize and discuss the consequences of threats to the generalizability of a quantitative study and describe potential solutions researchers may use to minimize these threats.

8. Discuss the analogous concerns about validity for qualitative research designs.

TERMS IN THIS CHAPTER

Assignment (also referred to as *allocation*): The process by which subjects are placed into two or more groups in a study; inadequate assignment procedures may threaten research validity (internal validity) by producing groups that are different from one another at the start of the study.

Attrition (also referred to as *dropout* or *mortality*): A term that refers to subjects who stop participation in a study for any reason; loss of subjects may threaten research validity (internal validity) by reducing the sample size and/or producing unequal groups.

Bias: Results or inferences that systematically deviate from the truth "or the processes leading to such deviation."[1(p.251)]

Compensatory equalization of treatments: A threat to research validity (internal validity) characterized by the purposeful or inadvertent provision of additional encouragement or practice to subjects in the control (comparison) group in recognition that they are not receiving the experimental intervention.

Compensatory rivalry: A threat to research validity (internal validity) characterized by subjects in the control (comparison) group who, in response to knowledge about group assignment, change their behavior in an effort to achieve the same benefit as subjects in the experimental group.

Construct underrepresentation: A threat to construct validity characterized by measures that do not fully define the variable or construct of interest.

Construct validity: The degree to which a measure matches the operational definition of the concept or construct it is said to represent.[2]

Diffusion (imitation) of treatments: A threat to research validity (internal validity) characterized by a change in subject behavior that may occur as a result of communication among members of different study groups.

Experimental design: A research design in which the behavior of randomly assigned groups of subjects is measured following the purposeful manipulation of an independent variable(s) in at least one of the groups; used to examine cause-and-effect relationships between an independent variable(s) and an outcome(s).[2,3]

External validity (also referred to as *applicability* or *generalizability*): The degree to which quantitative research results may be applied to other individuals and circumstances outside of a study.[2]

History: A threat to research validity (internal validity) characterized by events that occur during a study that are unrelated to the project but may influence its results.

Instrumentation: A threat to research validity (internal validity) characterized by problems with the tools used to collect data that may influence the study's outcomes.

Internal validity: In experimental and quasi-experimental research designs, the degree to which a change in the outcome can be attributed to the experimental intervention rather than to extraneous factors.[4]

Masked (also referred to as *blinded*): (1) In diagnostic test and clinical measure papers, the lack of knowledge about previous test/measure results; (2) in prognostic factor papers, the lack of knowledge about exposure status; and (3) in intervention papers, the lack of knowledge about to which group a subject has been assigned.

Maturation: A threat to research validity (internal validity) characterized by the natural processes of change that occur over time in humans that may influence a study's results independent of any other factors.

Nonexperimental design (also referred to as an *observational study*): A study in which controlled manipulation of the subjects is lacking[2]; in addition, if groups are present, assignment is predetermined based on naturally occurring subject characteristics or activities.[5]

Placebo: "An intervention without biologically active ingredients."[6(p.682)]

Power: The probability that a statistical test will detect, if it is present, a relationship between two or more variables (or scores) or a difference between two or more groups (or scores).[2,4]

Quasi-experimental design: A research design in which there is only one subject group or in which randomization to more than one subject group is lacking; controlled manipulation of the subjects is preserved.[7]

Reflexivity: A principle of qualitative research methods that suggests researchers should reflect on and continually test their assumptions in each phase of the study.[8]

Research validity: "The degree to which a study appropriately answers the question being asked."[6(p.225)]

Resentful demoralization: A threat to research validity (internal validity) characterized by subjects in the control (comparison) group who, in response to knowledge about group assignment, limit their efforts in the study.

Selection (also referred to as *sampling*): The process by which subjects are chosen from a potential candidate pool.

Statistical regression to the mean: A threat to research validity (internal validity) that may occur when subjects produce an extreme value on a single test administration[2]; mathematically the next test scores for these individuals mostly will move toward the mean value for the measure.

Testing: A threat to research validity (internal validity) characterized by a subject's change in performance due to growing familiarity with the testing or measurement procedure or to inconsistent implementation of the procedures by study personnel.

Transferability: The degree to which qualitative research results may be applied to other individuals and circumstances outside of a study.[8]

Triangulation: A method to confirm a concept or perspective as part of the qualitative research process.[4,8]

Introduction

A variety of research designs are used to answer questions about diagnostic tests, clinical measures, prognostic factors, interventions, clinical prediction rules, outcomes, and self-report outcomes measures as well as questions about individuals' perspectives and experiences. These designs have strengths and limitations that affect the extent to which the answers obtained in a study can be believed. "Believability" in quantitative research traditionally is referred to as *internal validity*; however, this term is defined specifically with reference to *experimental* and *quasi-experimental designs* that are used to

CLINICAL SCENARIO

Can I Trust These Study Results?

When Anne met with her physician, he expressed doubt regarding the usefulness of the research available about her elbow pain. She remembered from her college thesis work that there were study design mistakes that could result in misleading conclusions about an experiment. She assumed her physician was referencing similar problems. You have mentioned your interest in using evidence in your collaborative decision making about how to manage her situation.

What will you tell her about your analysis of the information to reassure her of your confidence in the credibility of results from studies you read?

study the efficacy or effectiveness of interventions. As a result, it is difficult to apply this concept to other types of research designs.[9] For the purposes of this text, the more general term *research validity* is used to characterize the extent to which a quantitative study of any type produces truthful results.[6] "Believability" in qualitative research is a more challenging notion because the underlying paradigm ascribes to the multiple realities of the participants involved. If the truth is grounded in each individual's point of view, how is a reader to judge whether the investigator has adequately captured the phenomenon of interest? Nevertheless, qualitative researchers strive to establish the trustworthiness of their work in ways that are consistent with the concept of research validity.[8]

A number of factors may threaten a project's research validity. Investigators should anticipate and address through their research plan the issues that may undermine the study's value. Furthermore, physical therapists reviewing evidence should make their own assessment about the degree to which research validity is supported by a study's design. This appraisal is a fundamental step in evidence-based physical therapist practice because weak research validity may suggest that a study's results cannot be trusted.

In addition to evaluating the accuracy of a study's results, therapists also must determine whether these findings are relevant to their particular patient or client. Relevance is established when the study includes subjects and circumstances that are similar to the therapist's patients or clients and clinical context. A quantitative study's relevance traditionally is referred to by the term *external validity*; however, *applicability* and *generalizability* are synonyms that are used routinely as well. *Transferability* is the analogous term in qualitative research.[8]

This chapter discusses factors that threaten a study's research validity, as well as potential design solutions investigators may apply to minimize the impact of these problems. The use of statistical adjustment to address some threats also is addressed. The chapter concludes with a brief discussion of potential threats to the external validity or transferability of quantitative and qualitative studies, respectively.

"Believability": Quantitative Studies

Research validity relates to the truthfulness, or accuracy, of a quantitative study's results and is determined based on how well the research design elements (1) focus on what the investigator wants to know and (2) prevent unwanted influences from contaminating the study's outcomes. A quick way to evaluate the research validity of a quantitative study is to ask the following question:

- Can a "competing" (alternative) explanation for this study's results be identified?[4]

If the answer is "no," then it may be possible to conclude that the study has strong research validity. This conclusion should be verified by reviewing the research design elements in more detail to confirm that they are sufficient to achieve objectives (1) and (2) just stated. If the answer is "yes," however, then these follow-up questions should be asked:

- What are the specific problems with the research design elements?
- What unwanted influences are introduced into the study as a result of these design problems?
- What alternative explanation(s) of the study's results are possible due to the introduction of these unwanted influences?

The answers to these questions will help determine whether the research validity of the study has been so compromised that a physical therapist cannot (or will not) use this piece of evidence in his or her patient/client management process.

Threats to Research Validity

The design problems that introduce unwanted influences into a quantitative study are referred to collectively as "threats to research validity." A research design can be undermined in a variety of ways. For evidence-based physical therapists the hope is that these threats have been anticipated by the investigator and addressed in such a way as to minimize their impact (keeping in mind of course that there is no such thing as a perfect research design!). The following sections of this chapter discuss the types of threats and potential solutions to avoid or minimize them, for which evidence-based practitioners should be watchful. Most of these threats are relevant only in intervention studies. Threats that also pertain to studies of diagnostic tests, clinical measures, prognostic factors, clinical prediction rules, outcomes research, and self-report outcomes measures are noted in a separate section, along with possible solutions to minimize them.

Threats to Research Validity of Intervention Studies

Imagine a study about school-based physical therapy for children with spastic diplegia that is investigating the comparative effectiveness of task-specific functional training versus a neurodevelopmental treatment (NDT)[10] approach for normalization of gait patterns. Spastic diplegia is a form of cerebral palsy in which individuals have excessive muscle tone in their lower extremities but normal motor tone in their upper extremities.[11] This hypothetical study has four possible outcomes:

1. The two approaches are equally effective;
2. The functional training approach is more effective than the NDT approach;
3. The NDT approach is more effective than the functional training approach; or
4. Neither approach improves the subjects' gait patterns.

No matter which answer is identified, a physical therapist reading this study should think about whether any of the following factors interfered with its accuracy.

Threats Related to the Subjects

Selection

The Problem *Selection* is a threat to research validity that arises when (1) access to the population of interest is limited and/or (2) the method used to choose participants results in a sample that is not representative of the population of interest. The need to wait until individuals first seek medical attention for a condition being investigated is an example of the first situation. Researchers have no control over the timing and volume of potential subject identification under those circumstances. Implementation of nonprobabilistic sampling approaches is an example of the second problem. Choosing participants through these methods increases the likelihood that some individuals who should be studied will not have the opportunity to participate.

Both situations may produce study results that do not represent the complete picture of a phenomenon. For example, children enrolled in the gait study that used a nonprobabilistic sampling method may have volunteered because of a higher motivation level than other eligible children. If the study participants also have less severe forms of spastic diplegia, then their success with functional training or NDT may be exaggerated because children with lower motivation levels and/or more pronounced impairments were not included.

Study Design Solutions Greater access to a population of interest often is achieved through research designs in which more than one location serves as a study site. These multicenter trials enhance the opportunity to identify and recruit potential subjects by virtue of the number and distribution of facilities (i.e., hospitals or clinics) in a region. The analogous approach in the gait study would be to include all of the schools in a district rather than just one. Use of random sampling methods is the obvious solution to remedy the second problem described above. Unfortunately, nonprobabilistic methods are more commonly implemented because of time and resource constraints. As a result, other research design methods must be used to overcome the biased representation that is likely in the study sample.

Assignment

The Problem *Assignment* (also referred to as *allocation*) is a threat to research validity that occurs when the process of placing subjects into groups results in differences in baseline characteristics between (or among) the groups at the outset of a study. Characteristics commonly of interest in clinical studies include subject age, gender, ethnic and racial background, education level, duration and severity of the clinical problem(s), presence of comorbidities, medication regimen, current functional status, and current activity habits, among others. In the gait study, it is possible to envision that children might be different in their age, gender, number and effect of other disease processes, current motor control abilities, and severity of spasticity. If the group allocation process is successful, then these characteristics will be distributed equally between the functional training group and the NDT group before either intervention is applied.

At a minimum, authors will provide descriptive statistics about the relevant attributes of each group. A more sophisticated approach is to test statistically for differences in these descriptive characteristics. Whether differences are identified by visual inspection of descriptive data or by statistical inference, the concern is the same: if the groups are unequal before the functional training and NDT is provided, then the investigators will have difficulty ascribing any change to the actual intervention. In other words, the study's outcome may be due to baseline differences between groups rather than to either treatment approach.

Study Design Solutions The most important solution to the assignment problem is to use a randomized allocation technique to put the subjects into groups. Randomized allocation techniques help distribute characteristics and influences equally to avoid extraneous influences created by the presence of imbalances between or among study groups. Keep in mind that equal groups are not guaranteed. When the random assignment process is unsuccessful, or when randomization to groups is not possible logistically (as in *nonexperimental designs*), then statistical adjustment for baseline differences should be implemented.

Attrition

The Problem   *Attrition* (also referred to as *dropout* or *mortality*) refers to the loss of subjects during the course of a study. Subjects may leave a study for any number of reasons, including recurrent illness, injury, death, job or family demands, progressive loss of interest in study participation, or a change of mind about the value of participating in the first place. In the gait study, children may withdraw because of competing school demands, boredom or frustration, a change in a parent's availability to bring them to the treatment session, and so on. When subjects withdraw from a study they reduce the sample size and, in the case of multiple groups, introduce the possibility of group inequality in terms of relevant characteristics. The reduction in sample size has implications for statistical analysis because of mathematical assumptions about the number and distribution of data points in a sample. In addition, the *power* of statistical tests to detect a difference among the groups may be lost. The group inequality issue is the same as described when assignment is a threat.

Study Design Solutions   In well-funded studies with the necessary administrative infrastructure and the availability of more study candidates, replacement of lost subjects may be possible. Absent that opportunity, investigators should at least document the characteristics and reasons for withdrawal of the subjects lost. A comparison of characteristics between the lost and remaining subjects might reveal that the dropouts were similar (a desirable result) or that they were somehow different and now are not represented in the sample (a less desirable result). In addition, a reexamination of the remaining groups would be warranted to determine if they had become different from each other as a result of the attrition. Investigators should not arbitrarily remove subjects to equalize the numbers between groups because this step introduces additional *bias* into the study. Statistical estimation of missing data is another strategy that may be used. Finally, an "intention-to-treat" analysis may be performed in cases when it is possible to collect outcomes data on study dropouts.

Maturation

The Problem   *Maturation* refers to changes over time that are internal to the subjects. A person's physical, psychological, emotional, and spiritual status progresses and declines as a result of, or in spite of, the events in the "outside world." These changes are reflected by age, growth, increased experience and familiarity with a particular topic or skill, healing, development of new interests and different motivations, and so on. Any of these situations may alter subjects' performance in a study and thereby introduce a competing explanation for the study's results. In other words, the results might indicate a change due to the variable of interest when in fact the change was due to maturation of the subjects. The length of time between measures will increase the possibility of a maturation effect occurring.

The children with spastic diplegia certainly will be changing as a result of their natural growth process. How that growth affects their muscle length and tone, their coordination, their understanding of the interventions applied to them, and so on may influence their ability and desire to improve their gait patterns. If the investigators cannot account for the reality of the children's growth, how can they conclude which, if either, intervention facilitated the subjects' normalization of gait?

The timing of events in a study also may result in maturation effects. Subjects may have a greater or lesser ability to perform a study-related task based on when the task is scheduled and/or how frequently it is performed. For example, fatigue may play a role in performance in children who receive their functional training followed by gait assessment later in the day as compared to children who participate earlier in the day. Similarly, if the study requires repeated measures of gait, then performance may decline over time as children lose energy (or interest). Finally, subject familiarity with the study's procedures is a form of maturation that may influence the results. Children who practice standing activities at the end of every session may feel more relaxed and comfortable walking than children who work on trunk control in sitting prior to the gait activity.

Study Design Solutions   Investigators may randomly assign subjects to a treatment and a control (comparison) group to equally distribute the effects of subjects' natural change over time, such that their impact is washed out. In this example, children would be assigned randomly to the functional training and NDT groups. In addition, the investigators may take several baseline measures of each subject's performance (i.e., gait) before starting the experiment. Baseline measures that are similar to one another would suggest that maturation is not occurring. Finally, investigators can reduce problems related to the timing and sequencing of interventions through a protocol designed to ensure that:

- The time of day for study participation is consistent;
- Adequate rest is provided in between repeated measures; and
- Specific intervention techniques are provided in random order to avoid the practice or familiarity effect.

Compensatory Rivalry or Resentful Demoralization

The Problem   If communication among study participants is not tightly controlled, then subjects may acquire knowledge about the different groups' activities. If members of the control (comparison) group learn details about the interventions in the experimental group, and if they perceive that these interventions are significantly better than what they are receiving, then these subjects may react in one of two ways:

1. *Compensatory rivalry*, or the "we'll show them" attitude; or
2. *Resentful demoralization*, or the "we're getting the short end of the stick so why bother" attitude.[2(p.85)]

In both cases, the control (comparison) group's knowledge about the experimental group results in an alteration in behavior such that potential differences due to the intervention might be diminished (rivalry), eliminated, or inflated (demoralization). Consider the children in the gait study. If they all attend the same school and are in the same classroom, they will have natural opportunities to interact with one another. A perception of inequality among members of the functional training group may trigger one of the responses described, thereby resulting in a change in behavior or effort by those children. As a result, the change in gait patterns of children in the NDT group may appear artificially worse or better than the changes achieved by the children in the functional group.

Study Design Solutions   One method by which investigators may avoid compensatory rivalry or resentful demoralization is to keep the subjects in each group separated such that communication is not possible. This strategy will be challenging to implement if all of the children in the gait study attend the same school. Social interaction is an integral part of the school day, so the likelihood of sharing information among study participants is high. The obvious alternative is to enroll students from different schools if it is logistically feasible to do so.

A second method is to *mask* (or *blind*) the subjects so they do not know to which group they belong. This is a standard approach in drug trials where an inert tablet can be used as a *placebo*. Most interventions physical therapists provide are more challenging to disguise because of the physical effort involved.

Clinicians providing treatment in the gait study won't be able prevent the children from recognizing or understanding the differences between the two movement-based approaches being compared.

A third option is to provide thorough, explicit instruction to subjects (or their caregivers) about the importance of adhering to their current routine or regimen. Changes in behavior during the study time frame should be avoided unless extreme or unexpected circumstances arise. Approaching parents, teachers, and the children themselves about the need to avoid changes in activity levels during the gait study would be the most feasible solution if interaction among members of the two treatment groups is anticipated.

Diffusion or Imitation of Treatment

The Problem *Diffusion or imitation of treatment* also may occur when subjects in different groups have contact with one another during the study. Either purposefully or unintentionally, these individuals may share aspects of the treatment in their group that prompts changes in behaviors by members in a different group. If the children in the functional training group describe the tasks they perform as part of their treatment, then children in the NDT group might start performing these same tasks at home in an effort to copy or try out these alternative activities. If this situation occurs, it will be difficult to attribute any changes to the NDT approach.

Study Design Solutions The solutions for diffusion of treatment are the same as those applied to compensatory rivalry and resentful demoralization.

Statistical Regression to the Mean

The Problem *Statistical regression to the mean* occurs when subjects enter a study with an extreme value for their baseline measure of the outcome of interest. For example, a few children in the gait study may have a crouched gait pattern composed of hip and knee flexion in excess of $100°$ when compared to the majority of children in the sample whose flexion at the same joints exceeds normal by only $10°$ to $25°$. As a result, the children with the crouched gait pattern may show improvement in their kinematics simply because a second measure of their hip and knee position is likely to show decreased flexion. This situation will cloud the true effects, if any, of the interventions.

Study Design Solutions Investigators have two options to help avoid statistical regression to the mean. The first option is to eliminate outliers from the baseline scores so the sample is limited to a distribution that is closer to the mean (i.e., within one standard deviation). This strategy is most useful when the researchers have access to a large population from which to draw a sample to study. The second option is to take repeated baseline measures and average them to reduce the extremes through the aggregation process. This solution is preferable when small samples must have their size and composition preserved.

Threats Related to Investigators
Compensatory Equalization of Treatments

The Problem *Compensatory equalization of treatments* occurs when the individuals providing the interventions in the study purposefully or inadvertently supplement the activities of subjects in the control (comparison) group to "make up for" what subjects in the experimental group are receiving. The potential for this situation may be stronger in studies in which multiple physical therapists are providing treatments outside the supervision of the investigator. In their quest to do the best for their patients, these therapists may feel compelled to work them a little harder, give them extra opportunities to practice, provide more encouragement, and so on. This extra effort by the physical therapists may dilute the differences in performance attributable to the intervention of interest. Put in the context of the gait study, children in the functional training group may walk just as well as children in the NDT group because the physical therapists provided additional training opportunities to the children who were performing task-specific skills.

Study Design Solutions The most direct method for dealing with compensatory equalization of treatments is to mask the investigator(s) or the therapist(s) such that they do not know which group is receiving which intervention. As noted previously, disguising the interventions in the gait study likely will be impossible.

A second step is to provide a clear and explicit protocol for intervention administration, including a script for instructions if indicated. A third step is to ensure that communication about the interventions between investigators or therapists is minimized or eliminated. In effect, the physical therapists in the gait study would know simply that they are to perform NDT techniques or task-specific skills according to the protocol provided to them. The details of the other intervention would be unavailable. If enough therapists in different clinics are involved in the study, then it may be possible to avoid cross-contamination by keeping children receiving NDT treatment in one clinic and children receiving functional training in another.

Threats Related to Study Logistics

History

The Problem *History* refers to events that occur outside of an intervention study that are out of the investigators' control. The label is misleading because the problem is due to concurrent events, not past incidents. This threat can be remembered with the phrase "life goes on." In other words, the activities of daily life proceed whether or not a research project is underway, thereby producing extraneous influences that may interfere with the study. The opportunity for a history effect to occur grows as the length of time between measures of the outcome increases. For example, children in the functional training versus NDT study may have changes in their physical education activities over the course of a school year that may enhance or diminish their ambulatory abilities during the study. If the investigators cannot control the timing of the study to avoid this natural alteration in a child's school agenda, then they will have to find another way to deal with this situation. Otherwise, any differences (or lack thereof) in gait performance noted might be attributed to changes in the schedule rather than to the interventions provided during the study.

Study Design Solutions Investigators have a couple of design options to deal with the threat of history to their study. First, they might use a control or comparison group in addition to their treatment group and then randomly assign subjects to each. Random assignment should distribute subjects most susceptible to "history threats" equally between the groups, thereby minimizing the influence of any changes as a result of the events occurring outside of the study. This would be a workable solution in the gait study because it already has two groups in its design.

Second, the investigators can try to schedule the study to avoid a predictable external event altogether. In this example, the researchers might contact the schools attended by their subjects and inquire as to the nature and timing of their physical education activities. The information provided by the schools may allow the investigators to organize the intervention and data collection timetable in such a way as to miss the changes in physical education activities that are planned over the course of the school year.

Instrumentation

The Problem The research validity of an intervention study may be challenged by problems with the tools used to measure the variable(s) of interest. Examples of *instrumentation* problems include selection of the wrong measurement approach or device, inherent limitations in the measurement, malfunction of the device, and inaccurate application of the device. For example, gait analysis of children with spastic diplegia might be performed through visual inspection by the physical therapist (less accurate), or it might be performed by progressively sophisticated technologic means, including a video and computer (more accurate). In the former case, the potential for inaccuracy rests in the normal variability that is part of all human activity. What one physical therapist sees in terms of a child's ability may not be what another therapist sees.

However, use of technology requires an understanding of how to use it properly and how to calibrate it (if possible) to ensure that the measures are reliable and valid. There also is a possibility for equipment malfunction (sometimes in subtle ways) that is not detected immediately by the researcher. Finally, instruments that are applied incorrectly may produce inaccurate measures. As a result of these issues, improvement of gait patterns may be an artifact of measurement rather than a true change in the subjects.

Study Design Solutions   First and foremost, investigators should consider carefully what it is they want to measure and the techniques available to do so. Measurement reliability, measurement validity, and responsiveness should be evaluated with an effort toward obtaining the most useful device or technique known.

Any technologic equipment should be calibrated against a known measure prior to use in the study whenever possible. Similarly, the authors should describe an orientation and training process during which individuals collecting data for the study learned and demonstrated the proper use of the measurement device and/or technique. Protocols for collection of measures also should be implemented. Statistical comparisons of their results may be offered to demonstrate stability of these measures within and across raters. Finally, the conditions under which the measurements are taken (e.g., temperature, humidity) should be maintained at a constant level throughout the study, if possible.

Testing

The Problem   *Testing* can threaten a study's research validity because subjects may appear to demonstrate improvement based on their growing familiarity with the testing procedure or based on different instructions and cues provided by the person administering the test. For example, children in the gait study may demonstrate improvement because of practice with the gait assessment process rather than because of the functional training or NDT. Similarly, investigators who encourage some children during their test but not others (e.g., "Come on, you can walk a little farther") may introduce the potential for performance differences due to extraneous influences rather than the interventions.

Study Design Solutions   In studies in which increasing experience with the testing procedures is the concern, investigators may give the subjects several practice sessions with a particular test or measure before collecting actual data on the assumption that the subjects' skill level will plateau. This leveling off would eliminate the practice effect once the actual data collection started. Alternatively, the authors might average the scores of multiple measures from one testing session to reduce the effect of changing skill level through a mathematical aggregation technique. To avoid introducing unwanted influences during the testing procedure itself, the investigators should describe a clearly articulated protocol for administering the test, including a script for instructions or coaching if indicated. Finally, competence performing the test to specification also should be verified in all test administrators prior to the start of the actual data collection.

Table 8-1 summarizes the threats to research validity, along with possible remedies, for studies about interventions physical therapists use.

TABLE 8-1   Threats to Research Validity of Intervention Studies and Possible Solutions

Threat	Nature of Threat	Possible Solutions
Threats Related to Subjects		
Selection	Nonrepresentative sample that produces inaccurate results relative to the population of interest	• Recruit subjects from multiple locations. • Randomize the subject selection process.
Assignment	Unequal baseline characteristics of groups that might influence the study's outcome	• Randomize the assignment of subjects to groups. • Perform statistical adjustment.
Attrition	Loss of subjects resulting in reduction of sample size and/or inequality of group baseline characteristics	• Replace subjects, if appropriate and feasible. • Perform statistical adjustment.
Maturation	Natural change in human behavior or function over the course of time that may influence the study's outcome	• Randomize the assignment to groups. • Time the study to minimize the effect. • Randomize the testing or treatment order. • Perform statistical adjustment.
Compensatory Rivalry or Resentful Demoralization	Changes in behavior that occur as a result of subjects learning they are members of the control or comparison group	• Keep subjects separated. • Mask the subjects to prevent knowledge of group assignment. • Ask all study participants to avoid behavior changes during the study time frame.
Diffusion or Imitation of Treatments	Changes in behavior that occur in the control or comparison group as a result of communication with subjects in the experimental group about the interventions they are receiving	• Keep subjects separated. • Mask the subjects to prevent knowledge of group assignment. • Ask all study participants to avoid behavior changes during the study time frame.
Statistical Regression to the Mean	Subjects who start the study with extreme scores for the outcome measure change as a result of the mathematical tendency for scores to move toward the mean value	• Trim extreme data values from the study. • Aggregate repeated baseline measures.

TABLE 8-1	Threats to Research Validity of Intervention Studies and Possible Solutions (*Continued*)	
Threat	**Nature of Threat**	**Possible Solutions**
Threats Related to Investigators		
Compensatory Equalization of Treatments	Purposeful or inadvertent supplementation of the control or comparison group's activities that influences these subjects' performance	• Mask the investigators to prevent knowledge of group assignment. • Implement and enforce protocols for the interventions. • Ask all study participants to avoid discussing their activities with anyone.
Threats Related to Study Logistics		
History	Concurrent events occurring outside the study that influence the study's outcome	• Randomize the assignment to groups. • Time the study to avoid the event(s). • Perform statistical adjustment.
Instrumentation	Inappropriate selection, application, or function of techniques or instruments used to collect data in a study	• Select appropriate technique or instrument. • Ensure user training and practice. • Have testers use specific protocols. • Calibrate instruments.
Testing	Change in the outcome that occurs as a result of a subject's increased familiarity with the testing procedure, or as a result of inappropriate cues provided by the tester	• Provide subjects with practice sessions. • Have testers use specific protocols, including scripts.

Threats to Research Validity in Quantitative Studies About Other Components of the Patient/Client Management Model

Many of the threats to research validity just described, as well as their potential solutions, are relevant only to studies about interventions. Assignment, compensatory rivalry, resentful demoralization, diffusion or imitation of treatment, and compensatory equalization of treatments do not apply to studies about diagnostic tests, clinical measures, prognostic factors, clinical prediction rules, outcomes, or self-report outcomes measures because (1) there is only one group in the study; (2) two or more groups in the study are naturally occurring; or (3) purposeful, experimental manipulation of one group differently from another group does not occur. In contrast, selection, attrition, and inclusion of subjects with extreme values of a characteristic (e.g., "too healthy" or "too sick") are concerns for any study for reasons previously stated.

TABLE 8-2   Threats to the Research Validity of Studies About Elements of the Patient/Client Management Model Other Than Interventions

Threat	Present (+)/Absent (–)	Affected Studies
Selection	+	• All study types
Assignment	–	N/A
Attrition	+	• All study types
Maturation	+	• Primarily longitudinal studies of prognostic factors, clinical prediction rules about prognosis, and outcomes
Compensatory Rivalry or Resentful Demoralization	–	N/A
Diffusion or Imitation of Treatments	–	N/A
Statistical Regression to the Mean	+	• All study types
Compensatory Equalization of Treatments	–	N/A
History	+	• Primarily longitudinal studies of prognostic factors, clinical prediction rules about prognosis, and outcomes
Instrumentation	+	• Primarily studies of diagnostic tests, clinical measures, and clinical prediction rules about diagnosis
Testing	+	• Primarily studies of diagnostic tests, clinical measures, and clinical prediction rules about diagnosis

Some threats to research validity are particularly concerning for investigations intent on answering specific types of questions. For example, studies about diagnostic tests, clinical measures, and clinical prediction rules related to diagnosis may be undermined completely by instrumentation and testing threats. The point of these studies is to establish the utility of the technique as a method to identify, quantify, and/or classify a clinical problem—an objective that will not be possible if there is doubt about the accuracy of the results obtained. Similarly, longitudinal research designs about prognostic factors, clinical prediction rules related to prognosis, and outcomes will be more susceptible to time-related threats such as maturation and history. These research validity issues are unlikely to be relevant in cross-sectional studies about diagnostic tests and clinical measures unless there is a significant delay between administration of the test or measure of interest and the reference standard test or measure. The same strategies available to minimize these various threats in intervention studies apply to research designs focused on other aspects of the physical therapist patient/client management model.

Table 8-2 summarizes threats to research validity of studies that pertain to diagnostic tests, clinical measures, prognostic factors, clinical prediction rules, outcomes, and self-report outcomes measures.

The Role of Investigator Bias

Investigator bias results when researchers purposefully or inadvertently design, or interfere with, the study's procedures such that the results systematically deviate from the truth. Some sources of investigator bias are relevant to all types of clinical research, whereas others are dependent on the type of question posed and the design used to study it.

Selection

Selection criteria that are defined too narrowly *relative to the question of interest* are an example of possible investigator bias that is concerning for all studies. Another issue is the purposeful selection or exclusion of some subjects rather than others based on characteristics not included in the criteria. In both situations, the resulting lack of representativeness in the sample means the question is answered incompletely and may provide a skewed representation of the phenomenon of interest. For example, imagine an outcomes study about individuals with acute low back pain in which the researchers (1) selectively enroll subjects with mild symptoms because they express greater motivation to engage in physical therapy, or (2) exclude potential subjects who are on the older end of the qualifying age range because they may not respond as quickly to intervention. The findings will not reflect the range of outcomes that are likely to be achieved across the spectrum of pain presentations, cooperation levels, or treatment responses.

Assignment

Assignment becomes a source of investigator bias when individuals responsible for enrolling subjects respond to additional information by changing the group to which a subject has been randomly assigned. For example, study personnel may decide to place some subjects originally intended for the NDT group into the functional training group because the children's parents have expressed skepticism about the value of an alternative therapeutic approach. This purposeful interference with the pre-established protocol for placing children into groups undermines the benefits achieved from a randomized allocation process and adds to the threat of "assignment."

Testing

Individuals responsible for the application of tests and measures may produce inaccurate results due to their knowledge of subjects' group classification (if relevant to the research design) or previous test results, or both. Prior knowledge of subject status may produce an expectation for a particular result that influences investigator interpretation of the measurement they are taking, a situation that adds to the "testing" threat to research validity. In both instances, the strategy to minimize these threats is to conceal the information from the study personnel so they are not influenced by, or tempted to respond to, knowledge about the subjects.

Investigator bias may threaten the validity of studies about diagnostic tests in an additional way. Imagine a hypothetical study evaluating a clinical test's ability to detect a torn ligament. Researchers may decide to apply a superior comparison test (e.g., magnetic resonance imaging [MRI]) only to subjects who have a positive finding on the ligament stress test. As a result, subjects who tested negative on the ligament stress test will not have their actual diagnosis verified, a situation that may overestimate the usefulness of the ligament stress test.

Table 8-3 summarizes threats related to investigator bias, as well as possible design solutions, in all studies.

TABLE 8-3   Threats to Research Validity from Investigator Bias

Threat	Type of Study Affected	Nature of Threat	Possible Solutions
Selection	• Diagnostic tests • Clinical prediction rules related to diagnosis	• Use of subjects who do not represent the population of interest defined by the research question. • Limits the ability to determine how well the diagnostic test or clinical prediction rule differentiates between or among different stages of the disorder of interest.	• Adequately define inclusion and exclusion criteria to create a sample that represents the spectrum of the disorder of interest.
Selection	• Prognostic factors • Clinical prediction rules related to prognosis	• Use of subjects who are "too healthy" or "too sick." • May result in misrepresentation of the timetable to recovery or adverse outcome, thereby undermining the usefulness of a prognostic factor(s).	• Enroll subjects at a common, early point in their condition.
Selection	• Interventions • Outcomes	• Use of subjects who do not represent the population of interest defined by the research question. • Limits the ability to determine the usefulness of the intervention for individuals with different levels of condition and/or different prognostic profiles.	• Adequately define inclusion and exclusion criteria to create a sample that represents the spectrum of the condition of interest.
Assignment	• Intervention	• Individuals responsible for enrolling subjects interfere with group assignment process. • May create unbalanced groups prior to the start of the study.	• Create a predetermined subject assignment list and conceal information about subject allocation.
Testing	• Diagnostic tests	• Investigators apply the superior comparison test only to subjects who test positive on the diagnostic test of interest. • May overestimate the usefulness of the diagnostic test.	• Apply the superior comparison test to all subjects regardless of the result of diagnostic test of interest.
Testing	• Diagnostic tests • Clinical measures • Prognostic factors • Interventions • Clinical prediction rules • Outcomes	• Individuals responsible for measurement of subjects are influenced in their interpretation by knowledge of current subject status or prior test or measurement results. • May produce inaccurate results due to investigator expectations.	• Conceal information about subject status or prior test results from individuals collecting measures.

Additional Solutions to Research Validity Threats

When investigators do not have a study design solution available to them to protect against threats to research validity, they do have two alternatives. First, they can compensate statistically for the threats through the use of control variables in their analyses. For example, "time" might be used as the control variable to reduce the effects of history or maturation. Problems with testing and instrumentation might be addressed by adjusting for the people who administered the test or used the instrument. When groups differ at the outset of a study, then specific subject characteristics, such as age or baseline functional status, might be used as control factors. An alternative statistical method to address unbalanced groups is the "intention to treat analysis." The point is that there may be a mathematical way to isolate the effects of these unwanted influences so that the investigators can more accurately determine the contribution of their intervention or other variable(s) of interest.

Second, the investigators can simply acknowledge that threats to research validity were present and need to be recognized as a limitation to the study. Reasons for the inability to control these issues at the outset of the study usually are presented in order for the reader to understand the logistical challenges the researchers faced and to help future investigators avoid similar problems.

Threats to Construct Validity

The "believability" of research results also depends on a clear and adequate definition of the variables used in the study. "The meaning of variables within a study" is characterized by the term *construct validity*.[2(p.85)] An evidence-based physical therapist assesses the integrity of construct validity by comparing the variable(s) with their measures to determine if the latter truly represent the former. For example, investigators may wish to examine the relationship between patients' socioeconomic status and their attendance in outpatient physical therapy. The researchers must decide how to measure the variable "socioeconomic status" to determine a result through statistical analysis. There are several options from which to choose in this example, including, but not limited to, a patient's

- Salary;
- Assets (e.g., home, car);
- Investments; and
- Family income.

All of these measures have a monetary basis that is consistent with the word "socioeconomic." To enhance the construct validity of their study, researchers may select one or more of these measures to define this variable.

Oftentimes the measure desired for a particular variable is not available to the researchers. Study design problems also may result in threats to construct validity of an independent, dependent, or control variable. One construct validity threat is the lack of sufficient definition of the variable, also referred to as *construct underrepresentation*. For example, a study of patient satisfaction with physical therapy may involve survey questions that ask patients to rate their experiences. If the questions only focus on issues related to making appointments, then an argument could be made that "satisfaction with physical therapy" was not completely addressed. Instead, the variable measured was satisfaction with the appointment-making process.

Another threat to construct validity occurs when subjects change their behavior in response to the perceived or actual expectations of the investigators (referred to by Carter et al. as "experimenter expectancies").[2(p.86)] In this situation, subjects respond to what they anticipate the investigator wants (also known as the Hawthorne effect)[4] or to subtle cues provided by the investigator as they perform a test or measure. Consider a hypothetical study in which an instructional method is being evaluated for its effectiveness in teaching the safest way to rise from a chair to patients following total hip replacement. Effectiveness would be judged by whether the patient complies with a motion restriction designed to protect the hip from dislocation. If the investigator frowns as subjects start to lean forward, then the subjects may modify their movement in response to this facial cue, especially if the investigator then smiles as a result of the correction. The effectiveness of the instructional method is misrepresented because the outcome variable is a reflection of the patients' response to the therapist's body language rather than their recall of the technique they were taught. Construct validity of the outcome variable is undermined in this situation.

Additional threats to construct validity occur when there are interactions between multiple treatments or when testing itself becomes a treatment. In the former case, independent variables initially defined as one treatment may in actuality reflect a combination of treatments that study subjects undergo. For example, a study looking at the effects of oral vitamin supplementation on aerobic exercise capacity may experience a construct validity problem if additional vitamins are obtained through subtle changes in diet not recognized by the subjects or the investigator. In the latter case, a study examining the effects of several stretching techniques on hamstring flexibility may experience a construct validity threat because the process of measuring the knee or hip range of motion also produces a stretching effect on the muscle group of interest.

Avoidance of construct validity problems starts with providing clearly stated operational definitions of all variables in the study. To the degree it is feasible, investigators should then select measures that are direct representations of these variables. In addition, masking investigators who are collecting measurements so as to minimize the effect of cues, as well as clearly differentiating and documenting treatments, are design steps to be considered. If all else fails, researchers should acknowledge where construct validity is in jeopardy and provide potential explanations for these problems so that future research may address these issues and readers may consider them when appraising the evidence for use with patients or clients.

"Believability": Qualitative Studies

Quantitative research designs assume that there is one objective truth that can be captured through properly designed and implemented methods. An investigator's ability to avoid or mitigate threats to research validity in his or her study determines the degree to which the findings are considered "believable." However, the concept of "believability" appears inconsistent with the paradigm upon which qualitative research designs are based. Reality and meaning depend on the unique perspective of each individual engaged in the investigation and, therefore, can take on multiple forms. Avoiding or minimizing threats to a study's validity in these designs seems unnecessary, if not counterproductive. However, the need to answer critics who discount the value of qualitative research findings as subjective and anecdotal has prompted qualitative researchers to develop strategies to affirm the trustworthiness of their designs.[8]

Triangulation is a method to confirm a concept or perspective generated through the qualitative research process.[4,8] Investigators have several options available to achieve this validation. First, they may use multiple sources of data, such as patients and caregivers, to describe a phenomenon. Second, they may use data collection methods such as interviews and direct observations that focus on the same issues or phenomena. Third, they may involve multiple researchers who, through discussion of the data they have collected, provide confirmatory or contradictory information. The consistency of concepts, themes, and perspectives gleaned using these different approaches lends credibility to the findings that are reported.

Reflexivity is a principle of qualitative designs that suggests researchers should reflect on and continually test their assumptions in each phase of the study.[8] Investigators who formally implement this principle in their work may document their preconceived notions about a phenomenon and the study participants, subject their analyses to repeated testing as new data are obtained, and challenge their interpretations from known theoretical perspectives. The intention is not to eliminate bias as would be attempted in quantitative research designs. Rather, reflexive scrutiny helps investigators place their biases in purposeful relationship to the context of their study and its participants.

Study Relevance

Once a study's "credibility" has been evaluated, physical therapists must determine whether the findings are relevant to their situation. *External validity* is the term used to describe the usefulness of a quantitative study with respect to the "real world." *Transferability* is the analogous term for qualitative research designs. In other words, a study has strong external validity or transferability when a reader can apply its results across groups (or individuals), settings, or times specific to his or her clinical situation. Threats to external validity or transferability include:

- Inadequate sample selection—subjects are different than, or they comprise only a narrowly defined subset of, the population they are said to represent;
- Setting differences—the environment requires elements of the study to be conducted in a manner different than what would happen in another clinical setting; and
- Time—the study is conducted during a period with circumstances considerably different from the present.[2]

To a certain extent, the logistics and resource (e.g., money) limitations with which all investigators must cope will introduce limitations to external validity or transferability in every study. For example, it may not be possible to recruit a diverse and large enough sample or to conduct the study in "real time," particularly when patients are the subjects. Individuals only become patients when they are affected by pathology or injury, the incidence and prevalence of which will determine the potential availability of subjects. However, the quest for a reasonable sample size may result in such a diverse subject pool that it cannot be said to represent anyone to any extent.

Researchers may try to control for external validity or transferability threats by randomly selecting a large sample in quantitative studies or recruiting participants with known differences in perspective in qualitative studies, conducting a study under "real-world" conditions, and/or studying a recent phenomenon and publishing the results as quickly as possible. Evidence-based practitioners must assess the extent and impact of threats to external validity or transferability of a study to determine whether its results can be applied to their patients or clients.

Summary

Research validity in quantitative designs addresses the extent to which a study's results can be trusted to represent the truth about a phenomenon. Construct validity refers to the degree to which variables are clearly defined and measured in a quantitative study. A variety of threats to research and construct validity may result in competing explanations for the study's findings, thereby challenging its believability. Qualitative researchers also must deal with issues related to the trustworthiness of their findings. External validity and transferability are terms that refer to the relevance of quantitative and qualitative studies, respectively. Limitations to external validity or transferability may restrict the degree to which a study's results can be applied to patients or clients outside of the study. Numerous design and statistical solutions are available to researchers to minimize threats to study believability and relevance. Evidence-based physical therapists must be aware of these threats and the design options used to decrease their impact when determining if evidence is useful and appropriate for the individuals with whom they work.

Exercises

1. Define *research validity*, *construct validity*, and *external validity*. What is the focus of each of these terms? Why are they important to a quantitative study's integrity?
2. Pick three threats to research validity and identify one cause and one quantitative research design solution for each. Provide examples of study scenarios relevant to physical therapist practice to support your answers.
3. Explain how investigators may introduce bias into a quantitative study. Provide an example of a study scenario relevant to physical therapist practice to support your answer.
4. Pick one threat to construct validity and identify one cause and one quantitative design solution. Provide an example of a study scenario relevant to physical therapist practice to support your answer.
5. Pick one threat to external validity and identify one cause and one quantitative design solution. Provide an example of a study scenario relevant to physical therapist practice to support your answer.
6. Describe methods of triangulation in qualitative research. How do they support the trustworthiness of the findings obtained with these designs? Provide an example of a study scenario relevant to physical therapist practice to support your answer.
7. Describe the principle of reflexivity in qualitative research. How does it support the trustworthiness of the findings obtained with these designs? Provide an example of a study scenario relevant to physical therapist practice to support your answer.
8. Pick one threat to transferability and identify one cause and one qualitative design solution. Provide an example of a study scenario relevant to physical therapist practice to support your answer.

References

1. Helewa A, Walker JM. *Critical Evaluation of Research in Physical Rehabilitation: Towards Evidence-Based Practice.* Philadelphia, PA: W.B. Saunders; 2000.
2. Carter RE, Lubinsky J, Domholdt E. *Rehabilitation Research: Principles and Applications.* 4th ed. St. Louis, MO: Elsevier Saunders; 2011.
3. Campbell DT, Stanley JC. *Experimental and Quasi-Experimental Designs for Research.* Boston, MA: Houghton Mifflin; 1963.
4. Portney LG, Watkins MP. *Foundations of Clinical Research: Applications to Practice.* 3rd ed. Upper Saddle River, NJ: Prentice Hall Health; 2009.
5. Straus SE, Richardson WS, Glaziou P, Haynes RB. *Evidence-Based Medicine: How to Practice and Teach EBM.* 3rd ed. Edinburgh, Scotland: Elsevier Churchill Livingstone; 2005.
6. Guyatt G, Rennie D. *Users' Guides to the Medical Literature: A Manual for Evidence-Based Clinical Practice.* 3rd ed. Chicago, IL: AMA Press; 2014.
7. Cook TD, Campbell DT. *Quasi-Experimentation: Design and Analysis Issues for Field Settings.* Boston, MA: Houghton Mifflin; 1979.
8. Green J, Thorogood N. *Qualitative Methods for Health Research.* 2nd ed. London, England: SAGE Publications; 2009.

9. Herbert R, Jamtvedt G, Hagen KB, Mead J. *Practical Evidence-Based Physiotherapy.* 2nd ed. Edinburgh, Scotland: Elsevier Butterworth-Heinemann; 2011.

10. Neuro-developmental treatment. Neuro-Developmental Treatment Association website. Available at: www .ndta.org. Accessed September 1, 2016.

11. Cerebral Palsy—Hope through Research: Glossary. National Institute of Neurologic Disorders and Stroke website, National Institutes of Health. Available at: www.ninds.nih.gov/disorders/cerebral_palsy/detail_cerebral_palsy .htm#238753104. Accessed September 1, 2016.

CHAPTER 9

UNRAVELING STATISTICAL MYSTERIES: DESCRIPTION

OBJECTIVES

Upon completion of this chapter, the student/practitioner will be able to do the following:
1. Discuss the following characteristics of selected descriptive statistical tools:

    a. Purpose;

    b. Indications for use;

    c. Method for use;

    d. Information provided by the statistics; and

    e. Limitations or caveats to their use.

2. Interpret and apply information provided by the statistical tools reviewed in this chapter.

TERMS IN THIS CHAPTER

Coefficient of variation (CV): The amount of variability in a data set expressed as a proportion of the mean.[1]

Effect size (ES): The magnitude of the difference between two mean values; may be standardized by dividing this difference by the pooled standard deviation to compare effects measured by different scales.[2]

Frequency: The number of times a phenomenon or characteristic occurs.

Interpercentile range: A measure of the spread from one percentile division point to the next; may be used to indicate the variability around the median.[3]

Interval level of measurement: A measure that classifies objects or characteristics in rank order with a known equal distance between categories but that lacks a known empirical zero point.

Mean: The sum of the data points divided by the number of scores (i.e., the average).

Median: The middle score in a data set.

Mode: The score that occurs most frequently in the data set.

Nominal level of measurement: A measure that classifies objects or characteristics but that lacks rank order and a known equal distance between categories.

Ordinal level of measurement: A measure that classifies objects or characteristics in rank order but that lacks the mathematical properties of a known equal distance between categories; may or may not have a natural zero point.

Percentiles: Division points in the data, such as quartiles or tertiles, that are used to identify where a certain percentage of the scores lie.[3]

Range: The spread of data points from the lowest to the highest score.

Ratio level of measurement: A measure that classifies objects or characteristics in rank order with a known equal distance between categories and a known empirical zero point.

Skew: A distortion of the normal bell curve that occurs as the result of extreme scores in the data set.

Standard deviation (SD): The average absolute distance of scores from the mean score of a data set.[4]

Standard error of the estimate (SEE): "The standard deviation of the difference between individual data points and the regression line through them."[2(p.482)]

Standard error of the mean (SEM): An estimate of the standard deviation of the population of interest; indicates the degree of error associated with repeated samples from the population.[3]

Standard error of measurement (SEM): "The standard deviation of measurement errors" obtained from repeated measures.[2(p.482)]

Variability: The degree to which scores in a data set are dispersed.[3]

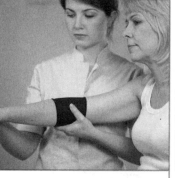

© Photographee.eu/Shutterstock

CLINICAL SCENARIO

How Big a Problem is Elbow Pain?

Anne found an article online by Sanders and colleagues.* The abstract summarized the results this way:

"In a cohort of 931 patients who had 2 or more clinical encounters for new-onset lateral epicondylosis during a 12-month period after initial diagnosis, 62% received a median of 3 physical therapy sessions (cost, $100/session) and 40% received a median of 1 steroid injection (cost, $82/injection). Only 4% of patients received surgical intervention with mean costs of $4000. The mean (median) total direct medical cost of services related to lateral epicondylosis for the entire cohort was $660 ($402) per patient over the 1-year period after diagnosis. Patients who continued to be treated conservatively between 6 and 12 months after diagnosis incurred relatively low median costs of $168 per patient."

Anne knew the definitions of terms such as *frequency, mean,* and *median.* How will you help her understand the application of the descriptive statistical results of this article to her?

*"Health Care Utilization and Direct Medical Costs of Tennis Elbow: A Population-Based Study" (*Sports Health*. 2016;8(4):355-358).

Introduction

The word "statistics" is intimidating to many researchers and clinicians, perhaps because of the frequently complex mathematical formulas used to create them, as well as the cryptic way in which they provide information. Yet statistics are simply a collection of tools that researchers use in the same way that physical therapists use clinical tools. For example, therapists can measure aerobic capacity with walking tests, treadmill tests, and cycle ergometer tests. Similarly, they can measure range of motion with manual goniometers, electronic goniometers, or inclinometers. All of these tools are meant to capture a particular phenomenon in an objective (unbiased) manner. In addition, they quantify what is measured so that changes in performance can be computed over the episode of physical therapy.

The tools that physical therapists use in the clinic have the following features in common with statistics:

1. A purpose for which they were specifically designed;
2. Indications for their use;
3. A defined method for their use;
4. A specific set of information they provide when used; and
5. Limitations beyond which the instruments cannot perform properly and/or there are important caveats to their use.

For example, a manual goniometer

1. Is designed to measure angles;
2. Is used when a physical therapist needs to quantify joint position and available range of motion during a physical examination;
3. Is applied with the pivot point over the axis of joint motion and the arms aligned with relevant bony landmarks;
4. Provides information in degrees; and
5. Has a standard error of measurement of plus or minus 4°.

When a physical therapist uses the goniometer properly, then information about joint position and range of motion is obtained and can be interpreted based on normative data about the way the healthy human body performs at a given age and gender. A physical therapist's interpretation of the value indicated by the goniometer may be expressed with terms such as "normal," "limited," "excessive," "improved," or "worsened."

When reading a study, it is helpful to think about the statistics the authors used in the same way that we think about the features of a goniometer. An evidence-based physical therapist's job is to consider whether the investigators selected the right statistical tools for their research question and applied the tools appropriately. A therapist then should consider what information the statistics have provided (i.e., the results of the study) and what he or she thinks about that information (i.e., whether the results provided are important and useful).

This chapter contains information about descriptive statistics commonly used in clinical research. The intent is to help the reader understand how descriptive statistics are used and how to interpret the information they provide.

Descriptive Statistics

Descriptive statistics do what their name implies: describe the data collected by the researchers. Researchers describe data for several reasons. First, they use descriptive statistics when the sole purpose of their study is to summarize numerically details about a phenomenon of interest. Common focus areas in these circumstances include, but are not limited to, the incidence and prevalence of a disease or disorder, characteristics of individuals with this problem, and associated diagnostic and intervention utilization rates. Studies in which description is the sole purpose often are intended to answer background questions physical therapists have about a clinical condition and its management.

Second, researchers use descriptive statistics in studies about relationships and differences to determine whether their data are ready for statistical testing. This step is necessary because inferential statistical tests are developed based on assumptions about the nature of the data and the patterns in which the data points lie. Violation of these assumptions likely will undermine the investigators' results.

Finally, investigators use descriptive statistics in studies about relationships or differences to provide information about relevant subject and/or environmental characteristics. These descriptions can help physical therapists determine whether a study includes subjects that resemble the patient or client for whom the evidence has been sought.

Distribution of the Data

Readiness for statistical testing is determined by examining the distribution of scores within the data set. Specifically, a researcher wants to know (1) the central point around which some of the data tend to cluster and (2) how far away from the central point all of the data lie. The first feature is referred to as a "measure of central tendency"[2] and may be characterized by the mean, the median, or the mode of the data. The most commonly used descriptive statistic is the *mean* (noted with the symbol $\bar{x}$), which represents the average of all the data points. The *median* represents the value that is in the middle of the data points, whereas the *mode* is the value that occurs most frequently in the data set. The mean traditionally is calculated with ratio or interval level data because it represents actual quantities of something with discrete increments between each value. Ordinal data in the form of "numbers" (e.g., 1–5 Likert scales to measure customer satisfaction) are symbols, not quantities. Many statisticians discourage calculating means with ordinal level data unless they were mathematically transformed first; however, there is considerable debate in the scientific and business communities about such a conservative approach.[5] As a result, physical therapists should be prepared to discover evidence that deviates from this recommendation. Both the median and the mode can be used with *ratio*, *interval*, and *ordinal level data*; however, the mode is the only measure of central tendency used to describe *nominal level data*.[2]

The second feature of a data set is its *variability*; that is, the degree to which scores are distributed around the central value. Variability most commonly is characterized by the range, the standard deviation, and/or the interpercentile range. The *range* identifies the lowest and highest score in the data set and may be expressed either by providing these values (e.g., 20 to 100) or by calculating the difference between them (e.g., 80). The limitation of using the range is that it does not provide information about each score. In contrast, the *standard deviation (SD)* is a value that summarizes the average absolute distance of all of the individual scores from the mean score.[6] Investigators typically report a mean value along with its SD to provide the most complete picture of the data. Bigger standard deviations indicate greater variability in the data set. *Interpercentile ranges* are created when data are divided into equal portions (i.e., tenths, quarters, thirds, and so on) to determine where an individual score lies relative to all of the other scores.[3] These divisions, referred to as *percentiles*, often are used to partition subjects into smaller groups for further comparison. Growth curves are familiar tools that implement interpercentile ranges to assist with assessment of an individual child's development relative to known typical values for healthy children of a given sex and age.

Researchers also may have an interest in comparing the variability among different measures of the same phenomenon (e.g., values obtained for body composition using a bioelectrical impedance device and calipers) or among the same measure from different samples (e.g., values obtained through repeated tests of grip strength). The descriptive statistic commonly used in these circumstances is the *coefficient of variation (CV)*. The coefficient of variation divides the standard deviation by its mean to create a measure of relative variability expressed as a percentage. The units of measurement cancel each other out in this calculation, allowing comparisons between or among different types of measures.

The measures of variability described to this point typically are used to evaluate data that have been collected one time. Researchers also may evaluate the variability that occurs when measures are performed, or samples are drawn, multiple times. Every measure is associated with some degree of error; the standard deviation of errors from multiple measures is a value referred to as the *standard error of measurement (SEM)*.[2] This statistic indicates by how much a measurement will vary from the original value each time it is repeated. The known variability in measurement error helps researchers and clinicians alike determine whether "true" change has occurred from one measure to the next.

For example, the standard error of measurement for a manual goniometer was noted previously to be plus or minus 4°. Consider the patient who is working to recover knee flexion after an operative procedure. Physical therapists commonly measure the affected joint before and after providing interventions. If the change in range of motion exceeds 4°, then an actual improvement in the patient's status may be documented. If the increase in range of motion is between 1° and 4°, then it is likely that measurement error is at work. In other words, the physical therapist cannot say with any certainty whether the patient actually improved or whether the new value was an artifact of the measurement process itself.

The *standard error of the mean (SEM)*, in contrast, provides an assessment of the variation in errors that occurs when repeated samples of a population are drawn. This value also may be referred to as an estimate of the variability around the mean for the population of interest in a study.[3] The lower the variation, the more likely it is that the mean value of a measure from the study sample represents the mean value of the same measure in the population from which it is drawn. Unfortunately, both measures of variability have the same abbreviation—SEM—which can be confusing when reading or listening to a research report. Evidence-based physical therapists should be mindful of the definition of the abbreviation, as well as of the context in which it is used, to avoid misinterpretation of the information provided.

Finally, researchers conducting studies about prognostic estimates may evaluate the variability around a line drawn through a collection of data points. The standard deviation of the distance between each data point and the line is referred to as the *standard error of the estimate (SEE)*. Smaller values for the SEE suggest more accurate predictions.

In addition to obtaining measures of central tendency and variability, researchers can quickly determine if data are ready for statistical testing by examining a visual display of the scores. Commonly used graphic displays include histograms (**Figure 9-1**) and line plots (**Figure 9-2**). Specifically, investigators want to know whether a plot of the data points results in a symmetrical bell-shaped curve (**Figure 9-3**).

Data that create a bell curve are said to be "normally distributed"[1] around a central value (usually the mean) for the group of scores. In addition, a predictable percentage of the scores can be located within 1, 2, or 3 SDs away from the mean score of normally distributed data. This feature of a bell curve is the foundation for a group of tests referred to as parametric statistics.

In the case of interval or ratio level data, extreme scores for the group can distort the curve or make it asymmetric in one direction or the other. Scores that pull the end (or "tail") of the curve farther out to the right (e.g., subjects with body mass indices that are markedly higher than the group average) result in a distribution that is "positively *skewed*." Scores that pull the end of the curve farther out to the left (e.g., subjects with ages that are markedly lower than the group average) result in a distribution that is "negatively skewed" (**Figure 9-4**).[4]

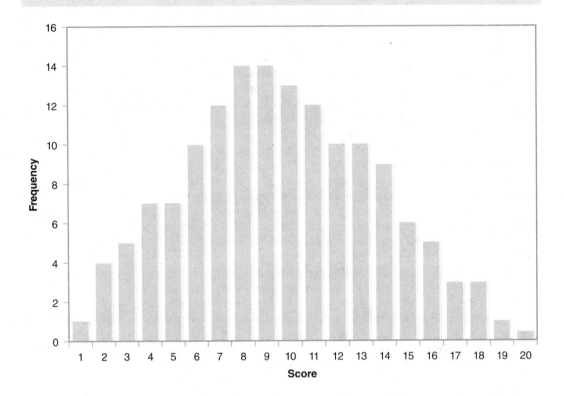

FIGURE 9-1 A histogram for a hypothetical set of data.

Note that extreme values also result in a shift in the mean toward the elongated tail, a situation that occurs because the mean is calculated using all values in the data set (including the extreme ones). The mode remains stationary because it is the value that occurs the most frequently; it is not a mathematical summary of all of the data set values. Finally, the median moves between the mean and mode because it is the value in the middle of a distribution that is now shifted in one direction or the other.

Subject Characteristics

An important feature of all clinical research is the description of subjects included in the study. This information is essential to the evidence-based physical therapist to determine how closely the subjects resemble the individual patient or client about whom the therapist has a question. A summary of subject characteristics also is important to investigators for two reasons. First, researchers wish to know the degree to which their sample represents the population of individuals from which it was drawn. Extreme differences between the sample and the population will limit the extent to which the results can be applied beyond the study itself. Second, investigators interested in comparing the

FIGURE 9-2   A line plot for a hypothetical set of data.

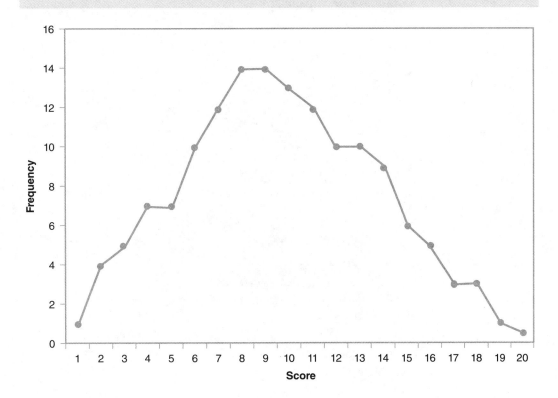

outcomes of an intervention between two or more groups need to know if relevant subject characteristics have been equally distributed among the groups at the start of the study. Unbalanced groups will make it difficult to isolate the effect of the experimental intervention from the potential influence of the participants' attributes, a situation that may undermine a quantitative study's research validity.

Patient or client characteristics commonly summarized using descriptive statistics include, but are not limited to the following:

- Demographic information:
  a. Age;
  b. Sex;
  c. Race/ethnicity;
  d. Education level;
  e. Socioeconomic status;
  f. Employment status;
  g. Marital status; and
  h. Presence and/or type of insurance coverage.

FIGURE 9-3   **Normal distribution of data (Bell Curve) with 1, 2, and 3 standard deviations.**

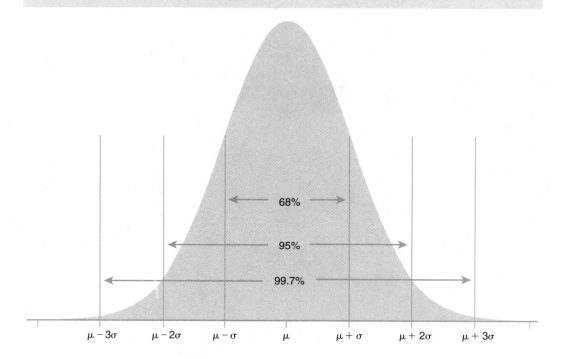

- Clinical information:
  a. Height;
  b. Weight;
  c. Diagnosis(es);
  d. Number and/or type of risk factors for disease or adverse event;
  e. Number and/or type of comorbidities;
  f. Health or functional status;
  g. Mental or cognitive status;
  h. Type of assistive device required for mobility;
  i. Number and/or type of medications;
  j. Number and/or type of diagnostic tests;
  k. Number and/or type of surgeries; and
  l. Type of referring physician.

Table 9-1 displays descriptive statistics for subject characteristics in a hypothetical study about risk factors for development of knee flexion contractures in elderly nursing home residents. Means, standard deviations, and ranges are presented for age, Mini Mental State Exam[7] score, and numbers

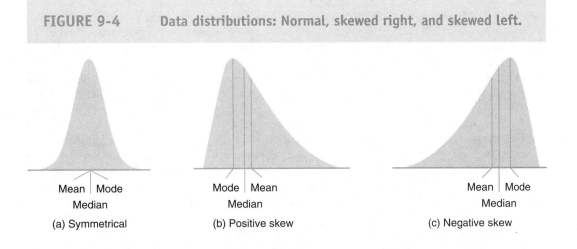

FIGURE 9-4   Data distributions: Normal, skewed right, and skewed left.

(a) Symmetrical — Mean | Mode / Median

(b) Positive skew — Mode | Mean / Median

(c) Negative skew — Mean | Mode / Median

TABLE 9-1   An Example of Descriptive Statistics in a Hypothetical Study of Risk Factors for Knee Flexion Contracture Development in Elderly Nursing Home Residents

Characteristic	Mean or %	Standard Deviation	Range
Age	84.4	4.5	77–92
Sex (% Female)	72	—	—
Mini Mental State Exam[7] Score	20.7	2.8	16–27
# of Comorbidities	2.75	1.2	1–5
# of Medications	3.75	1.1	2–6
Prior Knee Surgery (% Yes)	31	—	—

of comorbidities and medications because these variables are ratio level measures. The variables "sex" and "prior knee surgery" are nominal measures whose values require mathematical expression through frequencies. *Frequencies* may be stated as the actual number of subjects or as a proportion of the total number of subjects who have the characteristic. In this example, 72% of the subjects are female and 31% of the subjects had a prior knee surgery.

Effect Size

Physical therapists need quantitative evidence that does more than "describe" a phenomenon to answer many of their clinical questions. For example, a study about the utility of patient characteristics to predict discharge to home after an acute stroke will require an analysis of relationships. Similarly, a study about the effectiveness of an experimental intervention to alleviate lymphedema following mastectomy will require an analysis of differences between the group that received the new treatment and the group that did not. However, findings indicating a statistically important relationship or difference may not be sufficient to determine whether application of the information to an individual patient or client is warranted. Ideally, investigators also will include information about the size of the identified relationship or the difference. The descriptive statistic used to provide information about the magnitude of study findings is the *effect size (ES)*. This calculation may be performed in absolute or in relative terms.

For example, imagine an experimental study comparing two interventions to address shoulder pain in hair salon workers. One group of subjects receives body mechanics training plus exercise while the second group receives exercise alone. Outcomes in both groups are measured using the Disability of the Arm, Shoulder and Hand (DASH)[8] self-report survey. If the subjects in the body mechanics training plus exercise group achieved DASH scores 15 points higher, on average, than those achieved by the exercise-only group at the conclusion of the study, then the absolute magnitude of the effect is 15. The relative magnitude of the effect is derived when the variability in the data (i.e., the standard deviation) is included in the calculation. Often these relative effect sizes have values between 0 and 1. Several authors provide the following criteria for evaluating relative effect sizes:[2-4]

1. 0.20   minimal effect
2. 0.50   moderate effect
3. 0.80   large effect

Effect sizes that exceed 1 are even more impressive using these standards.

Summary

Statistics are tools researchers use to understand and evaluate the data they collect from subjects. As is true for clinical tools, statistical tests have defined purposes, indications for their use, specified methods for their application, and limitations or caveats regarding their performance. They also provide information in a particular form. The tools discussed in this chapter are designed to describe the data collected by identifying a central point and the variability around it. Evidence-based physical therapists use this information to determine, among other things, whether subject characteristics match the patient or client about whom they have a question. The magnitude of a measured relationship or difference between variables is another descriptive calculation that physical therapists may use to evaluate the usefulness of a predictive factor or intervention, respectively.

Table 9-2 summarizes the descriptive statistics commonly used in clinical research discussed in this chapter.[1-4,6]

TABLE 9-2   Descriptive Statistics

Statistic	Purpose	Indications for Use	Method for Use	Information Provided	Limitations or Important Caveats
Frequency	• To count things such as numbers of subjects, their characteristics, etc.	• In epidemiologic papers, to describe phenomena and their characteristics • In all other papers, to describe subjects, test results, and/or outcomes	• May be used with any level of data	• Numbers (counts) • Percentages	• None
Mean	• To summarize data • To determine the central point around which most of the data cluster	• In epidemiologic papers, to describe phenomena and their characteristics • In all other papers, to describe subjects, test results, or outcomes	• May be used with ratio and interval level data • Often used with ordinal data despite their lack of mathematical properties	• Average of all the values in the data set	• Influenced by extreme data values because all of the data points are used in the calculation
Median	• To summarize data • To determine the central point around which most of the data cluster	• Same indications as with the mean, especially when data set is skewed	• May be used with ratio, interval, and ordinal level data	• The middle value in the data set	• Not influenced by extreme values because no math is performed
Mode	• To summarize data • To determine the central point around which most of the data cluster	• Same indications as with the mean	• May be used with any level of data • Only summary statistic that may be used with nominal data	• The value(s) occurring most frequently in the data set	• Not influenced by extreme values because no math is performed • May have more than one mode in a data set

(continues)

TABLE 9-2   Descriptive Statistics (*Continued*)

Statistic	Purpose	Indications for Use	Method for Use	Information Provided	Limitations or Important Caveats
Range	• To describe the variability in a data set	• Often used to supplement information about the mean or median	• May be used with ratio, interval, or ordinal data	• The highest and lowest data values, or the difference between them	• Represents only two scores out of the entire data set; they may be outliers • The least helpful descriptor of variability

Standard Deviation (SD)	• To describe variability in the data set around the mean	• In papers that are purely descriptive in nature
		• In all other papers, to describe subjects, test results, or outcomes
			• Calculated as deviation of data from the mean	• Summary of individual data point deviations from the mean	• When data are normally distributed (bell shaped):
					  • 68% of data lie within ±1 SD
					  • 95% of data lie within ±2 SD
					  • 99% of data lie within ±3 SD

Interpercentile Range	• To describe the variability in a data set	• Often used to supplement information about the median	• May be used with any level of data • Division points may be tertiles, quartiles, etc.	• Ranges that contain a certain % of scores (e.g., the 25th percentile)	• Not greatly influenced by extreme values
Coefficient of Variation (CV)	• To measure variation relative to the mean (rather than variation "around" it)	• To compare variation among scores collected from tools with different units of measurement • To compare variation among repeated scores from the same tool	• Calculated as a ratio of the standard deviation over the mean	• % variation	• None

Statistic	Purpose	Indications for Use	Method for Use	Information Provided	Limitations or Important Caveats
Skewness	• To describe the shape of the curve created by the data points	• To determine whether the values in the data set are normally distributed	• Calculated as part of the summary description of the data	• Positive (right) or negative (left) value	• Will occur when there are outliers in the data set

Standard Error of Measurement (SEM)	• To determine the variability in repeated measures of an individual	• To differentiate between true change and error when measures are repeated in a study	• Estimated mathematically because it is logistically impractical to perform enough repeated measures to obtain this value	• Standard deviation of measurement errors	• Measurement errors are assumed to be normally distributed:
					  • 68% of data lie within ±1 SEM
					  • 95% of data lie within ±2 SEM
					  • 99% of data lie within ±3 SEM
					  • SEM is also the abbreviation for "standard error of the mean"

Standard Error of the Mean (SEM)	• To determine the variability in repeated samples from the same population	• May be reported in addition to, or instead of, the standard deviation	• Estimated mathematically because it is logistically impractical to draw repeated samples	• Standard deviation of the population mean (or sampling distribution)	• The larger the sample, the smaller the SEM
					• Sampling errors are assumed to be normally distributed:
					  • 68% of data lie within ±1 SEM
					  • 95% of data lie within ±2 SEM
					  • 99% of data lie within ±3 SEM
					  • SEM is also the abbreviation "standard error of measurement"

(continues)

TABLE 9-2　Descriptive Statistics (Continued)

Statistic	Purpose	Indications for Use	Method for Use	Information Provided	Limitations or Important Caveats
Standard Error of the Estimate (SEE)	• To determine the variability around a line through a collection of data points	• Studies about prognostic factors	• Calculated as distance of the data from the line	• Summary of the deviation of data points from the line	• The larger the sample, the smaller the SEE • Data deviations from the line are assumed to be normally distributed: 　• 68% of data lie within ±1 SEE 　• 95% of data lie within ±2 SEE 　• 99% of data lie within ±3 SEE
Effect Size	• To determine the extent of a relationship between or difference between variables	• Studies about prognostic factors, interventions, and outcomes	• Used with ratio or interval level measures	• Magnitude of a relationship or a difference	• Can be calculated in absolute and relative terms (by including the variability of the data)

Exercises

Questions 1, 2, and 3 pertain to the following scenario:

Study Purpose	"Describe patterns of calcium consumption in people with osteoporosis."
Results	(n = 75 subjects)
Sex	68% female
Subject Age (years)	Mean: 56.6
	Median: 61.2
	SD: 8.43
	Range: 32–97

1. Based on the range of ages in the subject pool, you would expect a plot of these data to create a curve that is
   a. normally distributed (bell shaped).
   b. skewed to the left.
   c. skewed to the right.
   d. bimodal.
2. The variable "sex" is quantified using which descriptive statistic?
   a. Frequency
   b. Mode
   c. Effect size
   d. Percentile
3. A sampling distribution of data indicates a mean of 63. The standard deviation of the error terms in this sampling distribution is referred to as the
   a. coefficient of variation.
   b. interpercentile range.
   c. standard error of the mean.
   d. standard error of the measure.

Questions 4, 5, and 6 pertain to the following scenario:

Study Question	"What is the effect of amount of daylight and depression level on frequency of exercise?"
Results:	Twenty-six percent of the subjects rated their depression level as moderate or higher. Subjects with less exposure to daylight indicated an average exercise frequency of 2.3 times per week (SD = ±0.5) compared to the group with more daylight exposure (mean = 3.8 times per week, SD = ±0.2).

4. What is the absolute effect size in this study?
   a. 1.5
   b. 0
   c. 3.4
   d. 1.9
5. What does the standard deviation of "±0.5" represent?
   a. Range of data points in the sample
   b. Variability of data points around the mean

    c. Standard error of the measure

    d. Relative effect size

6. The subjects rated their depression using the following scale: 0 = None, 1 = Mild, 2 = Moderate, 3 = Severe. The most frequent response selected was 1 (Mild). Which of the following does this result represent?

    a. The mean

    b. The median

    c. The mode

    d. The effect size

References

1. Polit DF, Beck CT. *Nursing Research: Principles and Methods.* 7th ed. Philadelphia, PA: Lippincott Williams & Wilkins; 2003.

2. Carter RE, Lubinsky J, Domholdt E. *Rehabilitation Research: Principles and Applications.* 4th ed. St. Louis, MO: Elsevier Saunders; 2011.

3. Portney LG, Watkins MP. *Foundations of Clinical Research: Applications to Practice.* 3rd ed. Upper Saddle River, NJ: Prentice Hall Health; 2009.

4. Batavia M. *Clinical Research for Health Professionals: A User-Friendly Guide.* Boston, MA: Butterworth-Heinemann; 2001.

5. MeasuringU. Available at: http://www.measuringu.com/blog/interval-ordinal.php. Accessed October 15, 2016.

6. Munro BH. *Statistical Methods for Health Care Research.* 5th ed. Philadelphia, PA: Lippincott Williams and Wilkins; 2005.

7. Mini Mental State Exam. Available at: https://en.wikipedia.org/wiki/Mini–Mental_State_Examination. Accessed September 1, 2016.

8. Disability of the Arm, Shoulder and Hand (DASH). Available at: http://www.dash.iwh.on.ca/. Accessed September 1, 2016.

CHAPTER 10

UNRAVELING STATISTICAL MYSTERIES: INFERENCE

OBJECTIVES

Upon completion of this chapter, the student/practitioner will be able to do the following:

1. Differentiate between:

   a. Parametric and nonparametric statistical tests;

   b. Tests of relationships and differences; and

   c. Independent and dependent data.

2. Discuss the following characteristics of selected inferential statistical tools:

   a. Purpose;

   b. Indications for use;

   c. Method for use;

   d. Information provided by the statistics; and

   e. Limitations or caveats to their use.

3. Interpret information provided by:

   a. The statistical tests reviewed in this chapter; and

   b. *p* values and confidence intervals.

4. Distinguish between statistical significance and clinical relevance.

5. Discuss the concept of statistical power.

TERMS IN THIS CHAPTER

Alpha (α) level (also referred to as *significance level*): A threshold set by researchers used to determine if an observed relationship or difference between variables is "real" or the result of chance.[1]

Benefit increase: The degree to which the chance of a positive outcome is increased as a result of an intervention; can be calculated in absolute and relative terms.[2]

Coefficient of determination: The amount of variance (expressed as a percentage) in one variable that can be accounted for by the value of another variable.

Confidence interval: A range of scores within which the true score for a variable is estimated to lie within a specified probability (e.g., 90%, 95%, 99%).[3]

Data transformation: A mathematical method by which researchers can convert their data into a normal distribution as required for parametric statistical tests.

Factorial design: An experimental research design in which the effects of two or more independent variables, and their interactions with one another, are evaluated.[3]

Inferential statistics: Statistical tests that permit estimations of population characteristics based on data provided by a sample.

Interrater reliability: The stability of repeated measures obtained by two or more examiners.

Interval level of measurement: A measure that classifies objects or characteristics in rank order with a known equal distance between categories but that lacks a known empirical zero point.

Intrarater reliability: The stability of repeated measures obtained by the same examiner.

Mean: The sum of the data points divided by the number of scores (i.e., the average).

Median: The middle score in a data set.

Multicollinearity: The degree to which independent variables in a study are related to one another.[4]

Negative likelihood ratio (LR–): The likelihood that a negative test result will be obtained in a patient or client with the condition of interest as compared to a patient or client without the condition of interest.[5]

Negative predictive value (NPV): The proportion of patients or clients with a negative test result who do not have the condition of interest.[2,5]

Nominal level of measurement: A measure that classifies objects or characteristics but that lacks rank order and a known equal distance between categories.

Nonparametric statistical tests (also referred to as *nonparametric statistics* and *nonparametric tests*): Statistical tests that are used with nominal and ordinal level data; also may be used with interval and ratio level data that are not normally distributed.

Number needed to treat (NNT): The number of subjects treated with an experimental intervention over the course of a study required to achieve one good outcome or prevent one bad outcome.[2]

Odds ratio (OR): The odds that an individual with a prognostic (risk) factor had an outcome of interest as compared to the odds for an individual without the prognostic (risk) factor.[2]

Ordinal level of measurement: A measure that classifies objects or characteristics in rank order but that lacks the mathematical properties of a known equal distance between categories; may or may not have a natural zero point.

Parametric statistical tests (also referred to as *parametric statistics* and *parametric tests*): Statistical tests that are used with interval and ratio level data that are normally distributed.

Positive likelihood ratio (LR+): The likelihood that a positive test result will be obtained in a patient or client with the condition of interest as compared to a patient or client without the condition of interest.[5]

Positive predictive value (PPV): The proportion of patients or clients with a positive test result who have the condition of interest.[2]

Power: The probability that a statistical test will detect, if it is present, a relationship between two or more variables (or scores) or a difference between two or more groups (or scores).[1,3]

p value: The probability that a statistical finding occurred due to chance.

Ratio level of measurement: A measure that classifies objects or characteristics in rank order with a known equal distance between categories and a known empirical zero point.

Risk reduction: The degree to which the risk of disease is decreased as a result of an intervention; can be calculated in absolute and relative terms.[2]

Sensitivity: The proportion of individuals with the condition of interest that have a positive test result. Also referred to as "true positives."[2]

Skew: A distortion of the normal bell curve that occurs as the result of extreme scores in the data set.

Specificity: The proportion of individuals without the condition of interest who have a negative test result. Also referred to as "true negatives."[2]

Standard deviation (SD): The average absolute distance of scores from the mean score of a data set.[6]

Standard error of the estimate (SEE): "The standard deviation of the difference between individual data points and the regression line through them."[3(p.482)]

Type I error: A result from a statistical test that indicates a significant relationship or difference exists when one does not exist (i.e., a false positive).[1]

Type II error: A result from a statistical test that indicates a significant relationship or difference does not exist when in fact one exists (i.e., a false negative).[1]

Variability: The degree to which scores in a data set are dispersed.[7]

CLINICAL SCENARIO

Which Treatment Will Be Most Helpful to Me?

© Photographee.eu/Shutterstock

Anne found an article online by Coombes and colleagues* in which the authors described their study as a 2 x 2 factorial design that examined the individual effects of injections and physical therapy as well as the effect of interactions between two intervention types. Primary outcome measures were global rating of change scores (measured on a 1–6 Likert scale) at various points in time and 1-year recurrence of the condition.

How will you explain the implications of these study design details for choices researchers can make for statistical analysis and their relevance to clinical decision making?

*Effect of Corticosteroid Injection, Physiotherapy, or Both on Clinical Outcomes in Patients with Unilateral Lateral Epicondylalgia. A Randomized Controlled Trial. *JAMA*. 2013;309(5):461-469.

Introduction

Descriptive statistics provide summary information about the variables of interest in a study. Analysis of the relationships between these variables, or the differences that occur because of them, requires more sophisticated statistical tools that allow researchers to make inferences about a phenomenon. *Inferential statistics* permit estimates of population characteristics based on data from the subjects available for study. This chapter focuses on inferential statistics commonly used in clinical research. The intent is to help you understand how these statistics are used and how to interpret the information they provide. A discussion about additional statistical methods relevant to evidence-based physical therapist (EBPT) practice follows. Finally, methods to determine the importance of statistical results are reviewed. Calculation of specific statistics and their practical application in research projects is beyond the scope of this textbook. Those of you with a desire to learn more should start with the sources itemized in the reference list at the end of the chapter to obtain additional details about these procedures.

Parametric Statistics

Parametric statistics are a form of inferential statistics that do more than describe; they help investigators and evidence-based physical therapists make decisions about what the data indicate relative to a clinical phenomenon of interest such as risk factors for a condition or the effectiveness of a new intervention.

Traditionally, these statistics are used for *ratio* or *interval level measures*. An advantage of these tests is that they provide detailed information about data that are continuous in form.[6] Investigators also use these tests with *ordinal level measures*.[1] This practice is somewhat controversial, but it is becoming more prevalent, especially in social sciences research. Remember that ordinal level measures use symbols (i.e., numerals) that are ordered in rank; however, the distance between each symbol is not known, so technically there is no way to "do math" with these data. For example, imagine a ruler with no hash marks on it and the numerals 1 to 12 written at random intervals along the face. In the absence of equal distances between each symbol, it would be impossible to quantify what is being measured. Despite these issues, parametric tests are viewed as "robust" enough to withstand their use with ordinal level data.[1]

A key assumption in parametric statistical tests is that the data are normally distributed.[3] If the distribution is not normal (e.g., the curve demonstrates a positive or negative *skew*), then several methods are available to transform the data to fix the problem. Options include logarithmic transformation, squaring the data, and taking the square root of the data, among others.[1] The decision to transform depends on how skewed the distribution is and whether *data transformation* will permit interpretation of the results. Authors will indicate which transformation technique they used, if any. An alternative to transformation is to use a nonparametric statistical test instead.[1]

Parametric tests can be categorized into one of two groups: tests of relationships and tests of differences. The following sections describe frequently encountered statistical tests in each category.

Parametric Tests of Relationships

Tests of relationships are used when an investigator wants to determine whether two or more variables are associated with one another. These tests have several functions in clinical research. First, association tests may be used in methodologic studies to establish the reliability and validity of measurement instruments. Second, investigators perform these tests to examine the *intrarater* or *interrater reliability* of data collectors prior to the start of a study. In both cases, the preferred outcome of the tests is to show a strong correlation or relationship indicating that the measures are stable and are capturing what they propose to capture. Third, association tests are used to evaluate whether all variables under consideration need to remain in the study. Variables that have overlapping qualities can add redundancy to statistical models, thereby causing some difficulties with the analysis. In cases where this interrelationship is strong, the variables in question are said to demonstrate *multicollinearity*.[4] Often researchers eliminate one variable in the associated pair to reduce this problem. Finally, the most sophisticated tests of association are used to model and predict a future outcome as is required in studies of prognostic factors.

Basic parametric association tests evaluate the relationship's strength, direction, and importance. "Strength" refers to how closely the values of one variable correspond to the values of the other variable(s) and is expressed by a correlation coefficient with a scale from 0 to 1. A coefficient that equals 1 indicates perfect association, whereas a coefficient that equals zero indicates no association at all. Portney and Watkins offer the following criteria by which to judge the strength of the correlation coefficient:[1(p.525)]

- 0.00–0.25   "little or no relationship"
- 0.26–0.50   "fair degree of relationship"
- 0.51–0.75   "moderate to good relationship"
- 0.76–1.00   "good to excellent relationship"

"Direction" is noted via the (–) or (+) sign in front of the correlation coefficient. The (–) indicates a negative or inverse relationship, as illustrated by the statement "bone density decreases as age increases." The (+) indicates a positive relationship and is illustrated by the statement "alertness decreases as caffeine levels decrease" (or "alertness increases as caffeine levels increase"). In other words, a negative correlation means that the values of the two variables change in opposite directions, whereas a positive correlation means that the values of the two variables change in the same direction.

Finally, the "importance" of the association is indicated by the amount of *variability* in the outcome (expressed as a percentage) that can be explained by the relationship. This variability is indicated by the *coefficient of determination*. For example, although age may account for some of the reduction in bone density over time, other factors such as diet, exercise, heredity, and smoking also may play a role. If age only explains 30% of the variability in bone density, then 70% is left over to explain with these other factors. However, if age explains 85% of the variability in bone density, then there are fewer factors to search out and evaluate.

More sophisticated tests of association are used to predict the value of a dependent variable based on the value(s) of the independent variable(s). The dependent variable usually is referred to as the "outcome"; the independent variables may be called "predictors" or "factors." Collectively known as regression equations or models, these tests of association provide information about the strength and direction of the relationship between the predictors and outcome, as well the proportion of variability in the outcome explained by each individual factor. Regression equations also calculate the extent to which individual data points vary from the predicted model, a value referred to as the *standard error of the estimate*.[3] Consider again the question about factors related to bone density in the preceding example. A regression equation could be used to determine whether, and to what degree, age, diet, exercise, heredity, and smoking predict the actual bone density values of individuals suspected of having osteoporosis. A regression equation also may be tested statistically to help a researcher determine whether it is an important method with which to model a particular phenomenon.

Table 10-1 itemizes parametric tests of association commonly used in clinical research:

- The Pearson product moment correlation (Pearson's r);
- The intraclass correlation coefficient (ICC);
- Multiple correlation;
- Linear regression; and
- Multiple linear regression.[1,3,4,6]

TABLE 10-1   Parametric Statistical Tests of Relationships

Statistical Test	Purpose	Indications for Use	Methods for Use	Information Provided	Limitations or Important Caveats
Pearson Product Moment Correlation (Pearson's r)	• To answer the question "Is there a relationship between two variables?"	• Studies that assess the reliability of measures • Studies that assess the association between two variables	• Designed for use with ratio or interval level measures	• Correlation coefficient (r); indicates the strength of the association from −1 to +1 (negative to positive) • Coefficient of determination (r^2); indicates the % variation in one variable that can be explained by the other variable • p value • Confidence interval (CI)	• Synonyms = correlation, association, relationship • Assumes the data are linearly related • Association does not equal causation
Intraclass Correlation Coefficient (ICC)	• To answer the question "Is there a relationship among three or more variables?"	• Studies that assess the reliability of repeated measures • Studies that assess the association among three or more pairs of variables	• Designed for use with ratio or interval level measures • Six formulas to choose from depending on the purpose of the analysis	• Reliability coefficient (ICC); indicates the strength of the association from −1 to +1 (negative to positive) • A value of 0 means the variation in the scores is due to measurement error • p value • Confidence interval (CI)	• Assumes the data are linearly related
Multiple Correlation	• To answer the question "Is there a relationship among three or more variables?"	• Studies that assess the association among three or more variables	• Designed for use with ratio or interval level measures	• Correlation coefficients; indicates the strength of the association from −1 to +1 (negative to positive) • Coefficient of determination; indicates the % variation in one variable that can be explained by the other variable • p value • Confidence interval (CI)	• Assumes the data are linearly related • Association does not equal causation

Statistical Test	Purpose	Indications for Use	Methods for Use	Information Provided	Limitations or Important Caveats
Linear Regression	• To answer the question "Can the value of an outcome (y) be predicted based on the value of a known factor (x)?"	• Studies about prognostic factors	• Dependent variable (y) is a ratio or interval level measure	• β = the amount of change in y per unit change in x • SE = standard error of the estimate • r = the strength of the relationship between x and y (-1 to $+1$) • r^2 = the percent of variance in y explained by x • F-statistic to determine if $r^2 > 0$ • p value for r^2 • Confidence interval for the predicted value of y	• Works best when the independent variable is highly correlated with the dependent variable
Multiple Linear Regression	• To answer the question "Can the value of an outcome (y) be predicted based on the value of two or more known factors (x_1, x_2, etc.)?"	• Studies about prognostic factors	• Predictions performed with two or more independent variables • Dependent variable (y) is a ratio or interval level measure • Independent variables (x) may be nominal, interval, or ratio level measures • Independent variables may be entered into the regression equation in several ways: • All together in a block • One at a time (forward step-wise) • All together with removal one at a time (backward step-wise)	• β = the amount of change in y per unit change in x • SE = standard error of the estimate • R = the strength of the relationship between x and y • R^2 = the percent of variance in y explained by the group of independent variables (x_1, x_2, etc.) • β = standardized regression coefficient that explains the percent of variance in y attributable to x; calculated for each independent variable • F- or t-statistic to determine if $\beta > 0$ and/or $R^2 > 0$ • p value for β and R^2 • Confidence interval for the predicted value of y	• Works best when the independent variable is highly correlated with the dependent variable • Assumes independent variables are not correlated with one another

Parametric Tests of Differences

Parametric tests of differences are used when an investigator wants to compare *mean* scores from two or more groups of subjects or repeated scores from the same subjects. Comparisons are indicated to evaluate whether the groups have equally distributed characteristics at the start of the study and in studies where a treatment approach is tested for its ability to produce a difference in one group as compared to the other(s).

Before conducting a parametric test of differences, investigators must determine whether the data points in each group are independent of one another. In other words, data either came from distinctly separate individuals or were gathered upon repeated measures of the same subjects. Statistical comparisons made using distinct groups of subjects are referred to as "between-group" tests, whereas comparisons made using repeated measures on the same subjects are referred to as "within group" tests.[6] **Table 10-2** illustrates a "between-group" comparison of subject characteristics at the start of a hypothetical study evaluating interventions for shoulder pain in hair salon workers. The outcome of interest is captured using the Disability of the Arm, Shoulder and Hand (DASH)[8] self-report questionnaire.

Data points in "between-group" analyses like this study are said to be independent of one another because they are obtained from different subjects. In other words, the DASH scores obtained from the subjects in the body mechanics plus exercise group do not influence the DASH scores in the exercise-only group.

A "within-group" version of this project would be to compare the DASH score at the end of the study with the score at the beginning of the study for individuals in only one of the groups (e.g., the body mechanics training plus exercise group). Data points within a group are said to be dependent on one another. In other words, the disability score a subject produced at the start of the study is related to the disability score the subject achieves at the end of the study because it came from the same person. This dependency must be acknowledged mathematically for statistical purposes. As a result, independent and dependent versions of the same tests of differences are available for use.

Selection of the appropriate statistical test of differences also depends on several other factors. First, the number of groups to be compared must be considered. The most simplistic versions of these tests

TABLE 10-2	A Comparison of Group Characteristics in a Hypothetical Study Investigating the Use of Body Mechanics Training Plus Exercise Versus Exercise Alone for the Management of Shoulder Pain in Hair Salon Workers

Characteristic	Body Mechanics Plus Exercise Group Mean (SD*) or %	Exercise Alone Group Mean (SD*) or %	p value
Age	35.8 (3.6)	29.2 (2.2)	0.04
Gender (% Female)	73	64	0.01
Income	$31,456.00	$30,598.00	0.48
DASH[8] Score at Start of Study[†]	73.4 (3.8)	71.6 (3.1)	0.27
# of Medications	1.8 (0.4)	2.0 (0.6)	0.34
Prior Surgery (% Yes)	15	16	0.15

*SD = standard deviation
[†]DASH = Disability of the Arm, Shoulder, and Hand

are designed to compare two groups only, whereas more sophisticated tests can compare three or more groups. A related issue is the number of variables used. *Factorial designs*, in which two or more variables are of interest, require analysis of the main effects resulting from each variable, as well as analysis of the effects that occur as a result of the interaction between or among variables. Second, the ability to control for extraneous variables may be desired. Only certain forms of tests of differences permit this adjustment. Third, more than one dependent variable or outcome will require yet another test. **Table 10-3** itemizes parametric tests of differences commonly used in clinical research:

- The *t*-test and its dependent measure counterpart, the paired *t*-test;
- The analysis of variance (ANOVA) test and its dependent measure counterpart, the repeated measures ANOVA test;
- The analysis of covariance (ANCOVA) test, used to adjust for confounding variables; and
- The multiple analysis of variance (MANOVA) test, used when there is more than one dependent variable.[1,3,4,6]

Nonparametric Statistics

Nonparametric tests are designed to deal with *nominal* and ordinal level measures. As such, they cannot extract as much information as parametric tests because the data are no longer continuous (i.e., the measures do not have a theoretically infinite set of values). An advantage to these tests is that they do not rely as heavily on normal distributions of the data; therefore, they also may be an appropriate choice when interval or ratio data are severely skewed and are not appropriate for transformation. Finally, these statistics do not depend on large sample sizes to have their assumptions met, so they may be an appropriate choice for interval or ratio data obtained from small groups of subjects.[1]

Nonparametric tests parallel their parametric counterparts in that there are tests of relationships and tests of differences. In addition, there are considerations related to the independence of the scores, the number of groups to be compared, the need to control extraneous variables, and the number of dependent variables included. **Table 10-4** itemizes nonparametric tests of relationships, and **Table 10-5** itemizes nonparametric tests of differences.[1,3,4,6]

Additional Statistics in Evidence-Based Therapist Practice

In addition to the traditional inferential statistics described here, several other calculations are used to evaluate the usefulness of diagnostic tests, prognostic indicators, interventions, clinical prediction rules, and self-report outcomes measures. An ideal diagnostic test is one that always correctly identifies patients with the disorder ("true positives") as well as those individuals free of it ("true negatives").[9] The degree to which a diagnostic test can meet these expectations is established by the values calculated for a test's *sensitivity, specificity, positive predictive value,* and *negative predictive value.*[2,5] A diagnostic test's usefulness also depends on the extent to which the result increases or decreases the probability of the presence of a disease or disorder in individual patients, as indicated by its *positive* or *negative likelihood ratios.*[2,5] Details about these calculations and their interpretation can be found elsewhere.

Prognostic indicators are useful when they can quantify via an *odds ratio* the probability that a patient or client will achieve a particular positive or adverse outcome.[5] Interventions, in contrast, may be evaluated by the degree to which they reduce the risk of a bad outcome (*risk reduction*) or increase the probability of a good outcome (*benefit increase*), as well as by the number of patients required for treatment (*number needed to treat*) before one good outcome occurs.[2,5] Details about these calculations and their interpretation can be found elsewhere.

TABLE 10-3   Parametric Statistical Tests of Differences

Statistical Test	Purpose	Indications for Use	Method for Use	Information Provided	Limitations or Important Caveats

Independent *t*-test	• To answer the question "Is there a difference between two groups?"	• Comparisons of characteristics between groups at start of study
		• Comparison of outcomes due to a prognostic (risk) factor or treatment
			• Examines differences between the means of two groups only
			• Designed for use with parametric data (interval, ratio)
				• *t*-statistic
				• *p* value
					• Assumes:
					  • Normally distributed data
					  • Equal variance between groups
					  • Independence of scores from one another

Paired *t*-test	• To answer the question "Is there a difference within the same group?"	• Pretest/posttest designs in which subjects act as their own controls	• Examines differences in mean values between the experimental condition and control condition • Designed for use with parametric data (interval, ratio)	• *t*-statistic • *p* value	• Assumes normally distributed data

Analysis of Variance (ANOVA)	• To answer the question "Is there a difference between two or more groups?"	• Designs in which the independent variable (e.g., the treatment) has two or more levels
		• Factorial designs with two or more independent variables
		• Used when there is only one dependent variable (outcome)
			• Examines differences between or among the means of each group
			• Designed for use with parametric data (interval, ratio)
			• Factorial designs:
			  • One independent variable = one-way ANOVA
			  • Two independent variables = two-way ANOVA
				• F-statistic
				• *p* value
				• For tests with two or more independent variables:
				  • Main effects for each variable
				  • Interaction effects between each variable
					• All assumptions listed under *t*-test apply
					• When comparing three or more groups, will only indicate that a difference exists—will NOT indicate where the difference is (i.e., which groups are different)
					• Requires additional ("post hoc") statistical tests to determine which groups are different from one another

Statistical Test	Purpose	Indications for Use	Method for Use	Information Provided	Limitations or Important Caveats

Repeated Measures Analysis of Variance (ANOVA)	• To answer the question "Is there a difference among repeated measures on subjects within the same group?"	• Repeated measures designs in which the independent variable (e.g., the treatment) has two or more levels AND subjects act as their own controls
		• Factorial designs with two or more independent variables
		• Used when there is only one dependent variable (outcome)
			• Examines differences in mean values among repeated measures
			• Designed for use with parametric data (interval, ratio)
			• Factorial designs:
			  • One independent variable = one-way repeated measures ANOVA
			  • Two independent variables = two-way repeated measures ANOVA
				• F-statistic
				• p value
				• For tests with two or more independent variables:
				  • Main effects for each variable
				  • Interaction effects between each variable
					• All assumptions listed under t-test apply
					• Will only tell you that a difference exists—will NOT indicate where the difference is (i.e., which groups are different)
					• Requires additional ("post hoc") statistical tests to determine which groups are different from one another

Analysis of Covariance (ANCOVA)	• To answer the question "Is there a difference among two or more groups while controlling for covariates (extraneous variables)?"	• Designs in which the independent variable (e.g., the treatment) has two or more levels • Used when there is only one dependent variable (outcome)	• Uses the covariate(s) to adjust the dependent variable, then examines differences among the means of each group • Designed for use with parametric data (interval, ratio)	• F-statistic • p value	• All assumptions listed under t-test apply • Covariates are not correlated with each other • Covariates are linearly related to the dependent variable • Covariates may be nominal, interval, or ratio level measures
Multivariate Analysis of Variance (MANOVA)	• To answer the question "Is there a difference in two or more outcomes among two or more groups?"	• Designs in which the independent variable (e.g., the treatment) has two or more levels • Factorial designs with two or more independent variables • Used if more than one dependent variable (outcome)	• Accounts for the relationship among multiple dependent variables during group comparisons • Designed for use with parametric data (interval, ratio)	• Wilks' lambda • F-statistic • p value	• All assumptions listed under t-test apply • Will only tell you that a difference exists—will NOT indicate where the difference is (i.e., which groups are different) • Requires additional ("post hoc") statistical tests to determine which groups are different from one another

TABLE 10-4   Nonparametric Statistical Tests of Relationships

Statistical Test	Purpose	Indications for Use	Method for Use	Information Provided	Limitations or Important Caveats
Chi-Squared Test of Independence	• To answer the question "Is there a relationship between two variables?"	• Epidemiologic studies (e.g., case-control designs)	• Compares actual to expected frequencies of the variables • Designed for use with nominal level measures	• Chi-square (χ^2) statistic • p value	• This procedure is designed to test whether two sets of data are independent of each other • A significant result indicates that the variables are not independent (i.e., they have an association)
Spearman Rank Correlation Coefficient	• To answer the question "Is there a relationship between two variables?"	• Studies that assess the reliability of measures • Studies that assess the association between two variables	• Designed for use with ordinal level measures	• Correlation coefficient (ρ); indicates the strength of the association from –1 to +1 (negative to positive) • p value	• Synonyms = correlation, association, relationship • Assumes the data are linearly related • Association does not equal causation
Kappa	• To answer the question "Is there a relationship among three or more variables?"	• Studies that assess the reliability of repeated measures • Studies that assess the association among three or more pairs of variables	• Designed for use with nominal level measures	• Reliability coefficient (κ); indicates the strength of the association from –1 to +1 (negative to positive) • p value	• Synonyms = correlation, association, relationship • Assumes the data are linearly related

Statistical Test	Purpose	Indications for Use	Method for Use	Information Provided	Limitations or Important Caveats
Logistic Regression	• To answer the question "What is the probability of an event occurring based on the value of a known factor?"	• Studies about prognostic factors	• Dependent variable (y) is nominal (dichotomous) level data • Predictor (x) [independent variable] may be nominal, interval, or ratio level measures	• β = the amount of change in y per unit change in x • SE = standard error of the estimate • r = the strength of the relationship between x and y (-1 to $+1$) • r^2 = the percent of variance in y explained by x • F-statistic to determine if $r^2 > 0$ • p value for r^2 • Confidence interval for the predicted value of y	• Works best when the independent variable is highly correlated with the dependent variable
Multiple Logistic Regression	• To answer the question "What is the probability of an event occurring based on the value of two or more known factors?"	• Studies about prognostic factors	• Predictions performed with two or more independent variables • Dependent variable (y) is nominal (dichotomous) • Predictor (x) [independent variable] may be nominal, interval, or ratio level measures • Independent variables may be entered into the regression equation in several ways: • All together in a block • One at a time (forward step-wise) • All together with removal one at a time (backward step-wise)	• β = the amount of change in y per unit change in x • SE = standard error of the estimate • R = the strength of the relationship between x's and y • R^2 = the percent of variance in y explained by x's • Exp (β) = odds ratio • F- or t-statistic to determine if Exp (β) > 0 and/or $R^2 > 0$ • p value for Exp (β) and R^2 • Confidence interval for the predicted value of y and Exp (β)	• Works best when the independent variable is highly correlated with the dependent variable • Assumes independent variables are not correlated with one another

TABLE 10-5   Nonparametric Statistical Tests of Differences

Statistic	Purpose	Indications for Use	Method for Use	Information Provided	Limitations or Important Caveats
Mann-Whitney U	• To examine differences between two groups	• Comparisons of characteristics between groups at start of study • Comparison of outcomes due to prognostic (risk) factor or treatment	• Designed for use with nonparametric data or problematic parametric data (e.g., non-normally distributed)	• Ranks the data for each group • U-statistic • *p* value	• Does not assume normal distribution of data • Can be used with small sample sizes
Wilcoxon Rank Sum	• To examine differences between two groups	• Comparisons of characteristics between groups at start of study • Comparison of outcomes due to prognostic (risk) factor or treatment	• Designed for use with nonparametric data or problematic parametric data (e.g., non-normally distributed)	• Rank sum of the data for each group • *z*-score • *p* value	• Does not assume normal distribution of data • Can be used with small sample sizes
Wilcoxon Signed Rank Test	• To examine differences within the same group	• Pretest/posttest designs in which subjects act as their own controls	• Examines differences in the *median* values between the experimental condition and control condition • Designed for use with nonparametric data (ordinal, nominal)	• Ranks the difference between each pair of numbers • *z*-score • *p* value	• None
Chi-Squared Goodness-of-Fit Test	• To examine differences between two groups	• To determine "goodness of fit" between data from sample and data estimated from population	• Compares actual to expected frequencies • Typically used with nominal level measures	• Chi-square statistic (χ^2) • *p* value	• In goodness-of-fit tests it is preferable that the actual frequencies match the expected frequencies; this match will be indicated by a **nonsignificant** result

Statistic	Purpose	Indications for Use	Method for Use	Information Provided	Limitations or Important Caveats
Kruskal-Wallis H	• To examine the difference between three or more groups (control group and experimental groups)	• Factorial designs in which the independent variable (e.g., the treatment) has three or more levels • Used when there is only one dependent variable (outcome) • May be used with parametric data if it is not normally distributed	• Designed for use with nonparametric data (ordinal, nominal)	• Ranks • H-statistic • *p* value	• Does not assume normal distribution of data • Can be used with small sample sizes • Will only tell you that a difference exists—will NOT tell you where the difference is (i.e., which groups are different) • Requires additional ("post hoc") statistical tests to determine which groups are different from one another
Friedman's ANOVA	• To examine differences among repeated measures on subjects within the same group	• Repeated measures designs in which subjects act as their own controls • Used when there is only one dependent variable (outcome)	• Examines differences in rank sums among repeated measures • Designed for use with nonparametric data (ordinal, nominal)	• Rank sums • F-statistic, or Friedman's chi-square statistic • *p* value	• Does not assume normal distribution of data • Can be used with small sample sizes • Will only indicate that a difference exists—will NOT indicate where the difference is (i.e., which groups are different) • Requires additional ("post hoc") statistical tests to determine which groups are different from one another

The development and validation of clinical prediction rules may be evaluated with the same calculations used in studies about diagnostic tests and prognostic indicators. Finally, self-report outcomes measures such as the DASH[8] are assessed for their reliability and validity, as well as for their responsiveness to change.

Investigators often use these calculations in combination with inferential statistical tests and provide the results for readers to consider. Physical therapists reviewing the evidence also may be able to calculate these values from data provided by authors who use traditional statistics alone.

Statistical Importance

As noted at the outset of this chapter, the goal of statistical testing in quantitative studies is to evaluate the data in an objective fashion. Two methods by which investigators assess the importance of their statistical results are the *p* value and the confidence interval. In both instances, researchers must choose a threshold that indicates at what point they will consider the results to be "significant," rather than a chance occurrence. A declaration of statistical significance is synonymous with rejection of the null hypothesis (i.e., "there is no difference [relationship]").

p Values

The *p value* is the probability that a study's findings occurred due to chance.[1] For example, a *p* value equal to 0.10 is interpreted to mean that there is a 10% probability that a study's findings occurred due to chance. The statistics software program used to perform the inferential test of relationships or differences also calculates this probability. Authors provide information about this "obtained" *p* value with the rest of their results. The *alpha* (α) *level*, or *significance level*, is the term used to indicate the threshold the investigators selected to detect statistical significance when they designed their study, the traditional value of which is 0.05.[10] Obtained *p* values lower than the a priori 0.05 threshold indicate even lower probabilities of the role of chance. Authors may identify their chosen alpha level in the methods section of their study or they simply may indicate in their results that the *p* values calculated as part of the statistical tests were lower than a critical value. In either case, investigators select alpha levels to reduce the opportunity of making a *type I error*—that is, identifying a relationship or difference that really does not exist (a false positive).[3] The lower the alpha level (and resulting obtained *p* value), the lower the opportunity for such an error.

The limitation of a *p* value is that it is a dichotomous, "yes–no" answer to the question about significance. This approach leaves no room for finer interpretations based on an assessment that uses continuous level information. Sterne and Smith argue that this approach to determining the importance of a statistical test result is limited for two reasons:

1. A predetermined threshold value (e.g., $\alpha = 0.05$) is arbitrary.
2. There are other means by which to evaluate the importance of a study's result using continuous values—specifically, the confidence interval.[10]

These authors contend that the context of the study, along with other available evidence, is as important as the *p* value for determining whether the results are meaningful. Furthermore, *p* values considerably lower than 0.05 (e.g., 0.001) are more convincing with respect to rejection of the null hypothesis.

Confidence Intervals

By comparison, the *confidence interval* is a range of scores within which the true score for a variable is estimated to lie within a specified probability.[3] Narrower intervals mean less variability in the data. The thresholds for confidence intervals are the probability levels within which they are calculated, the typical values of which are 90%, 95%, and 99%. If investigators select a 95% confidence interval (95% CI), the traditional value used, then they are indicating the range within which there is a 95% probability that the true value for the population is located.

Sim and Reid point out that a confidence interval provides information about statistical significance while also characterizing a statistical result's precision and accuracy.[11] An interval that includes the value "zero" indicates that the null hypothesis—"there is no relationship (difference)"—cannot be rejected. Furthermore, a narrow interval range (e.g., 95% CI) indicates that the result obtained is close to the true value (precision), whereas a wider interval range (e.g., 99% CI) increases the chance the population value will be included (accuracy). These CIs are consistent with p values of 0.05 and 0.01, respectively. In both instances, an evidence-based physical therapist can read the information provided and accept or reject the importance of the result based on its statistical significance; however, the CI provides the additional information about the range of possible population values.

The debate about the appropriateness of p values likely will continue for the foreseeable future. An evidence-based physical therapist's job is to understand the information provided about p values and/or confidence intervals because the relative objectivity of these values is an important counterbalance to the subjective human appraisal of the same results.

Power

Statistical significance depends in part on a study's sample size. Investigators have a vested interest in determining the number of subjects that are required to detect a significant result. *Power* is the probability that a statistical test will detect, if present, a relationship between two or more variables or a difference between two or more groups.[1,3] Failure to achieve adequate power will result in a *type II error,* a situation in which the null hypothesis is accepted incorrectly (a false negative). Fortunately, investigators can identify the minimum sample size required for their study by conducting a power analysis. This technique requires investigators to select their desired alpha level, effect size, and power. The threshold for power often is set at 0.80, which translates into a 20% chance of committing a type II error.[7] Software programs designed to perform these analyses calculate the number of subjects required to achieve these criteria. Essentially, larger sample sizes increase the opportunity to detect a meaningful relationship or difference if it is present. The p values will be lower and confidence intervals will be narrower when adequate sample sizes are obtained.

Clinical Relevance

As noted, statistical tests along with their obtained p values and confidence intervals help researchers and evidence-based physical therapists objectively evaluate the data collected from subjects. The next challenge is to determine whether the study's results are useful from a clinical perspective. As an example, imagine a study in which investigators examine the effectiveness of a new aerobic exercise program on the functional exercise capacity of elderly subjects as measured using a graded treadmill test. One possible result of the study is that a statistically significant difference (e.g., $p = 0.03$) is found between subjects in the exercise group as compared to subjects in a "usual activity" group. If the change in performance in the exercise group amounts to 8 additional minutes on the treadmill, then most people would probably agree that a clinically meaningful improvement occurred. But if the exercise group only gains 1.5 additional minutes on the treadmill, then this finding may not translate into an improvement in subjects' ability to perform daily tasks, despite the statistical significance of the finding. In other words, the results would not be clinically relevant.

An alternative scenario is that the study's results produce a p value greater than the threshold for significance (e.g., $\alpha = 0.05$). If the exercise group increased its treadmill time by 8 minutes but the p value equaled 0.07, then evidence-based physical therapists might still be inclined to try the aerobic exercise program with their patients. In other words, therapists might be willing to accept an increased probability (7% versus 5%) that the study's results occurred due to chance because an additional 8 minutes of exercise capacity might translate into improved household mobility. Researchers sometimes acknowledge the potential for this type of scenario by using the phrase "a trend toward significance." As noted in the previous section, debate continues regarding which α level represents the best threshold for statistical significance. A confidence interval may provide additional insights if the researchers provide this information[12]; however, the statistical result is the same (e.g., 0.05 and 95% CI). Ultimately, evidence-based physical therapists must weigh all the information in their own minds to make a decision about applying the evidence during patient/client management.

Summary

Inferential statistics are tools researchers use to make estimates related to a population of interest from data they collect from a sample of individuals. These tools are designed to answer questions about relationships and differences using data derived from different levels of measurement. They also provide insight into the usefulness of diagnostic tests, prognostic indicators, interventions, clinical prediction rules, and self-report outcomes measures. The importance of statistical results is evaluated through the use of probabilities and confidence intervals. Evidence-based physical therapists must use their clinical expertise and judgment to determine whether statistical findings are clinically meaningful and appropriate to incorporate into patient/client management.

Exercises

Questions 1, 2, and 3 pertain to the following scenario:

Study Hypothesis	"Calcium consumption is associated with osteoporosis in postmenopausal women."
Alpha Level	≤ 0.05
Results	($n = 75$ subjects)
Subject Age (years)	Mean 56.6
	Median 61.2
	SD 8.43
	Range 32–97
Statistical Analysis	$\chi^2 = 5.46$ $p = 0.07$

	Osteoporosis (+)	Osteoporosis (−)
<1000 mg CA^{2+}	25	22
>1000 mg CA^{2+}	12	16

1. What type of statistical test is being used in this scenario?
   a. Chi-square test
   b. Spearman rank correlation
   c. Two-way analysis of variance
   d. Wilcoxon rank sum test

2. Based on the statistical results reported, you would expect the study's authors to:
   a. accept the hypothesis.
   b. consider the hypothesis proven.
   c. reject the hypothesis.
   d. none of the above.
3. These results conflict with numerous other studies using larger sample sizes. What type of error most likely occurred to cause this discrepancy?
   a. Math error
   b. Test choice error
   c. Type I error
   d. Type II error

Questions 4 and 5 pertain to the following scenario:

Study Question   "Does patient gender predict the use of thrombolytic therapy ("clot busters") for patients presenting to the emergency department with signs of stroke?"

Variables and Measures   Gender = male or female; Age = years; Clot busters = yes or no

4. What category of statistical analysis should be used to answer the actual question posed?
   a. Nonparametric tests of differences
   b. Parametric tests of differences
   c. Nonparametric tests of relationships
   d. Parametric tests of relationships
5. Which specific statistical test would be most appropriate to analyze the question posed?
   a. Logistic regression
   b. Linear regression
   c. Pearson product moment correlation
   d. Spearman rank correlation coefficient

Questions 6, 7, and 8 pertain to the following scenario:

Study Question   "Will weight decrease in mildly obese teenagers as a result of an 8-week high-protein, low-carbohydrate diet, plus exercise?"

Alpha Level ≤ 0.05

Results $(n = 10)$

weight = pounds

Subject	Weight 1	Weight 2
1	211	194
2	173	169
3	186	170
4	165	172
—	—	—
—	—	—
—	—	—
10	201	195
	$\bar{x}_1 = 188.2$	$\bar{x}_2 = 180$

6. Which statistical test is most appropriate to analyze this data?
   a. Independent t-test
   b. One-way ANOVA test
   c. Paired t-test
   d. Two-way ANOVA test

7. The statistical test returns an obtained p value of 0.243. Based on *these results*, you would conclude which of the following?
   a. Diet plus exercise affects weight.
   b. Diet plus exercise does not affect weight.
   c. The findings are not generalizable.
   d. The findings are not plausible.

8. This study represents which of the following?
   a. Between-groups analysis with dependent measures
   b. Between-groups analysis with independent measures
   c. Within-group analysis with dependent measures
   d. Within-group analysis with independent measures

Questions 9, 10, and 11 pertain to the following scenario:

Study Question	"What is the effect of amount of daylight and depression on exercise frequency?"
Depression	"Depressed" or "not depressed" based on inventory score threshold
Daylight	Number of hours
Exercise Frequency	Number of exercise bouts per week
Alpha Level	≤ 0.01
Results	($n = 100$)

	F	p value
Daylight Hours	10.62	0.001
Depression	.89	0.263
Hours $\times$ Depression	13.21	0.031

9. What type of statistical test is used in this study?
   a. One-way ANOVA
   b. Two-way ANOVA
   c. Three-way ANOVA
   d. None of the above

10. How would you interpret the results presented above?
    a. Depression affects exercise frequency.
    b. The amount of daylight affects exercise frequency.
    c. There is no interaction between daylight hours and depression.
    d. Both b and c.

11. The threshold for statistical significance in this study is a
    a. 1% probability that the results occurred due to chance.
    b. 5% probability that the results occurred due to chance.
    c. 95% probability that the results occurred due to chance.
    d. 99% probability that the results occurred due to chance.

Questions 12, 13, and 14 pertain to the following scenario:

Study Question   "Can length of hospital stay following total hip replacement be predicted by patient demographic and clinical characteristics?"

Subjects $n = 200$ total hip replacement cases from one Boston hospital

Predictor Variables

Patient Demographics	Patient Clinical Characteristics
Age (# of years)	Postoperative hemoglobin (deciliters)
Gender (1 = female, 0 = other)	Postoperative white blood cell count (deciliters)
Race (1 = white, 0 = other)	Nausea (1 = yes, 0 = no)

Outcome

Length of stay (LOS) Number of days in the hospital

Alpha Level   ≤0.05

(β)		Std. β	p value
0.417	AGE	0.251	0.020
−0.103	GENDER	0.102	0.171
0.893	RACE	0.015	0.082
−1.430	HEMOGLOBIN	0.269	0.050
2.590	WHITE BLOOD CELLS	0.182	0.001
0.960	NAUSEA	0.003	0.040
Constant = 3.9			

12. The statistical test used in this study is a
    a. multiple linear regression.
    b. multiple logistic regression.
    c. simple linear regression.
    d. simple logistic regression.

13. The negative sign in front of the unstandardized β for hemoglobin implies which of the following?
    a. As hemoglobin goes down, length of stay goes down.
    b. As hemoglobin goes up, length of stay goes down.
    c. As hemoglobin goes up, length of stay goes up.
    d. Hemoglobin is not related to length of stay.

14. How would you interpret the p value and standardized beta results for nausea?
    a. Not statistically significant but an important influence on LOS
    b. Not statistically significant and an unimportant influence on LOS
    c. Statistically significant with maximal influence on LOS
    d. Statistically significant with minimal influence on LOS

Questions 15 and 16 pertain to the following scenario:

Study Question   "Is a figure-of-8 tape measuring technique (in millimeters) a reliable and valid method for quantifying edema following an acute ankle sprain?"

Study Setting   1 local sports medicine physical therapy clinic

Data Collectors   5 staff physical therapists

Methods   The physical therapists practiced the technique together on the first 5 subjects.

15. Which of the following statistical tests will allow the researchers to evaluate the physical therapists' interrater reliability with the figure-of-8 technique?

   a. Kappa

   b. Intraclass correlation coefficient

   c. Pearson's r

   d. Spearman's ρ

16. The scores with the figure-of-8 technique were compared statistically with scores from a water volume displacement technique, a measure with established validity. The obtained correlation coefficient was 0.68 ($p = 0.04$). What do these results suggest about the validity of the figure-of-eight technique?

   a. There is no evidence of validity.

   b. There is poor evidence of validity.

   c. There is moderate evidence of validity.

   d. There is unquestionable evidence of validity.

References

1. Portney LG, Watkins MP. *Foundations of Clinical Research: Applications to Practice.* 3rd ed. Upper Saddle River, NJ: Prentice Hall Health; 2009.

2. Straus SE, Richardson WS, Glaziou P, Haynes RB. *Evidence-Based Medicine: How to Practice and Teach EBM.* 3rd ed. Edinburgh, Scotland: Elsevier Churchill Livingstone; 2005.

3. Carter RE, Lubinsky J, Domholdt E. *Rehabilitation Research: Principles and Applications.* 4th ed. St. Louis, MO: Elsevier Saunders; 2011.

4. Munro BH. *Statistical Methods for Health Care Research.* 5th ed. Philadelphia, PA: Lippincott Williams and Wilkins; 2005.

5. Herbert R, Jamtvedt G, Hagen KB, Mead J. *Practical Evidence-Based Physiotherapy.* 2nd ed. Edinburgh, Scotland: Elsevier Butterworth-Heinemann; 2011.

6. Batavia M. *Clinical Research for Health Professionals: A User-Friendly Guide.* Boston, MA: Butterworth-Heinemann; 2001.

7. Polit DF, Beck CT. *Nursing Research: Principles and Methods.* 7th ed. Philadelphia, PA: Lippincott Williams & Wilkins; 2003.

8. Disability of the Arm, Shoulder and Hand (DASH). Available at: http://www.dash.iwh.on.ca. Accessed September 1, 2016.

9. Helewa A, Walker JM. *Critical Evaluation of Research in Physical Rehabilitation: Towards Evidence-Based Practice.* Philadelphia, PA: W.B. Saunders; 2000.

10. Sterne JAC, Smith GD. Sifting the evidence—what's wrong with significance tests? *BMJ.* 2001;322(7280):226–231.

11. Sim J, Reid N. Statistical inference by confidence intervals: issues of interpretation and utilization. *Phys Ther.* 1999;79(2):186–195.

12. Stratford PW. The added value of confidence intervals. *Phys Ther.* 2010;90(3):333–335.

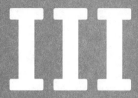

PART

III

APPRAISING THE EVIDENCE

CHAPTER 11

APPRAISING EVIDENCE ABOUT DIAGNOSTIC TESTS AND CLINICAL MEASURES

OBJECTIVES

Upon completion of this chapter, the student/practitioner will be able to do the following:

1. Discuss the purposes and processes of diagnosis and differential diagnosis in physical therapist practice.

2. Critically evaluate evidence about diagnostic tests and clinical measures, including:

   a. Important questions to ask related to research validity; and

   b. Measurement properties of reliability and validity.

3. Interpret and apply information provided by the following calculations:

   a. Sensitivity and specificity;

   b. Receiver operating characteristic curves;

   c. Positive and negative predictive values;

   d. Positive and negative likelihood ratios;

   e. Pre- and posttest probabilities; and

   f. Test and treatment thresholds.

4. Evaluate p values and confidence intervals to determine the potential importance and meaningfulness of reported findings.

5. Discuss considerations related to the application of evidence about diagnostic tests and clinical measures to individual patients or clients.

TERMS IN THIS CHAPTER

Bias: Results or inferences that systematically deviate from the truth "or the processes leading to such deviation."[1(p.251)]

Concurrent validity: A method of criterion validation that reflects the relationship between a test or measure of interest and a measure with established validity ("criterion measure"), both of which have been applied within the same time frame.[2]

Confidence interval: A range of scores within which the true score for a variable is estimated to lie within a specified probability (e.g., 90%, 95%, 99%).[2]

Criterion validity: The degree to which a test or measure of interest relates to a measure with established validity ("criterion measure").[3]

Diagnosis: A process of "integrating and evaluating the data that are obtained during the examination to describe the individual condition in terms that will guide the physical therapist in determining the prognosis and developing a plan of care."[4]

Differential diagnosis: A process for distinguishing among "a set of diagnoses that can plausibly explain the patient or client's presentation."[5(p.673)]

Face validity: A subjective assessment of the degree to which an instrument appears to measure what it is designed to measure.[6]

Gold standard (also referred to as *reference standard*) test or measure: A diagnostic test or clinical measure that provides a definitive diagnosis or measurement. A "best in class" criterion test or measure.[1]

Index test or measure: The diagnostic test or clinical measure of interest, the utility of which is being evaluated through comparison to a gold (or reference) standard test or measure.[7]

Instrumentation: A threat to research validity (internal validity) characterized by problems with the tools used to collect data that may influence the study's outcomes.

Masked (also referred to as *blinded*): (1) In diagnostic test and clinical measure papers, the lack of knowledge about previous test/measure results; (2) in prognostic factor papers, the lack of knowledge about exposure status; and (3) in intervention papers, the lack of knowledge about to which group a subject has been assigned.

Measurement reliability: The extent to which repeated test results or measurements agree with one another. Also referred to as "stability," "consistency," and "reproducibility."[6]

Measurement validity: The degree to which a measure captures what it is intended to measure.[6]

Minimal detectable change (MDC): The amount of change that just exceeds the standard error of measurement of an instrument.[6]

Negative likelihood ratio (LR–): The likelihood that a negative test result will be obtained in an individual with the condition of interest as compared to an individual without the condition of interest.[8]

Negative predictive value (NPV): The proportion of individuals with a negative test result who do not have the condition of interest.[9]

Positive likelihood ratio (LR+): The likelihood that a positive test result will be obtained in an individual with the condition of interest as compared to an individual without the condition of interest.[8]

Positive predictive value (PPV): The proportion of individuals with a positive test result who have the condition of interest.[9]

Posttest probability: The odds (probability) that an individual has a condition based on the result of a diagnostic test.[9]

Pretest probability: The odds (probability) that an individual has a condition based on clinical presentation before a diagnostic test is conducted.[9]

Prevalence: The proportion of individuals with a condition of interest at a given point in time.[10]

p value: The probability that a statistical finding occurred due to chance.

Responsiveness: The ability of a measure to detect change in the phenomenon of interest.[6]

Sensitivity (Sn): The proportion of individuals with the condition of interest that have a positive test result. Also referred to as "true positives."[9]

Specificity (Sp): The proportion of individuals without the condition of interest who have a negative test result. Also referred to as "true negatives."[9]

Standard error of measurement (SEM): The extent to which observed scores are disbursed around the true score; "the standard deviation of measurement errors" obtained from repeated measures.[2(p.482)]

Standardized response mean (SRM): An indicator of responsiveness based on the difference between two scores (or the "change score") on an outcomes instrument.

Test threshold: The probability below which a physical therapist determines that a suspected condition is unlikely and forgoes diagnostic testing.[10]

Treatment threshold: The probability above which a physical therapist determines that a diagnosis is likely and forgoes further testing in order to initiate treatment.[10]

CLINICAL SCENARIO

Does That Test Provide Additional Useful Information?

© Photographee.eu/Shutterstock

When Anne was discussing management options with the orthopedic surgeon, he mentioned several imaging tests that some physicians use to confirm a lateral epicondylitis diagnosis. She reported that he was skeptical that they provided enough additional information to justify their time and expense. He cited an article* that indicated high sensitivity and specificity for detecting increased tendon thickness using ultrasound. However, the authors concluded, "further prospective study is necessary to determine whether quantitative ultrasound with these cutoff values can improve the accuracy of the diagnosis of lateral epicondylitis." Based on that statement, the physician determined his clinical examination was sufficient. Anne agreed that testing that does not improve a clinician's diagnostic accuracy is wasteful on multiple levels. She was curious about the article though, so downloaded it, and brought it to you for review.

How will you explain what the authors did and what their findings (e.g., sensitivity, specificity, etc.) mean?

*Lee MH, Cha JG, Wook J, et al. Utility of sonographic measurement of the common tensor tendon in patients with lateral epicondylitis. *AJR*. 196(6);1363-1367.

Introduction

The *Guide to Physical Therapist Practice, 3.0* describes examination as the step in the patient/client management model during which physical therapists gather information about an individual's problem or concern. Examination includes review of available health-related records, interviews with the patient or client, performance of a systems review, and application of diagnostic tests and clinical measures.[4] In today's busy health care environment, physical therapists strive to collect the most relevant data as efficiently and effectively as possible. With that goal in mind, this chapter focuses on the evaluation of evidence that informs physical therapists' choices regarding diagnostic tests and clinical measures.

Diagnostic Tests

Diagnosis is a process in which patient data are collected and evaluated to classify a condition, determine prognosis, and identify possible interventions.[4] *Differential diagnosis* is the method by which doctors (of medicine, physical therapy, and so on) use information to make decisions between two or more alternatives to explain why an individual has a set of signs and symptoms.[5] In both cases, the conclusions reached are informed by results from the patient's history, clinical examination, and associated diagnostic tests.

Diagnostic tests have three potential purposes in physical therapist practice: (1) to help focus the examination on a particular body region or system, (2) to identify potential problems that require referral to a physician or other health care provider, and (3) to assist in the classification process.[11] The decision to perform a diagnostic test rests on a clinician's estimation of the probability that an individual has the condition that is suspected based on clinical examination findings and relevant subjective history. In **Figure 11-1**, Hayden and Brown describe a continuum of probabilities from 0% to 100% along which are two decision points: the "test threshold" and the "treatment threshold."[10]

The *test threshold* is the probability below which a diagnostic test will not be performed because the possibility of the particular diagnosis is so remote. The *treatment threshold* is the probability above which a test will not be performed because the possibility of the particular diagnosis is so great that immediate treatment is indicated. Fritz and Wainner refer to this decision point as the "action threshold."[11] In between these two decision points are the probabilities for which administering a test or tests is indicated to rule in or rule out the suspected diagnosis.

FIGURE 11-1   Diagnostic test and treatment thresholds.

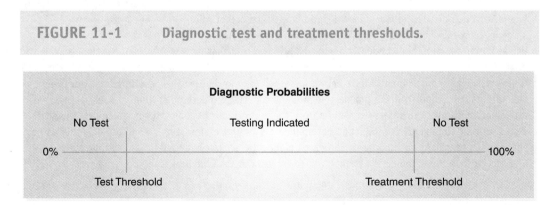

Reprinted from *Annals of Emergency Medicine,* 33(5), Hayden, SR, Brown, MD, Likelihood Ratio: A Powerful Tool for Incorporating the Results of a Diagnostic Test Into Clinical Decisionmaking, 575-580, Copyright 1999, with permission from American College of Emergency Physicians. Published by Mosby, Inc. All rights reserved.

TABLE 11-1	Examples of Studies About Diagnostic Tests Relevant to Physical Therapist Practice

- Sman AD, et al. Diagnostic accuracy of clinical tests for ankle syndesmosis injury. *Br J Sports Med.* 2015;49(5):323-329.
- Bjerkefors J, et al. Diagnostic accuracy of common clinical tests for assessing abdominal muscle function after complete spinal cord injury above T6. *Spinal Cord.* 2015;53(2):114-119.
- Hanchard NC, et al. Physical tests for shoulder impingements and local lesions of bursa, tendon, or labrum that may accompany impingement. *Cochrane Database Syst Rev.* 2013; 30(4):CD007427.
- Hutting N, et al. Diagnostic accuracy of premanipulative vertebrobasilar insufficiency tests: a systematic review. *Man Ther.* 2013;18(3):1770182.
- Kasai Y, et al. A new evaluation method for lumbar spinal instability: passive lumbar extension test. *Phys Ther.* 2006;86(12):1661-1667.

Successful diagnosis and differential diagnosis depend, in part, on the availability and use of diagnostic tests that are reliable, valid, and provide persuasive information. A test that has demonstrated *measurement reliability* produces stable results over time, whereas a test that has demonstrated *measurement validity* is said to capture correctly what it is supposed to be testing. The ability to provide persuasive information is reflected by the extent to which the test results change estimates about the presence of a suspected disorder or condition.

Physical therapists primarily use clinical (or "special") tests to examine their patients or clients, although the latitude to order imaging studies and diagnostic laboratory procedures may be granted to those in military practice. Civilian therapists also may have opportunities to recommend diagnostic tests during consultations. In all cases, a physical therapist should consider the evidence about diagnostic tests to improve the quality, safety, and efficiency of care and to support the patient's or client's values and preferences.

Table 11-1 provides some examples of studies about diagnostic tests physical therapists use to rule in or rule out the presence of a suspected condition.

Study Credibility

Evidence pertaining to diagnostic tests that physical therapists use first should be evaluated with an assessment of research validity. Higher research validity provides greater confidence that a study's findings are reasonably free from *bias*. In other words, the results are believable. Appraisal of evidence about diagnostic tests starts with the questions itemized in **Table 11-2**. These questions are modeled after critical appraisal worksheets developed by the Centre for Evidence Based Medicine at the University of Oxford and the revised Quality Assessment of Diagnostic Accuracy Studies (QUADAS-2) appraisal tool.[7,12] Their purpose is to help physical therapists determine whether there are problems with a study's design that may have biased the results with respect to the utility of the diagnostic test of interest (i.e., the *index test*).[9]

1. Did the investigators include subjects with all levels or stages of the condition being evaluated by the index test?
This question focuses on the utility of the index test in various clinical scenarios. For example, different levels of severity may characterize the condition of interest such that the identification

TABLE 11-2	Questions to Assess the Validity of Evidence About Diagnostic Tests

1. Did the investigators include subjects with all levels or stages of the condition being evaluated by the index test?
2. Did the investigators evaluate (or provide a citation for) the reliability of the index diagnostic test?
3. Did the investigators compare results from the index test to results from a gold standard comparison diagnostic test?
4. Did all subjects undergo the comparison diagnostic test?
5. Were the individuals performing and interpreting each test's results unaware of the other test's results (i.e., were they masked, or blinded)?
6. Was the time between application of the index test and the gold standard comparison diagnostic test short enough to minimize the opportunity for change in the subjects' condition?
7. Did the investigators confirm their findings with a new set of subjects?

and/or quantification of each level is essential to guide prognosis and treatment. A diagnostic example relevant to physical therapist practice is the use of grades to rank the severity of ligament damage that has occurred during a lateral ankle sprain. Grade I represents minimal tearing with maintenance of full function and strength. Grade II reflects a partial ligament tear with mild joint laxity and functional loss. Grade III indicates a full-thickness ligament tear with complete joint laxity and functional loss.[13] Each of these levels requires a progressively greater treatment intensity and recovery time; therefore, it is preferable that a diagnostic test be evaluated for its ability to differentiate among all three of these grades. The ability of the test to distinguish between those who have been treated for the ankle sprain and those who have not also is helpful to assess the patient's progress. Finally, a test that can discriminate among other similar conditions (e.g., fracture, tendinopathy) will be useful in the differential diagnostic process.[1,11]

Readers should understand that the extent to which an index test is evaluated is determined by the research question posed by the investigators. A study that only evaluates the accuracy of a ligament stress test in patients with a grade III ankle sprain is not necessarily weaker from a research validity standpoint. However, the ability to apply the study's findings to patients with grade I and grade II ankle sprains is limited.

2. Did the investigators evaluate (or provide a citation for) the reliability of the index diagnostic test?

The validity of a diagnostic test depends, in part, on its ability to obtain the same results under the same conditions within the same time frame. A test's reliability may be evaluated at the same time its validity is assessed. However, it is more common for this measurement attribute to be tested in a separate investigation. In that case, authors seeking to determine whether an index diagnostic test is valid will reference previously published works to verify the precondition of reliability.

3. Did the investigators compare results from the index test to results from a gold standard comparison diagnostic test?

This question addresses the need to verify measurement validity of the index test with a superior reference standard. Ideally, the comparison test will be the *gold standard*, or "best in class," instrument or method. For physical therapists, relevant gold standard diagnostic tests commonly are radiographic images, laboratory results, or surgical or autopsy findings. The choice of a comparison test ultimately depends on the research question being investigated as well as the investigator's prerogative. As a result, comparison tests that are not "best in class" may be used.

In all cases, a comparison test should have superior capability because of its technologic features and/or its own track record of reliability and validity. In addition, the purpose and potential outcomes of the comparison test should be consistent with the purpose and outcomes of the index test.[11] Performing an x-ray to assess the usefulness of a functional balance scale would not be a meaningful comparison despite the technologic superiority of radiography. Comparison to a superior reference standard allows researchers to verify the extent to which the index test correctly classifies individuals who have the condition (i.e., "true positives") and individuals who do not (i.e., "true negatives"). Readers should be aware, however, that the actual usefulness of a gold standard itself often cannot be confirmed because a reference against which to compare it does not exist. At a minimum, face validity of the comparison test is essential in these cases. The possibility that the comparison will be replaced over time as technology evolves also should be acknowledged.[8]

4. Did all subjects undergo the comparison diagnostic test?

This question clarifies the degree to which the investigators may have introduced bias into the study by administering the comparison test to a select group of subjects previously evaluated by the index test. This selective evaluation may occur in situations in which the comparison method is expensive and/or when subjects are judged to have a low probability of having the condition of interest.[11] In studies about diagnostic tests, the specific concern is application of the comparison test (e.g., an x-ray) only to subjects who produce positive results on the index test (e.g., a ligament stress test). In this example, the diagnostic accuracy of the ligament stress test will be misleading because there will be no information about the extent to which true and false negative results occurred when the index test was applied.

5. Were the individuals performing and interpreting each test's results unaware of the other test's results (i.e., masked, or blinded)?

Ideally, the index test and the comparison test will be applied to subjects by examiners who are *masked* (or *blinded*). Masking the individuals responsible for administering the different tests further enhances validity by minimizing tester bias. In other words, the possibility is reduced that a particular finding will occur on one test as a result of knowledge of another test's result.

6. Was the time between application of the index test and the gold standard comparison diagnostic test short enough to minimize the opportunity for change in the subjects' condition?

The concern for studies about diagnostic tests is that the condition of interest will evolve if too much time elapses between administration of the index test and administration of the gold standard test. A change in a subject's status may lead to misclassification such that the accuracy of the index test is called into question. For example, the severity of a ligament sprain may be underestimated if enough time has passed to allow sufficient healing.

7. Did the investigators confirm their findings with a new set of subjects?

This question alludes to the possibility that the research findings regarding an index test occurred due to unique attributes of the sample. Repeating the study on a second group of subjects who match the inclusion and exclusion criteria outlined for the first group provides an opportunity to evaluate the consistency (or lack thereof) of the test's performance. Often this step is not included in a single research report due to insufficient numbers of subjects and/or lack of funds. As a result, evidence-based physical therapists may have to read several pieces of evidence about the same diagnostic test if they wish to verify its usefulness to a greater degree.

Additional Considerations

The previous questions serve as an initial screening of the evidence to determine its potential usefulness—that is, its research validity. From an evaluative standpoint, a "no" answer to questions 2 through 6 may indicate a "fatal flaw" in the research design related to unacceptable levels of bias in the results. Readers may use more latitude in their analysis with respect to questions 1 and 7 given that researchers have the prerogative to frame a research question how they wish and to study it within their resource limitations. Herbert et al. suggest that research articles that fail to meet many of the criteria indicated by these questions should be set aside and a new evidence search initiated when possible.[8] In the absence of this opportunity, the evidence should be considered carefully in light of its limitations, especially when an index test is associated with a significant degree of risk to the patient or client.

Finally, there are additional concerns pertaining to research design in evidence about diagnostic tests. Specifically, readers should note the presence or absence of a detailed description of the following:

1. The setting in which the research was conducted;
2. The protocol for the test(s) used, including scoring methods; and
3. The characteristics of the sample obtained.

This information allows evidence-based physical therapists to determine if the diagnostic test of interest is applicable and feasible in their environment (1, 2) and if the subjects included resemble the patient or client about whom there is a question (3). Well-designed studies may have limited usefulness when these details are lacking.

Study Results

Reliability

Evidence-based physical therapist practice relies on tests of relationships to determine the reliability of diagnostic tests. Verification of reliability is an acknowledgment that the data captured during a test is composed of the "true value" and error. Error may be the result of the subject, the observer, the instrument itself, and/or the environment in which the test was performed.[2,6] An accurate diagnosis depends, in part, on the ability to minimize error during the testing process to avoid a false-positive or false-negative result. Investigators also use tests of relationships to demonstrate the intrarater or interrater reliability of their test administrators. The need to demonstrate that those collecting the data can do so in a reproducible manner over many subjects is driven by the threat to research validity known as *instrumentation*.

Examples of statistics commonly used to evaluate the reliability of diagnostic tests include the Pearson's product moment correlation (r), the intraclass correlation coefficient (ICC), Spearman's rho (ρ), and kappa (κ). All of these tests assess the strength of the association between measures collected on patients or research subjects. The first two tests are designed for use with interval or ratio level measures; the second two are designed for use with ordinal and nominal data, respectively. Pearson's r and Spearman's ρ compare only two measures, whereas the ICC and kappa (κ) can be used to compare multiple pairs of measures simultaneously. Portney and Watkins offer the following criteria by which to judge the strength of the correlation coefficient:[6(p.525)]

- 0.00–0.25   "little or no relationship"
- 0.26–0.50   "fair degree of relationship"
- 0.51–0.75   "moderate to good relationship"
- 0.76–1.00   "good to excellent relationship"

The *standard error of measurement (SEM)* also may be used to assess the variability in repeated measurements.

A *p* value or confidence interval also may be used to assess the statistical significance and clinical usefulness of the relationship tested.

Validity

The validity of diagnostic tests may be evaluated from several perspectives. The first approach is to consider the *face validity* of the instrument or technique. A test evaluating lower extremity muscle performance would not have face validity for assessing ligament integrity. The second approach is to assess statistically the relationship between results from the index test and the results from the comparison test. The statistical tests described in the previous section also apply here. Higher correlation coefficients indicate greater correspondence between the results of the different tests. In other words, the test of interest provides essentially the same information as the comparison test. This statistical approach is used to verify *criterion validity* or *concurrent validity*, or both.[2,3]

Finally, measurement validity of a diagnostic test may be evaluated through mathematical calculations based on a two-by-two (2 × 2) table (**Figure 11-2**). A 2 × 2 table is the basis for the chi-square test of association and is a traditional method of classifying nominal data in epidemiologic studies that are evaluating the association between a risk factor and disease. The classic public health example is the association between cigarette smoking and lung cancer.

Figure 11-2 should be interpreted in the following manner:

- Cell (a) represents the individuals who smoked and who developed lung cancer;
- Cell (b) represents individuals who smoked and did not develop lung cancer;
- Cell (c) represents people who did not smoke and who developed lung cancer; and
- Cell (d) represents people who did not smoke and who did not develop lung cancer.

The 2 × 2 table is easily adapted for evaluation of diagnostic tests by changing the labels for the rows to reflect a positive diagnostic test result and a negative diagnostic test result, respectively.

FIGURE 11-2   **A 2 x 2 table used for epidemiologic research on smoking and lung cancer.**

	+ Lung Cancer	− Lung Cancer
+ Smoking	(a)	(b)
− Smoking	(c)	(d)

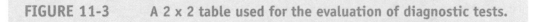

FIGURE 11-3   A 2 x 2 table used for the evaluation of diagnostic tests.

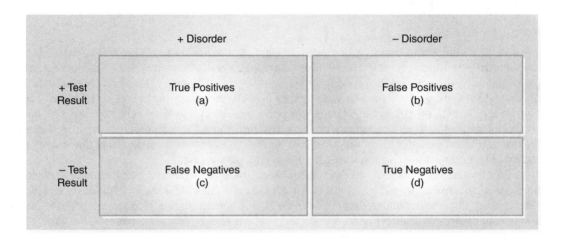

	+ Disorder	− Disorder
+ Test Result	True Positives (a)	False Positives (b)
− Test Result	False Negatives (c)	True Negatives (d)

A valid diagnostic test consistently produces true positives or true negatives, or both.[1] In addition, the test produces information that allows the physical therapist to adjust his or her estimate of the probability that a patient has the condition of interest. The following mathematical calculations based on the data in the 2 × 2 table in **Figure 11-3** are used to determine whether a diagnostic test meets these standards.

Sensitivity (Sn)

A diagnostic test is said to be *sensitive* when it is capable of correctly classifying individuals with the condition of interest (true positives).[9] This information allows evidence-based physical therapists to determine which test may be most appropriate to use when a particular condition is suspected. Most authors provide the value for sensitivity (0% to 100%) of the test they evaluated; however, the sensitivity also can be calculated using the following formula:

$$Sensitivity = \frac{Patients\ with\ the\ condition\ who\ test\ positive\ (a)}{All\ patients\ with\ the\ condition\ (a + c)}$$

There is an important caveat for tests that are highly sensitive (good at detecting people with a condition): when a negative result is obtained using a highly sensitive test, then a clinician can say with confidence that the condition can be ruled out. In other words, false negatives are so unlikely that the test will catch most, if not all, of those individuals with the condition. Therefore, a negative test result for a highly sensitive test indicates the person is condition free. Sackett et al. developed the mnemonic **SnNout** (Sn = highly sensitive test, N = negative result, out = rule out disorder) to help remember this caveat.[14]

Figure 11-4 provides a graphic illustration of this concept. The (+) and (−) symbols represent individuals in whom the condition of interest is present and absent, respectively. The hypothetical diagnostic test has high sensitivity as demonstrated by its ability to correctly identify those who are

FIGURE 11-4   A graphic illustration of SnNout.

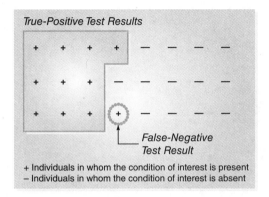

True-Positive Test Results

False-Negative Test Result

\+ Individuals in whom the condition of interest is present
− Individuals in whom the condition of interest is absent

positive (+ symbols surrounded by the dark green line). Only one individual was missed because the test produced a false-negative result. The overall likelihood of false negatives is so small in this example that a negative test result is believable and rules out the disorder when this test is used.

Specificity (Sp)

A diagnostic test is said to be specific when it is capable of correctly classifying individuals without the condition of interest (true negatives).[9] As with sensitivity, *specificity* indicates which test may be appropriate to use for a suspected condition. Most authors provide the value for specificity (0% to 100%) of the test they evaluated; however, the specificity also can be calculated from the 2 × 2 table using the following formula:

$$Specificity = \frac{Patients\ without\ the\ condition\ who\ test\ negative\ (d)}{All\ patients\ without\ the\ condition\ (b + d)}$$

There is an important caveat for tests that are highly specific (good at detecting people without the condition): when a positive result is obtained using this test, then a clinician can say with confidence that the condition can be ruled in. In other words, false positives are so unlikely that the test will catch most, if not all, of those individuals without the condition. Therefore, a positive test result for a highly specific test indicates a person has the condition. The mnemonic **SpPin** (Sp = highly specific test, P = positive test result, in = rule in disorder) is the reminder about this situation.[14]

Figure 11-5 provides a graphic illustration of this concept. The (+) and (−) symbols represent individuals in whom the condition of interest is present and absent, respectively. The hypothetical diagnostic test has high specificity as demonstrated by its ability to correctly identify those who are negative (− symbols surrounded by dark green line). Only one individual was missed because the test produced a false-positive result. The likelihood of false positives is so small in this example that a positive test result is believable and rules in the disorder when this test is used.

FIGURE 11-5 A graphic illustration of SpPin.

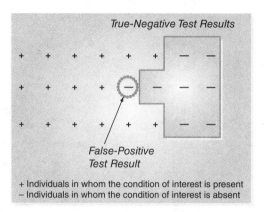

+ Individuals in whom the condition of interest is present
− Individuals in whom the condition of interest is absent

Receiver Operating Characteristic Curves

Unfortunately, sensitivity and specificity have limited usefulness for two reasons: (1) they indicate a test's performance in individuals whose status is known (i.e., they have or do not have the condition) and (2) they reduce the information about the test to a choice of two options based on the threshold, or cut point, according to which a result is classified as positive or negative. Different test cut points require recalculation of sensitivity and specificity, a situation that is inefficient when a range of test scores may indicate a range of severity of a condition.[1]

One way to improve the usefulness of sensitivity and specificity calculations is the creation of a receiver operating characteristic (ROC) curve. An ROC curve is a graphic way to evaluate different test scores with respect to the number of true-positive and false-positive results obtained at each threshold or cut point. In effect, the curve allows an investigator to identify the signal-to-noise ratio of any score the diagnostic test can produce.[6] This approach is more efficient than creating a 2 × 2 table for each possible diagnostic test value.

An ROC curve is plotted in a box, the y-axis of which represents the test's sensitivity, or true-positive rate, and the x-axis of which represents 1 − specificity, or the false-positive rate. A perfect test will only have true-positive results, so it will not matter what test score is selected as a threshold to determine the presence of a condition. When that happens, the ROC curve essentially stays along the y-axis (**Figure 11-6**).

Diagnostic tests are rarely perfect—an ROC curve typically starts along the y-axis but eventually bends away from it and trails out along the x-axis. In these cases, a curve that reflects more true positives than false positives, or greater signal to noise, will fill the box (**Figure 11-7**).

If the curve is a perfect diagonal line, then the diagnostic test produces the same number of true-positive and false-positive results for any score and the determination of a diagnosis is reduced to a coin flip (**Figure 11-8**).

Investigators examine the curve to determine its area and to identify the most useful cut point or points among the available diagnostic test scores. The area under the curve simply represents the true and false positives for each and every score obtained from the diagnostic test or for specific cut points that the investigators wish to evaluate. A higher true-positive rate results in a bigger area under

FIGURE 11-6   A receiver operating characteristic (ROC) curve for a perfect test.

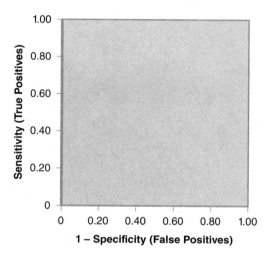

FIGURE 11-7   A receiver operating characteristic (ROC) curve for an imperfect but useful test.

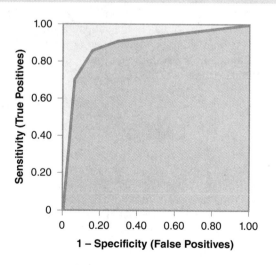

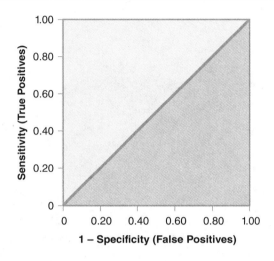

FIGURE 11-8 A receiver operating characteristic (ROC) curve for a test with results equal to chance.

the curve. Assuming an imperfect test, the threshold score is the point at which the curve starts to bend away from the *y*-axis because that is the point when the false-positive rate starts to increase. In other words, that is the point at which the diagnostic test provides the most information about people who have the problem and people who do not.

Positive Predictive Value

The *positive predictive value (PPV)* describes the ability of a diagnostic test to correctly determine the proportion of patients with the disease from all of the patients with positive test results.[9] This value is consistent with clinical decision making in which a test result is used to judge whether or not a patient has the condition of interest.[11] Most authors provide the PPV (0% to 100%) of the test they evaluated; however, the PPV also can be calculated from a 2 × 2 table using the following formula:

$$PPV = \frac{Patients\ with\ the\ condition\ who\ test\ positive\ (a)}{All\ patients\ with\ positive\ test\ results\ (a + b)}$$

Negative Predictive Value

The *negative predictive value (NPV)* describes the ability of a diagnostic test to correctly determine the proportion of patients without the disease from all of the patients with negative test results.[9] This value also is consistent with the clinical decision-making process. Most authors provide the NPV (0% to 100%) of the test they evaluated; however, the NPV also can be calculated from a 2 × 2 table using the following formula:

$$NPV = \frac{Patients\ without\ the\ condition\ who\ test\ negative\ (d)}{All\ patients\ with\ negative\ test\ results\ (c + d)}$$

An important caveat regarding the positive and negative predictive values of diagnostic tests: these values will change based on the overall *prevalence* of the condition. In other words, the PPV and NPV reported in a study will apply only to clinical scenarios in which the proportion of individuals with the condition is the same as that used in the study. Prevalence may change over time as preventive measures or better treatments are implemented. For these reasons, the PPV and NPV generally are not as useful as other measures of diagnostic test validity.[15]

Likelihood Ratios

Likelihood ratios are the mathematical calculations that reflect a diagnostic test's ability to provide persuasive information. Their values will help determine the extent to which a physical therapist will change his or her initial estimate regarding the presence of the disorder of interest. There are three advantages to using likelihood ratios in the diagnostic process. First, the ratios can be calculated for all levels of test results (not just positive and negative). Second, they are not dependent on the prevalence of the condition in the population.[9] Third, the ratios can be applied to individual patients or clients, whereas sensitivity, specificity, and positive and negative predictive values refer to groups of people.

A *positive likelihood ratio (LR+)* indicates the likelihood that a positive test result was obtained in a person with the condition as compared to a person without the condition. A *negative likelihood ratio (LR−)* indicates the likelihood that a negative test result was observed in a person with the condition as compared to a person without the condition.[8] Likelihood ratios have values greater than or equal to zero. An LR+ will have values greater than one (>1). An LR− will have values less than one (<1). A test with a likelihood ratio equal to one (= 1) is said to produce a result that is no better than chance (i.e., a coin flip) in terms of identifying whether a person is likely to have, or not have, the condition.[15]

Most authors provide the likelihood ratio of the test they evaluated; however, the ratio also can be calculated from a 2 × 2 table, or when authors provide sensitivity and specificity information, using the following formulas:

$$LR+ = \frac{Sensitivity}{1 - Specificity} \ or \ \frac{(a/a + c)}{[1-(d/b + d)]}$$

$$LR- = \frac{1 - Sensitivity}{Specificity} \ or \ \frac{[1-(a/a + c)]}{(d/b + d)}$$

Nomograms

A diagnostic test's likelihood ratio can be applied in clinical practice with the use of a nomogram, as depicted in **Figure 11-9**.[16]

The nomogram helps a clinician determine whether performing the test will provide enough additional information to be worth the risk and expense of conducting the procedure on a specific individual. Use of a nomogram involves the following steps:

- **Determine the patient or client's *pretest probability* of the condition.**

This step requires physical therapists to estimate the proportion of individuals who have the condition they suspect based on the data gathered during the examination. This estimate is a percentage value and can be determined by the following:

1. The known prevalence of the condition in the population (per epidemiologic studies);
2. The known prevalence of the condition in patients or clients referred to the therapist's clinic; or
3. Gut instinct about the probability this individual has the problem.

FIGURE 11-9 A nomogram.

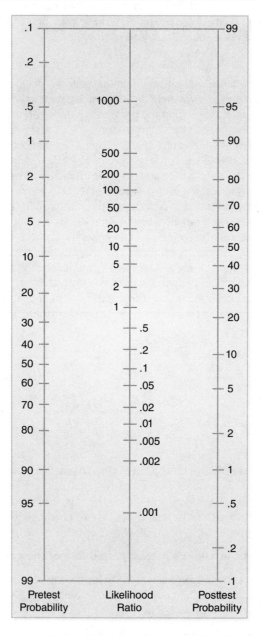

The proportion should be identified on the line on the left-hand side of the nomogram labeled "pretest probability."

- **Identify the likelihood ratio for the test.**

The likelihood ratio is identified from the best available evidence and should be identified on the middle line of the nomogram.

- **Connect the dots.**

A straight edge should be used to draw a line from the pretest probability through the likelihood ratio for the test to the line on the right of the nomogram entitled *"posttest probability."* This value also is expressed as a percentage and indicates the probability that the patient or client has the condition of interest now that a test result has been obtained. Guyatt and Rennie provide the following guidelines for interpreting likelihood ratios:[5(pp.128-129)]

- LR+ > 10 or LR− < 0.10 = large and conclusive change from pre- to posttest probability;
- LR+ = 5 − 10 or LR− = 0.10 − 0.20 = moderate change from pre- to posttest probability;
- LR+ = 2 − 5 or LR− = 0.20 − 0.50 = small but sometimes important change from pre- to posttest probability; and
- LR+ = 1 − 2 or LR− = 0.50 − 1.0 = negligible change in pretest probability.

Evaluating a Diagnostic Test: Calculations Based on Study Results

The following is an illustration of the use of a 2 × 2 table and nomogram with results from an actual study about a diagnostic test. Van Dijk et al. examined the usefulness of delayed physical examination for the diagnosis of acute inversion ankle sprains resulting in ligament rupture (*n* = 160).[17] Confirmation of the diagnosis was obtained through arthrography. One of the clinical procedures performed to assess the integrity of the anterior talofibular ligament was the anterior drawer test. **Figure 11-10** is a 2 × 2 table with results from the anterior drawer test and the arthrography.

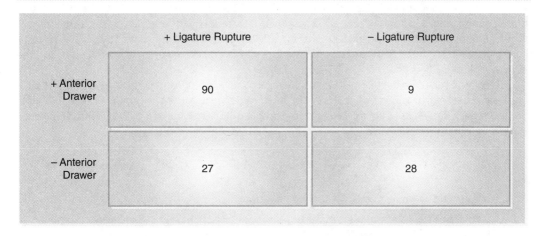

FIGURE 11-10   **Anterior drawer test and arthrography results from Van Dijk et al.**

	+ Ligature Rupture	− Ligature Rupture
+ Anterior Drawer	90	9
− Anterior Drawer	27	28

Data from Van Dijk CN, Lim LSL, Bossuyt PMM, Marti RK. Physical examination is sufficient for the diagnosis of sprained ankles. *J Bone Joint Surg.* Essential Surgical Techniques, 1996;78(6):958-962.

Calculations using these data produce the following values for sensitivity, specificity, positive and negative predictive values, and likelihood ratios.

Sensitivity	$90/117 = 0.77$
Specificity	$28/37 = 0.76$
Positive predictive value	$90/99 = 0.91$
Negative predictive value	$28/55 = 0.51$
+ Likelihood ratio	$0.77/1 - 0.76 = 3.21$
− Likelihood ratio	$1 - 0.77/0.76 = 0.30$

The authors concluded that, based on these results and data from other examination procedures, a delayed physical examination was sufficient to diagnose an ankle ligament rupture and was less invasive (and presumably less costly) than arthrography.

Figure 11-11 illustrates an application of the likelihood ratios from Van Dijk et al. using a nomogram. The prevalence of ligament rupture in the study was 76%; therefore, this value serves as the pretest probability in this example. The light green line indicates that a positive likelihood ratio of 3.2 increases the probability that an individual has a ligament tear to just over 90%; the dark green line indicates that a negative likelihood ratio of 0.30 decreases the probability that an individual has a ligament tear to approximately 38%. Assuming this study's research validity is sound, these changes in the pretest probability are large enough to suggest that the anterior drawer test is a worthwhile procedure to perform when a lateral ankle sprain is suspected.

Practical Use of Likelihood Ratios

Using a nomogram may be helpful in medical practice because the diagnostic tests physicians order often are expensive, invasive, and/or potentially risky to the patient. Deciding whether there is value added to clinical decision making by conducting another test makes sense under these circumstances. Civilian physical therapist practice often does not have to confront concerns about cost and invasiveness of diagnostic tests because therapists usually are prohibited from ordering and/or performing these procedures. However, clinical examination techniques often cause pain and, in some circumstances, have a high enough level of risk associated with them that their added value also should be considered. In addition, the contribution of a diagnostic test to accurate classification of the patient's condition should be acknowledged in an effort to direct treatment. Under these circumstances, a nomogram may be useful as illustrated by the anterior drawer test example. Physical therapists with diagnostic test ordering privileges, as well as those who perform diagnostic electrophysiologic and ultrasound examinations, will have even greater opportunities to put this simple tool to use.

Evidence-based physical therapists also may determine the shift from pretest to posttest probabilities via calculations provided by Sackett et al.[14] The procedure requires conversion of probabilities to odds and back again using the following steps (as illustrated with the use of the positive likelihood ratio data from the ankle study):

1. Pretest odds $= \dfrac{Pretest\ probability}{1 - Pretest\ probability} = 0.76/0.24 = 3.16$

2. Posttest odds = Pretest odds × +Likelihood ratio = $3.16 \times 3.2 = 10.11$

3. Posttest probability $= \dfrac{Posttest\ odds}{Posttest\ odds + 1} = 10.11/11.11 = 91\%$

FIGURE 11-11   Likelihood ratios for the anterior drawer test for ankle ligament rupture from Van Dijk et al.

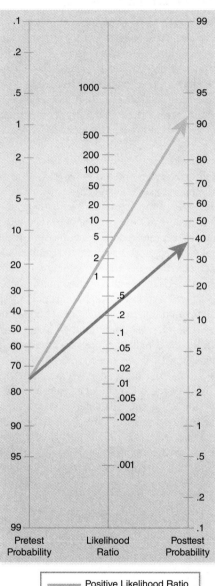

Positive Likelihood Ratio
Negative Likelihood Ratio

From New England Journal of Medicine, Fagan TJ. Nomogram for Bayes's Theorem, 293(5):257. Copyright © 1975 Massachusetts Medical Society. Reprinted with permission from Massachusetts Medical Society.

Whether using the nomogram or doing the math, therapists should evaluate the final posttest probability against the identified treatment threshold to determine if intervention, or further diagnostic testing, is warranted.[11]

The Statistical Importance of Study Results

In addition to the correlation coefficients, sensitivity, specificity, predictive values, and likelihood ratios reported in studies of diagnostic tests, investigators also provide information to determine the "meaningfulness"—or potential importance—of their results. The two primary ways to convey potential importance are via the *p* value and the confidence interval. A *p value* indicates the probability that the result obtained occurred due to chance. The smaller the *p* value (e.g., <0.05), the more important the result is statistically because the role of chance is so diminished, although not eliminated. In most cases *p* values are reported when correlation coefficients are calculated to evaluate the association between: (1) repeated scores from the index test and/or (2) scores from the index test and scores from the comparison test.

A *confidence interval* represents a range of scores within which the true score for a variable is estimated to lie within a specified probability (e.g., "I am [90%, 95%, 99%] confident the true value for this variable lies within this range of values I have calculated from my data").[2] Confidence intervals commonly are reported to indicate the precision of the estimate of sensitivity, specificity, predictive values, and likelihood ratios. For example, a likelihood ratio is meaningful if it lies within the confidence interval; however, a narrow range or interval is preferred for the purposes of validity. In other words, a narrow confidence interval suggests that the likelihood ratio obtained from data in the study is close to the "true" likelihood ratio if it could be calculated from the entire population (within the identified probability [e.g., 95%]). Unfortunately, there are no criteria by which to judge whether a confidence interval is "too wide." Remember that if a confidence interval around a likelihood ratio contains the value "1," then the true value includes chance (a coin flip), a finding that invalidates the result obtained by the researchers.[14] Authors may acknowledge this situation by stating that their result was not statistically significant.

Usually authors report the relevant confidence interval; however, readers also may calculate the interval for different estimates when they are not reported. Remember also that authors choose what their threshold values for statistical significance will be. In the case of *p* values, the traditional threshold is alpha (α) ≤ 0.05. In the case of confidence intervals, the traditional probability is 95%. Ultimately, these are arbitrary choices; therefore, evidence-based physical therapists must use their clinical judgment and expertise to determine the clinical meaningfulness or importance of a study's findings. This challenge will be apparent when results just miss significance (e.g., $p = 0.07$) or when confidence intervals are wide. Nevertheless, a study that minimizes bias and that demonstrates strong statistical significance with narrow confidence intervals should be taken seriously in terms of the information it provides.

Final Thoughts About Diagnosis in Physical Therapy

The need for evidence about diagnostic tests is intuitive in military physical therapist practice where test-ordering privileges are granted and in civilian outpatient physical therapist practice in states with direct access to physical therapist services. Home health physical therapists also may find themselves using this type of information when they encounter a patient whose signs and symptoms differ from those exhibited at the last visit.

Physical therapists working in inpatient settings, however, may wonder if the concept of diagnosis even applies to their practice. After all, the patient has been admitted with a diagnostic label such as "stroke," "myocardial infarction," or "hip fracture." Physical therapists do not need to decide which tests to perform to rule in or rule out these conditions. However, each of these patients requires physical therapy for a movement-related impairment, the classification of which must be determined from a variety of potential options. For example, exercise intolerance after myocardial infarction may be due to diminished aerobic capacity and/or due to peripheral muscle weakness. Physical therapists must perform clinical examination procedures to determine which of these problems underlies the poor exercise response in order to design and execute the most effective plan of care;[10] therefore, they must decide which procedures are the most useful to obtain the necessary information. In that sense, evaluation of evidence about diagnostic tests is relevant to physical therapists in all practice settings.

Clinical Measures

Clinical measures are distinct from diagnostic tests in that they are not used to detect the presence of, or put a label on, a suspected condition per se. Instead, they are more commonly used to quantify and/or describe in a standardized fashion a patient's impairments in body functions and structures as well as activity limitations and participation restrictions. When applied appropriately they provide objective, often performance-based, indications of the extent of a problem. Scores on clinical measures also may help distinguish among different levels of severity of a problem. Clinical measures obtained during the initial patient or client visit often serve as the foundation for goal development in the physical therapist's plan of care. The baseline values are used for comparison to subsequent measures to evaluate what progress, if any, the individual is making toward those goals.[4,6]

Successful clinical measurement depends, in part, on the availability and use of instruments and procedures that are reliable, valid, and responsive. As is the case with diagnostic tests, a measure that has demonstrated reliability produces stable results over time, whereas a measure that has demonstrated validity is said to capture correctly what it is supposed to be measuring. *Responsiveness* is the ability of a clinical measure to detect change in the phenomenon of interest.[6]

Clinical measurement is an essential component of the examination process in any practice setting. As a result, physical therapists should consider the evidence about clinical measures, such as the examples listed in **Table 11-3**, to select those that provide the most accurate information under a given set of circumstances.

TABLE 11-3	**Examples of Methodologic Studies About Clinical Measures**

- Hidding JT, et al. Measurement properties of instruments for measuring lymphedema: systematic review. *Phys Ther.* 2016;96(12);1965-1981.
- Jacome C, et al. Validity, reliability, and ability to identify fall status of the Berg Balance Scale, the BESTest, the Mini-BESTest, and Brief BESTest in patients with COPD. *Phys Ther.* 2016;96(11):1807-1815.
- Sommers J, et al. de Morton mobility index is feasible, reliable, and valid in patients with critical illness. *Phys Ther.* 2016;96(10):1658-1666.
- Aertssen WFM, et al. Reliability and structural and construct validity of the functional strength measurement in children aged 4–10 years. *Phys Ther.* 2016;96(6):888-897.
- O'Shea A, et al. Reliability and validity of the measurement of scapular position using the protractor method. *Phys Ther.* 2016;96(4):502-510.

Study Credibility

Evaluation of evidence about clinical measures (commonly referred to as methodologic studies) follows a similar process used to evaluate research about diagnostic tests. The first step is to consider whether the index measure is being evaluated across the spectrum of the disorder to which it is being applied. For example, patients with different grades of ankle sprain are likely to present with different degrees of movement restriction. The utility of a goniometer is best understood if the accuracy of its measures is evaluated for patients with all grades of ankle sprain, not just patients in one category. Once the context of the index measure's utility is established, then appraisal of the research validity of the study itself may be accomplished using the remaining questions itemized in **Table 11-4**. The intent and interpretation of the questions is the same as that for evidence about diagnostic tests.

Researchers may investigate the reliability of an index measure as the primary purpose of their study. Alternatively, they may cite published studies that have established this measurement property previously. Verification of the index clinical measure's validity requires comparison to a superior, preferably gold standard, clinical measure. Gold standard clinical measures often are electronic versions of manual instruments such as goniometers, strength testing devices, and physiologic assessment methods. Similarly, investigators should compare all subjects with both the index clinical measure and the comparison measure to ensure that complete information about the index measure's performance is obtained. Tester bias also should be minimized by masking individuals from prior measurement results so as not to influence their interpretation of the data they are collecting. Finally, the index clinical measure and the gold standard measure should be applied within the same examination session or other suitably short time frame to minimize the possibility of change in the impairment, activity limitation, or participation restriction. The validity of the index measure will be challenged if a notably different result is obtained by the comparison technique.

TABLE 11-4	Questions to Assess the Validity of Evidence About Clinical Measures

1. Did the investigators include subjects with all levels or stages of the condition being evaluated by the index clinical measure?

2. Did the investigators evaluate (or provide a citation for) the reliability of the index clinical measure?

3. Did the investigators compare results from the index clinical measure to results from a gold standard clinical measure?

4. Did all subjects undergo the comparison clinical measure?

5. Were the individuals performing and interpreting each measure's results unaware of the other measure's results (i.e., were they masked, or blinded)?

6. Was the time between application of the index clinical measure and the gold standard comparison measure short enough to minimize the opportunity for change in the subjects' condition?

7. Did the investigators confirm their findings with a new set of subjects?

As is the case with any research endeavor, investigators determine the focus of their inquiry. That means that evidence about clinical measures may be limited to evaluation of reliability or validity, rather than both properties simultaneously. A similar challenge exists with respect to the lack of confirmation of study findings with a new set of subjects. As a result, evidence-based physical therapists may need to review several articles to get complete information about a clinical measure's utility.

Study Results

The reliability and validity of a clinical measure can be confirmed statistically using correlation coefficients. In addition, the responsiveness of a clinical measure is commonly evaluated through the calculation of the *minimal detectable change (MDC)* score. The MDC is the amount of change that just exceeds the standard error of measurement of the instrument.[6] The *standardized response mean (SRM)*, a reflection of the difference in scores between two measures over time, also may be reported. An SRM = 1.0 is a commonly stated threshold criteria for establishing responsiveness.

Calculations used to evaluate the accuracy of diagnostic tests (i.e., sensitivity, specificity, etc.) often are not reported in methodologic studies about the validity of clinical measures. The reason is that a technique or device designed to quantify weakness, movement restriction, or pain usually does not provide information that identifies the underlying diagnostic reason for these problems. For example, you cannot rule in or rule out a ligament tear simply by measuring the available range of motion of the ankle joint complex with a goniometer.

The exceptions to this situation are studies that evaluate whether a score from a clinical measure can predict a future outcome. Riddle and Stratford calculated sensitivity, specificity, predictive values, and likelihood ratios to determine the extent to which scores on the Berg Balance Test could predict future fall risk in elderly individuals.[18] As noted previously, the diagnostic process in its most general sense is a classification exercise. Although the Berg Balance Test cannot specify the pathologic process that may result in a fall, its ability to correctly classify elders at risk based on the score obtained is an important attribute of this clinical measure. Physical therapists may discover other studies about traditional clinical measures that mimic Riddle and Stratford's design. In those cases, the usefulness of the index measure should be considered in light of results that usually are associated with assessment of diagnostic test accuracy.

The Statistical Importance of Study Results

Investigators evaluating the usefulness of clinical measures also use *p* values and confidence intervals to assess the potential importance of their study's results. The same interpretive guidelines apply. The smaller the *p* value (e.g., <0.05), the more important the result is statistically because the role of chance is so diminished, although not eliminated. Similarly, a narrow confidence interval suggests that the correlation coefficient, MDC value, or SRM value in the study is close to the "true" value within the identified probability (e.g., 95%).

Evidence and the Patient or Client

Once the validity of a study about a diagnostic test or clinical measure is established and the importance of its results confirmed, the final step is to determine whether the evidence is appropriate for use with an individual patient or client. This is the point in the process during which the physical therapist must add his or her clinical expertise and judgment, along with the individual's preferences and values, to the information gleaned from the research.

There are several practical considerations before putting the evidence into practice. First, the diagnostic test or clinical measure of interest should be available, practical, and safe in the setting in which the physical therapist practices. For example, a measure that requires an immobile piece of expensive equipment, such as a Biodex System 4 Pro,[19] likely will be more appropriate for use in an outpatient clinic than in a skilled nursing facility.

Second, the test or measure should have demonstrated performance on patients or clients that resemble the individual with whom the physical therapist is working. These commonalities may include age, gender, signs, symptoms, previous activity or functional levels, comorbidities, and so on. Clinically important differences may indicate a need to discard the test or measure in favor of another option.

Third, in the case of diagnostic testing, the therapist must consider whether he or she can estimate pretest probabilities for his or her patient or client. Rarely encountered diagnoses may make this step difficult both in terms of the therapist's experience and available epidemiologic data. A reasonable pretest probability is essential to determining whether the test's results will add information by revising the probability of a diagnosis upward or downward. Evidence that provides ambiguous answers to these considerations will demand more of the physical therapist in terms of his or her clinical judgment about the usefulness and safety of a diagnostic test.

In addition to addressing these practical issues, the physical therapist also must take into account his or her patient or client's preferences and values with respect to his or her health status and its management. Exploration of these issues occurs during the initial interview and continues throughout the episode of care. Areas of interest or concern for an individual may include, but are not limited to[20,21] the following:

1. The potential risk of injury or pain involved with the procedure;
2. Whether sufficient benefit will occur once the test or measure results are known;
3. Cost (financial, as well as time away from work, school, or family);
4. Confidence in the test or measure and/or the examiner; and
5. Appreciation of and belief in the value of scientific evidence.

Individual cultural and social norms will shape the discussion of these issues for the patient or client as well as for family members or other caregivers involved in the situation.

Ideally, both the physical therapist and the individual seeking rehabilitation services will agree on the optimal course of action. However, the ethical principle of autonomy dictates that the patient or client must decide whether the diagnostic test or clinical measure is worth the effort and risk to undergo the procedure. Reluctance may translate into suboptimal performance that further confounds results of the clinical examination, a situation that the physical therapist must take into account as he or she considers the data obtained.

Evidence Appraisal Tools

Table 11-5 provides a checklist to guide the evaluation of evidence about diagnostic tests for use in any practice setting.[7,12,22] **Table 11-6** provides a comparable checklist for evidence about clinical measures. Alternatively, readers might consider accessing online appraisal resources. A strategy worth considering is the creation of reference notebooks that contain completed checklists or worksheets along with their associated research articles. These compendia could facilitate the use of evidence regarding diagnostic tests or clinical measures for all physical therapists in a particular setting (as long as there is a commitment to keeping them up to date).

TABLE 11-5	Evidence About Diagnostic Tests: Quality Appraisal Checklist

Research Validity of the Study

Did the investigators include subjects with all levels or stages of the condition being evaluated by the index diagnostic test?	___ Yes ___ No ___ Insufficient detail
Did the investigators evaluate (or provide a citation for) the reliability of the index diagnostic test?	___ Yes ___ No ___ Insufficient detail
Did the investigators compare results from the index test to results from a gold standard diagnostic test?	___ Comparison to a gold standard test was performed ___ Comparison to another test was performed ___ Comparison was performed but the description is inadequate ___ No comparison was made
Were all subjects evaluated with the comparison diagnostic test?	___ Yes ___ No ___ Insufficient detail
Were the individuals performing and interpreting each test's results unaware of the other test's results (i.e., were they masked, or blinded)?	___ Yes ___ No ___ Insufficient detail
Was the time between application of the index test and the gold standard comparison diagnostic test short enough to minimize the opportunity for change in the subjects' condition?	___ Yes ___ No ___ Insufficient detail
Did the investigators confirm their findings with a new set of subjects?	___ Yes ___ No ___ Insufficient detail
Do you have enough confidence in the research validity of this paper to consider using this evidence with your patient or client?	___ Yes ___ Undecided ___ No

Relevant Study Findings

Results reported that are specific to your clinical question:

Sensitivity _____

Specificity _____

(continues)

TABLE 11-5	Evidence About Diagnostic Tests: Quality Appraisal Checklist (*Continued*)

Positive predictive value(s) _____

Negative predictive value(s) _____

+ Likelihood ratio(s) _____

− Likelihood ratio(s) _____

Correlation coefficient(s) _____

Other _____

Statistical significance and/or precision of the relevant study results:

Obtained *p* values for each relevant statistic reported by the authors: _____

Obtained confidence intervals for each relevant statistic reported by the authors: _____

Is the index diagnostic test reliable?	___ Yes
	___ No
	___ Mixed results
	___ Insufficient detail
Is the index diagnostic test valid? If yes, continue below.	___ Yes
	___ No
	___ Mixed results
	___ Insufficient detail
What is the pretest probability that your patient or client has the condition of interest?	_____
What is the posttest probability that your patient or client has the condition of interest if you apply this test?	_____

Application of the Evidence to Your Patient or Client

Are there clinically meaningful differences between the subjects in the study and your patient or client?	___ Yes
	___ No
	___ Mixed results
	___ Insufficient detail
Can you perform the index diagnostic test safely and appropriately in your clinical setting given your current knowledge and skill level and your current resources?	___ Yes
	___ No
	___ Insufficient description of the techniques used
Does the index diagnostic test fit within this patient or client's expressed values and preferences?	___ Yes
	___ No
	___ Mixed results
Will you use the index diagnostic test for this patient or client?	___ Yes
	___ No

TABLE 11-5   Evidence About Diagnostic Tests: Quality Appraisal Checklist (*Continued*)

Sample Calculations

Target Disorder

Biceps Pathology and SLAP Lesion

From Holtby and Razmjou[22]

		Present	Absent	Totals
Diagnostic test result (Yergason's)	Positive (pain in bicipital groove or glenohumeral [GH] joint)	**a** 9	**b** 6	**a + b** 15
	Negative (no pain in bicipital groove or GH joint)	**c** 12	**d** 22	**c + d** 34
	Totals	**a + c** 21	**b + d** 28	**a + b + c + d** 49

Sensitivity = a/(a + c) = 9/21 = 43%

Specificity = d/(b + d) = 22/28 = 79%

Positive predictive value = a/(a + b) = 9/15 = 60%

Negative predictive value = d/(c + d) = 22/34 = 65%

Likelihood ratio for a positive test result = LR+ = sens/(1 − spec) = 43%/21% = 2.05

Likelihood ratio for a negative test result = LR− = (1 − sens)/spec = 57%/79% = 0.72

Change in Probabilities If Test Is Performed

Positive Test Result

Pretest probability (prevalence) = (a + c)/(a + b + c + d) = 21/49 = 43%

Pretest odds = prevalence/(1 − prevalence) = 43%/57% = 0.75

Posttest odds = pretest odds × LR+ = 0.75 × 2.05 = 1.54

Posttest probability = posttest odds/(posttest odds + 1) = 1.54/2.54 = 61%

Negative Test Result

Pretest probability (prevalence) = (a + c)/(a + b + c + d) = 21/49 = 43%

Pretest odds = prevalence/(1 − prevalence) = 43%/57% = 0.75

Posttest odds = pretest odds × LR− = 0.75 × 0.72 = 0.54

Posttest probability = posttest odds/(posttest odds + 1) = 0.54/1.54 = 35%

Your Calculations

Target Disorder

		Present	Absent	Totals
Diagnostic test result	Positive	**a**	**b**	**a + b**
	Negative	**c**	**d**	**c + d**
	Totals	**a + c**	**b + d**	**a + b + c + d**

These questions were adapted from the Oxford Centre for Evidence-Based Medicine and applied to physical therapist practice.

TABLE 11-6	Evidence About Clinical Measures: Quality Appraisal Checklist

Research Validity of the Study

Did the investigators include subjects with all levels or stages of the condition being evaluated by the index clinical measure?	___ Yes ___ No ___ Insufficient detail
Did the investigators evaluate (or provide a citation for) the reliability of the index clinical measure?	___ Yes ___ No ___ Insufficient detail
Did the investigators compare results from the index measure to results from a gold standard measure?	___ Comparison to a gold standard measure was performed ___ Comparison to another measure was performed ___ Comparison was performed but the description is inadequate ___ No comparison was made
Were all subjects evaluated with the comparison measure?	___ Yes ___ No ___ Insufficient detail
Were the individuals performing and interpreting each measure's results unaware of the other measure's results (i.e., were they masked, or blinded)?	___ Yes ___ No ___ Insufficient detail
Was the time between application of the index clinical measure and the gold standard measure short enough to minimize the opportunity for change in the subjects' condition?	___ Yes ___ No ___ Insufficient detail
Did the investigators confirm their findings with a new set of subjects?	___ Yes ___ No ___ Insufficient detail
Do you have enough confidence in the research validity of this paper to consider using this evidence with your patient or client?	___ Yes ___ Undecided ___ No

Relevant Study Findings

Results reported that are specific to your clinical question:

Correlation coefficient(s) _____

Minimal detectable change _____

TABLE 11-6	Evidence About Clinical Measures: Quality Appraisal Checklist (*Continued*)

Standardized response mean _____

Other _____

Statistical significance and/or precision of the relevant study results:

Obtained *p* values for each relevant statistic reported by the authors: _____

Obtained confidence intervals for each relevant statistic reported by the authors: _____

Is the index clinical measure reliable?

   ___ Yes

   ___ No

   ___ Mixed results

   ___ Insufficient detail

Is the index clinical measure valid?

   ___ Yes

   ___ No

   ___ Mixed results

   ___ Insufficient detail

Is the index clinical measure responsive?

   ___ Yes

   ___ No

   ___ Mixed results

   ___ Insufficient detail

Application of the Evidence to Your Patient or Client

Are there clinically meaningful differences between the subjects in the study and your patient or client?

   ___ Yes

   ___ No

   ___ Mixed results

   ___ Insufficient detail

Can you perform the index clinical measure safely and appropriately in your clinical setting given your current knowledge and skill level and your current resources?

   ___ Yes

   ___ No

   ___ Insufficient description of the techniques used

Does the index clinical measure fit within this patient or client's expressed values and preferences?

   ___ Yes

   ___ No

   ___ Mixed results

Will you use the index clinical measure for this patient or client?

   ___ Yes

   ___ No

These questions were adapted from the Oxford Centre for Evidence-Based Medicine and applied to physical therapist practice.

Summary

Diagnostic tests and clinical measures are an essential component of physical therapist practice in any setting. The most useful diagnostic tests or clinical measures are those that have demonstrated reliability and validity and provide persuasive information. Reliability is demonstrated through statistical tests of relationships among repeated test results. Validity is demonstrated through statistical and mathematical comparisons to results from another test or measure, preferably a gold standard whose application will provide a definitive diagnosis or measurement.

A receiver operating characteristic (ROC) curve may be used to identify important thresholds or cut points in a diagnostic test's scoring system. The ability of a diagnostic test's result to change estimates about the presence of a disorder or condition is expressed through likelihood ratios. Likelihood ratios are the most flexible diagnostic test property for clinical use because they can be calculated for a spectrum of diagnostic test results and applied to individual patients or clients.

The most useful clinical measures are those that also are reliable and valid as well as responsive to change over time. Responsiveness of clinical measures may be indicated by the minimal detectable change or the standardized response mean.

Evidence about diagnostic tests and clinical measures should be evaluated to verify research validity and to determine if the results are useful and important for application with an individual patient or client. The final decision should reflect both the therapist's clinical expertise and judgment and the patient or client's preferences and values.

Exercises

1. Differentiate between a test threshold and a treatment threshold. Provide a clinical example relevant to physical therapist practice to illustrate your point.
2. Differentiate between the reliability and validity of a diagnostic test or clinical measure. Provide a clinical example relevant to physical therapist practice to illustrate your point.
3. Explain why a masked comparison to a superior diagnostic test or clinical measure is a necessary step in establishing the validity of an index test or measure. Provide a clinical example relevant to physical therapist practice to illustrate your point.
4. Differentiate between the sensitivity and specificity of a diagnostic test. What does it mean when sensitivity is low but specificity is high? What does it mean when sensitivity is high but specificity is low? Provide clinical examples relevant to physical therapist practice to illustrate your points.
5. Explain why positive and negative predictive values for diagnostic tests are limited in their usefulness. Provide a clinical example relevant to physical therapist practice to illustrate your point.
6. Differentiate between a positive and negative likelihood ratio. What does it mean when a likelihood ratio equals 1.0?
7. Differentiate between pretest and posttest probabilities. How does a likelihood ratio interact with these two values?

8. Use the following 2 × 2 table to calculate the sensitivity, specificity, positive and negative predictive values, and positive and negative likelihood ratios for a hypothetical diagnostic test:

	+ Condition	− Condition
+ Test	138	108
− Test	35	238

Interpret the results for each of the calculations.

9. Assume that a patient has a pretest probability of 30% for the diagnosis of interest in question 8. Use the nomogram in Figure 11-9 and determine the posttest probabilities for the positive and negative likelihood ratios obtained in question 8. How would you explain these posttest probabilities to the person on whom you have performed this diagnostic test?

10. A study regarding the diagnostic test in question 8 provides the following confidence intervals for the positive and negative likelihood ratios:

LR+ 95% CI (0.87, 6.8)

LR− 95% CI (0.20, 0.74)

What do these confidence intervals indicate about the usefulness of each likelihood ratio?

References

1. Helewa A, Walker JM. *Critical Evaluation of Research in Physical Rehabilitation: Towards Evidence-Based Practice.* Philadelphia, PA: W.B. Saunders; 2000.

2. Carter RE, Lubinsky J, Domholdt E. *Rehabilitation Research: Principles and Applications.* 4th ed. St. Louis, MO: Elsevier Saunders; 2011.

3. Polit DF, Beck CT. *Essentials of Nursing Research: Principles and Methods.* 7th ed. Philadelphia, PA: Lippincott Williams & Wilkins; 2003.

4. American Physical Therapy Association. Guide to Physical Therapist Practice. *3.0.* Available at: http://guidetoptpractice.apta.org. Accessed July 16, 2016.

5. Guyatt G, Rennie D. *Users' Guides to the Medical Literature: A Manual for Evidence-Based Clinical Practice.* 3rd ed. Chicago, IL: AMA Press; 2014.

6. Portney LG, Watkins MP. *Foundations of Clinical Research: Applications to Practice.* 3rd ed. Upper Saddle River, NJ: Pearson; 2009.

7. Whiting PF, Rutjes AWS, Westwood ME, et al. QUADAS-2: A revised tool for the quality assessment of diagnostic accuracy studies. *Ann Intern Med.* 2011;155(8):529–536.

8. Herbert R, Jamtvedt G, Hagen KB, Mead J. *Practical Evidence-Based Physiotherapy.* 2nd ed. Edinburgh, Scotland: Elsevier Butterworth-Heinemann; 2011.

9. Straus SE, Richardson WS, Glaziou P, Haynes RB. *Evidence-Based Medicine: How to Practice and Teach EBM.* 3rd ed. Edinburgh, Scotland: Elsevier Churchill Livingstone; 2005.

10. Hayden SR, Brown MD: Likelihood ratio: a powerful tool for incorporating the results of a diagnostic test into clinical decision making. *Ann Emerg Med.* 1999;33(5):575–580.

11. Fritz JM, Wainner RS. Examining diagnostic tests: an evidence-based perspective. *Phys Ther.* 2001;81(9):1546–1564.

12. Critically Appraising the Evidence. Worksheets for Diagnosis. Centre for Evidence Based Medicine. Oxford website. Available at: www.cebm.net. Accessed October 1, 2016.

13. Safran MR, Benedetti RS, Bartolozzi AR III, et al. Lateral ankle sprains: a comprehensive review: part 1: etiology, pathoanatomy, histopathogenesis, and diagnosis. *Med Sci Sports Exerc.* 1999;31(7):429S–437S.

14. Sackett DL, Straus SE, Richardson WS, et al. *Evidence-Based Medicine: How to Practice and Teach EBM.* 2nd ed. Edinburgh, Scotland: Churchill Livingstone; 2000.

15. Davidson M. The interpretation of diagnostic tests: a primer for physiotherapists. *Aust J Physiother.* 2002;48(3):227–233.

16. Fagan TJ. Nomogram for Bayes's theorem. *N Engl J Med.* 1975;293(5):257.

17. Van Dijk CN, Lim LSL, Bossuyt PMM, Marti RK. Physical examination is sufficient for the diagnosis of sprained ankles. *J Bone Joint Surg.* 1996;78(6):958–962.

18. Riddle DL, Stratford PW. Interpreting validity indexes for diagnostic tests: an illustration using the Berg Balance Test. *Phys Ther.* 1999;79(10):939–948.

19. Biodex System 4. Biodex Medical Systems website. Available at: http://www.biodex.com/physical-medicine/products/dynamometers/system-4-pro. Accessed October 1, 2016.

20. King M, Nazareth I, Lampe F, et al. Conceptual framework and systematic review of the effects of participants' and professionals' preferences in randomized controlled trials. *Health Technol Assess.* 2005;9(35):1–191.

21. Davey HM, Lim J, Butow PN, et al. Consumer information materials for diagnostic breast tests: women's views on information and their understanding of test results. *Health Expect.* 2003;6(4):298–311.

22. Holtby R, Razmjou H. Accuracy of the Speed's and Yergason's tests in detecting biceps pathology and SLAP lesions: comparison with arthroscopic findings. *Arthroscopy.* 2004;20(3):231–236.

CHAPTER 12

APPRAISING EVIDENCE ABOUT PROGNOSTIC (RISK) FACTORS

OBJECTIVES

Upon completion of this chapter, the student/practitioner will be able to do the following:

1. Discuss the three uses of prognosis in physical therapist practice.

2. Critically evaluate evidence about prognostic (risk) factors, including:

   a. Important questions to ask related to research validity; and

   b. Statistical approaches for identification of predictive indicators.

3. Interpret and apply information provided by:

   a. Survival curves;

   b. Odds ratios;

   c. Relative risks; and

   d. Hazard ratios.

4. Evaluate *p* values and confidence intervals to determine the potential importance of reported findings.

5. Discuss considerations related to the application of evidence about prognostic (risk) factors to individual patients or clients.

TERMS IN THIS CHAPTER

Bias: Results or inferences that systematically deviate from the truth "or the processes leading to such deviation."[1(p.251)]

Case-control design: A retrospective epidemiologic research design used to evaluate the relationship between a potential exposure (e.g., risk factor) and an outcome (e.g., disease or disorder); two groups of subjects—one of which has the outcome (i.e., the case) and one which does not (i.e., the control)—are compared to determine which group has a greater proportion of individuals with the exposure.[2]

Cohort design: A prospective epidemiologic research design used to evaluate the relationship between a potential exposure (e.g., risk factor) and an outcome (e.g., disease or disorder); two groups of subjects—one of which has the exposure and one of which does not—are monitored over time to determine who develops the outcome and who does not.[2]

Confidence interval: A range of scores within which the true score for a variable is estimated to lie within a specified probability (e.g., 90%, 95%, 99%).[3]

Hazard ratio (HR): An estimate of the relative risk of developing the problem of interest over the course of the study, weighted by the number of subjects available.[2]

Inception cohort: A group of subjects that are followed over time starting early in the course of their disease or disorder.[4]

Masked (also referred to as *blinded*): (1) In diagnostic test and clinical measure papers, the lack of knowledge about previous test/measure results; (2) in prognostic factor papers, the lack of knowledge about exposure status; and (3) in intervention papers, the lack of knowledge about to which group a subject has been assigned.

Odds ratio (OR): The odds that an individual with a prognostic (risk) factor had an outcome of interest as compared to the odds for an individual without the prognostic (risk) factor.[2,4]

Primary prevention: "Prevents a target condition in a susceptible or potentially susceptible population through such specific measures as general health promotion efforts."[5]

Prognosis: "The determination of the predicted optimal level of improvement in function and the amount of time needed to reach that level and also may include a prediction of levels of improvement that may be reached at various intervals during the course of therapy"."[5]

Prognostic factor: A sociodemographic, diagnostic, or comorbid characteristic of a patient or client that confers increased or decreased chances of positive or adverse outcomes from a disease/disorder or from interventions.[2,4]

***p* value**: The probability that a statistical finding occurred due to chance.

Relative risk (RR): The ratio of the risk of developing a disorder in patients with a prognostic (risk) factor compared to the risk in patients without the prognostic (risk) factor.[2,4]

Risk factor: A sociodemographic, diagnostic, or comorbid characteristic of a patient or client that confers increased or decreased chances of development of an adverse outcome.[2,4]

Secondary prevention: "Decreases duration of illness, severity of disease, and number of sequelae through early diagnosis and prompt intervention."[5]

Survival curve: A graphic representation of the frequency of an outcome of interest over time created by plotting the percentage of individuals who are free of the outcome at successive points in time.[2,4]

Tertiary prevention: "Limits the degree of disability and promotes rehabilitation and restoration of function in patients with chronic and irreversible diseases."[5]

Introduction

Prognosis is the process of predicting the future about a patient or client's condition. Physical therapists develop prognoses about (1) the risk of developing a future problem; (2) the ultimate outcome of an impairment in body structures or functions, an activity limitation, or a participation restriction; and (3) the results of physical therapy interventions.[5,6] Prognostic estimates are formulated in response to questions posed by patients or clients and their families, as well as to indicate the purpose of the therapist's plan of care. In both instances the predicted outcome includes a time frame for its development[5] to satisfy patient or client expectations as well as to address payer interests with respect to the duration and intensity of the physical therapy episode of care. This chapter focuses on the evaluation of evidence that informs physical therapists' prognoses for their patients or clients.

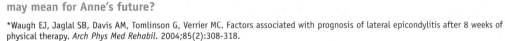

CLINICAL SCENARIO

What Factors Will Influence My Success in Physical Therapy?

Anne knows that a positive response to treatment of any kind is not guaranteed. She is curious about what may influence her outcome and whether any of those factors are under her (or your) control. You have uncovered an article* that addresses this question. In their conclusion, the authors state "Women and patients who report nerve symptoms are more likely to experience poorer short-term outcome after PT management of lateral epicondylitis."

How will you explain what the authors studied and what their findings (e.g., regression models) may mean for Anne's future?

*Waugh EJ, Jaglal SB, Davis AM, Tomlinson G, Verrier MC. Factors associated with prognosis of lateral epicondylitis after 8 weeks of physical therapy. *Arch Phys Med Rehabil.* 2004;85(2):308-318.

Risk of a Future Adverse Event

Physical therapists' concerns about the risk for developing future problems generally are focused on individuals for whom a primary medical diagnosis or impairment already is established. Risk mitigation is employed as part of *secondary* and *tertiary prevention* strategies in these situations.[5] Common examples of potential future problems patients may develop include:

- Skin breakdown as a result of sensation loss (as in diabetes and stroke) and/or immobility (as in spinal cord injury and casting);
- Re-injury with return-to-work or athletic activities following joint sprain or muscle strain; and
- Falls as a result of neurologic insult (as in stroke or brain injury).

As physical therapists have moved into health promotion and wellness, their focus has broadened to include *primary prevention* efforts with clients, such as addressing the risk for development of cardiovascular disease, osteoporosis, or arthritis as a result of inactivity. The goal in all of these examples is to prevent adverse events that may occur sometime in the future. The ability to identify (i.e., predict) different levels of risk among different individuals helps physical therapists tailor their plans of care and prioritize their resources accordingly.

Ultimate Outcomes

Physical therapists formulate prognoses related to the ultimate outcome of movement-related impairments in body structures and functions, activity limitations, and participation restrictions. In addition, they often are asked what the ultimate outcome of a condition will be. Unlike the risk for future adverse events, the ultimate outcome of an impairment or condition is easier to conceptualize in some respects because of the many clinical observations that have been catalogued about the natural course of various diagnoses.[6] Prognostic questions regarding ultimate outcomes that physical therapists may encounter (or have themselves) resemble these examples:

- Will I always need oxygen for activity?
- Will I walk without a walker again?
- Will my shoulder always be painful when I pitch?
- Will my child be able to attend school like other children?

These are the questions raised by patients and caregivers, as well as by students and professionals with limited experience with various clinical problems. In addition, there are questions about the time line for change that both patients and therapists wonder about, including

- How long will it take for this patient's incision (bone, tendon, ligament) to heal?
- When will this patient regain sensation in his hand after carpal tunnel surgery?
- How long before this patient can resume driving?

Identifying the ultimate outcome of a condition, impairment, limitation, or restriction in terms of progress, regression, death, or cure provides the context in which the plan of care is formulated and treatment-related prognostic estimates are determined.

Results from Physical Therapy Interventions

Predictions about the results produced by interventions are reflected in the goals physical therapists write in collaboration with their patients or clients. Whether directed toward remediation of impairments in body functions and structures, activity limitations, or participation restrictions, goals indicate what therapists expect in terms of responses to treatment.[5] In addition, this information is tied to a time line such as the number of days, weeks, or visits that is anticipated to achieve the specified outcome(s). The therapist's challenge is to consider the likelihood of achievement, within the specified time line, of the outcomes identified for a given individual. For example, a patient's ability to learn a home exercise program prior to hospital discharge following total knee arthroplasty may depend on the individual's cognitive abilities and support from family or caregivers. The status of each of these factors may alter the therapist's estimate of the likelihood of goal attainment. As noted earlier, prognoses about treatment responses are subsets of the prediction of ultimate outcomes.

Table 12-1 provides some examples of studies across the range of predictions that physical therapists make daily in their practices.

Elements of Prognosis

The preceding examples make the point that prognoses have three elements: (1) the outcome (or outcomes) that are possible, (2) the likelihood that the outcome (or outcomes will) occur, and (3) the time frame required for their achievement.[4] Identification of patient or client characteristics that may influence the outcomes identified are of particular interest. As illustrated in **Figure 12-1**, relevant characteristics may be demographic factors, disease-specific factors, medical comorbidities, and/or biobehavioral comorbidities.[7] The general term that describes characteristics predictive of any type of future outcomes is *prognostic factors*. Predictors of future adverse events usually are referred to as *risk factors*.[2,4] In both cases, the challenge is to identify which of the many pieces of information available about an individual are most predictive of the potential outcomes.

Because making predictions is an integral part of physical therapist patient/client management, it is important for therapists to be familiar with evidence about prognostic (risk) factors for the individuals

TABLE 12-1	Examples of Studies About Prognostic Estimates Relevant to Physical Therapist Practice

- Begnoche DM, et al. Predictors of independent walking in young children with cerebral palsy. *Phys Ther.* 2016;96(2):183-192.
- Fisher SR, et al. Predictors of 30-day readmission following inpatient rehabilitation for patients at high risk for hospital readmission. *Phys Ther.* 2016;96(1):62-70.
- Mulroy S, et al. Shoulder strength and physical activity predictors of shoulder pain in people with paraplegia from spinal injury. *Phys Ther.* 2015;95(7):1027-1038.
- French HP, et al. Predictors of short-term outcome to exercise and manual therapy for people with hip osteoarthritis. *Phys Ther.* 2014;94(1):31-39.
- Verkerk K, et al. Prognosis and course of disability in patients with chronic nonspecific low back pain: a 5- and 12-month follow-up cohort study. *Phys Ther.* 2013;93(12):1603-1614.

FIGURE 12-1	Types of characteristics that may serve as prognostic factors.

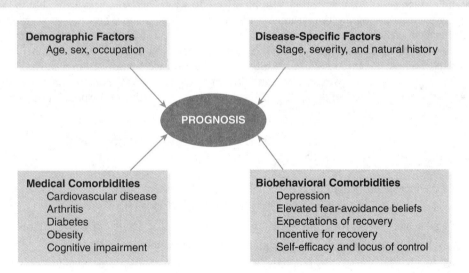

Reprinted from Beattie, P.; Nelson, R., Evaluating research studies that address prognosis for patients receiving physical therapy care: A Clinical Update, *Phys Ther.* 2007; 87:1527-1535 with permission from the American Physical Therapy Association. Copyright © 2007 American Physical Therapy Association.

receiving their services. This is especially true because daily practice often limits therapists' ability to follow up with patients or clients over a long enough period of time to determine if the outcomes they predicted really came true. In addition, they only see a limited, nonrepresentative set of individuals with a particular disorder, which adds a great deal of bias to their prediction estimates.[6,7] Evaluation of the best available evidence can help physical therapists overcome these natural practice limitations and improve their prognostic abilities.

Study Credibility

Evidence pertaining to prognostic factors first should be evaluated with an assessment of its research validity. Higher research validity provides greater confidence that a study's findings are reasonably free from *bias*. In other words, the results are believable. Appraisal of evidence about prognostic (risk) factors starts with the questions itemized in **Table 12-2**. These questions are modeled after critical appraisal worksheets developed by the Centre for Evidence-Based Medicine—Oxford.[8] Their purpose is to help physical therapists determine whether there are problems with a study's design that may have biased the results.[2,4]

1. Did the investigators operationally define the sample in their study?

One of the first concerns investigators must address with respect to their sample is its definition. Clearly articulated inclusion and exclusion criteria should be used to ensure that subjects fit the definition of individuals who have, or who are at risk for, the outcome of interest. For example, a study examining risk factors for the development of "arthritis" should specify whether the origin of the disorder of interest is systemic (i.e., rheumatoid arthritis) or biomechanical (i.e., osteoarthritis). The pathologies associated with these two forms of joint disease are sufficiently different from one another that risk factors are likely to differ to some degree. An operational definition of the disorder and the criteria by which it will be recognized will improve the validity of any associated risk factors.

2. Were the subjects representative of the population from which they were drawn?

The issue of representativeness pertains to the degree to which investigators were able to capture all eligible subjects during the time frame of the study. Enrolling some individuals (e.g., individuals in their 50s with osteoarthritis) and not others (e.g., individuals in their 70s with osteoarthritis) may result in systematic differences between participants and nonparticipants, the consequence of which is different prognostic estimates for each group.[6] Of course, investigators cannot force all eligible individuals to participate; however, they can perform statistical comparisons between participants and nonparticipants to determine whether the sample is representative of the population of interest.

TABLE 12-2	Questions to Assess the Validity of Evidence About Prognostic (Risk) Factors

1. Did the investigators operationally define the sample in their study?
2. Were the subjects representative of the population from which they were drawn?
3. Did all subjects enter the study at the same (preferably early) stage of their condition?
4. Was the study time frame long enough to capture the outcome(s) of interest?
5. Did the investigators collect outcome data from all of the subjects enrolled in the study?
6. Were outcome criteria operationally defined?
7. Were the individuals collecting the outcome measures masked (or blinded) to the status of prognostic factors in each subject?
8. Did the sample include subgroups of individuals for whom prognostic estimates will differ? If so, did the investigators conduct separate subgroup analyses or statistically adjust for these different prognostic factors?
9. Did investigators confirm their findings with a new set of subjects?

Statistically significant differences between the groups suggest that biased prognostic estimates may have resulted.

3. Did all subjects enter the study at the same (preferably early) stage of their condition?
This question is particularly salient for longitudinal *cohort designs*. Investigators must determine at what point individuals should be gathered for study. This decision depends in part on the nature of the outcome of interest and in part on the research question. Prognostic factors for resolution of an acute issue, such as muscle soreness after initiation of a new exercise routine, would require study immediately at the start of the exercise program because muscle soreness is self-limiting within a few days. In contrast, predictors of reduced mortality in a chronic disorder such as heart failure may be studied at several points along the disease progression depending on what the investigators want to know relative to prognosis from a given point in time. Understandably, patients too far along in the course of their disorder (i.e., advanced heart failure) may achieve the outcome of interest (i.e., death) early in the study and give a false sense of the time frame involved in its evolution.[4] The preferred starting point for studies of prognostic factors is just after a condition becomes clinically apparent. Subjects assembled at this point are referred to as an *inception cohort*.[4] Regardless of the starting point selected, the goal is to avoid a sample that is so heterogeneous that predicting future outcomes and their associated factors and time frames becomes unworkable.

4. Was the study time frame long enough to capture the outcome(s) of interest?
The length of follow-up time of a study will depend on which outcomes or events are being anticipated. The time frame identified must be long enough for the human body to achieve the outcome from a physiologic or psychological standpoint. If the time is too short, then a possible outcome will be missed.[4] However, studies requiring long time frames often require significant resources to support when conducted in real time. As a result, studies of rare events usually use a retrospective *case-control design* because of the low likelihood of an individual developing the problem in a prospective fashion.

5. Did the investigators collect outcome data from all of the subjects enrolled in the study?
The ability to capture the outcomes for all subjects is important because attrition for any reason (e.g., death, injury/illness, withdrawal of consent, logistic challenges, etc.) may provide a skewed representation of which outcomes occurred and when. Ideally, investigators will be able to determine what happened to subjects who left the study in order to evaluate whether the outcomes were truly different from for those who remained. Differences between subjects who remained and subjects who dropped out indicate that bias likely has been introduced to the prognostic estimates. Straus et al. describe a "5 and 20 rule" in which the loss of 5% of subjects likely has little impact, whereas the loss of 20% (or more) of subjects will undermine study validity to a considerable extent. Investigators also may conduct sensitivity analyses in which they calculate "best case" and "worst case" scenarios to determine the degree to which outcomes are affected by attrition.[4] Evidence-based physical therapists may then make their own decisions about whether the worst-case scenario reflects bias that undermines the study's value.

6. Were outcome criteria operationally defined?
This question addresses the validity of the measures used to capture the outcome(s) of interest. A clear definition of the outcome(s) is necessary to avoid misidentification (e.g., differentiating between wounds due to arterial insufficiency and pressure ulcers). Investigators should articulate specific clinical and/or testing criteria prior to the start of data collection. They also should verify that individuals collecting the information are appropriately trained and that their measures are reliable.

7. Were the individuals collecting the outcome measures masked (or blinded) to the status of prognostic factors in each subject?

Ideally, those measuring the outcome(s) will be *masked*, or ignorant of the subjects' prognostic (risk) factors. Prior knowledge of subject status may introduce tester bias into the study because expectations about the outcomes may influence application and interpretation of the measures used to capture them.

8. Does the sample include subgroups of individuals for whom prognostic estimates will differ? If so, did the investigators conduct separate subgroup analyses or statistically adjust for these different prognostic factors?

A subgroup is a smaller cluster of subjects who have a characteristic that distinguishes them from the larger sample. This characteristic is anticipated to influence the outcome of interest such that a different prognostic estimate is likely to be identified. Consider a hypothetical study about risk factors for the development of knee pain in individuals who are at least 80 years old. Age, along with associated ailments such as osteoarthritis, might be reasonable predictors of this outcome. However, if some of the subjects also are obese, then their development of knee pain may be influenced by their weight in addition to the other relevant characteristics. This difference in outcome development and expression for the subgroup of obese individuals may confound the results for the total sample.

Ideally, investigators will identify these additional prognostic (risk) factors and isolate them in some fashion. The simplest approach is to conduct separate analyses—in this case, for elderly subjects who are obese and for elderly subjects who are not. However, this method requires a sufficient sample size to have enough statistical power for the analysis. An alternative approach is to test a statistical model to predict the knee pain using the entire sample while adjusting for body weight or body mass index.[9] In either case, an evidence-based physical therapist should consider what additional factors specific to some of the subjects may predict or influence the outcome of interest for the entire group and review the evidence to determine whether the investigators accounted for these factors.

9. Did investigators confirm their findings with a new set of subjects?

This question alludes to the possibility that the research findings regarding prognostic (risk) factors occurred due to unique attributes of the sample. Repeating the study on a second set of subjects who match the inclusion and exclusion criteria outlined for the first set provides an opportunity to evaluate whether the same predictive factors are present. One strategy is to assemble a group of subjects and randomly select half of them to create the prognostic model, which then can be retested on the remaining half. This step often is not included in a single research report due to insufficient numbers of subjects and/or lack of funds. As a result, evidence-based physical therapists may need to read several pieces of evidence about the same prognostic (risk) factors if they wish to verify the factors' usefulness to a greater degree.

Additional Considerations

The previous questions serve as an initial screening of the evidence to determine its potential usefulness—that is, its research validity. From an evaluative standpoint, a "no" answer to any of questions 1 to 8 may indicate a "fatal flaw" in the research design related to unacceptable levels of bias. Readers may use more latitude in their analysis with respect to question 9, given that researchers must conduct their studies within their resource limitations.

Additional concerns pertaining to research design in evidence about prognostic (risk) factors include the presence or absence of a detailed description of the:

1. Characteristics of the sample obtained; and
2. Operational definitions, protocols, reliability, and validity of measures used to identify the prognostic (risk) factors.

This information allows evidence-based physical therapists to determine if the subjects included resemble the patient or client about whom there is a question (1) and if the predictive factors are identifiable and measurable in their clinical setting (2).

Study Results

Prognosis research uses both descriptive statistics as well as tests of relationships to identify prognostic (risk) factors. The descriptive statistics usually are reported as proportions, such as the percentage of subjects with a particular risk factor who developed a pressure ulcer or the percentage of subjects with a certain prognostic factor who returned to work. These values may be reported over time or at a certain point in time (commonly the median).[4] Another descriptive approach is the creation of a *survival curve* that plots the number of events or outcomes over time. Survival curves are calculated most commonly when investigators are evaluating the development of adverse events such as death, side effects from treatment, and loss of function. However, any dichotomous outcome may be depicted in this fashion. **Figure 12-2** is a survival curve from a study investigating whether the documented loss of muscle mass, and associated decrease in strength, in people undergoing hemodialysis was related to their mortality.

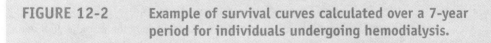

FIGURE 12-2   **Example of survival curves calculated over a 7-year period for individuals undergoing hemodialysis.**

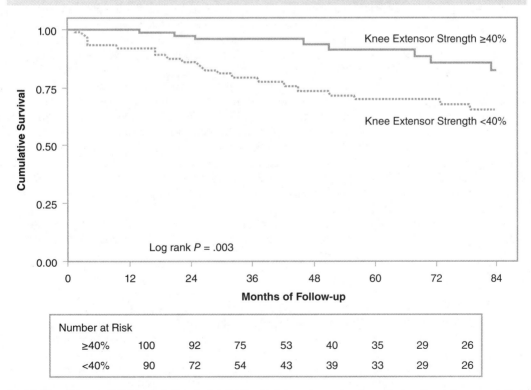

Reprinted from Matsuzawa R, Matsunaga A, Wang G, et al. Relationship between lower extremity muscle strength and all-cause mortality in Japanese patients undergoing dialysis, *Phys Ther.* 2014;94(7):947–956, by permission of Oxford University Press.

Subjects represented in the lower curve were those who had knee extensor strength below a cut-point established by the study authors; subjects represented in the upper curve had knee extensor strength at or above the selected threshold.[10] The slope of these curves gives an immediate visual idea regarding how quickly (or slowly) the outcome of interest occurred.[4,11] Both the data points and the slope indicate a poorer prognosis for subjects represented by the lower curve as compared to those represented by the upper curve. By the 7-year mark, 25% of the subjects (n = 22) with the risk factor of interest (i.e., knee extensor strength <40%) had died compared to only 8% of subjects (n = 8) without the risk factor. Clearly, these results suggest a contribution for physical therapists with respect to measuring baseline musculoskeletal strength in individuals requiring dialysis.

Statistical tests related to prognosis may take the form of simple associations or more sophisticated predictions via regression analyses. Association tests such as Pearson's r, Spearman's ρ, and chi square (χ^2) may be used in situations where a new relationship between a predictive factor and an outcome is being explored to determine whether further investigation is indicated. These tests provide the least amount of information because they only evaluate an association between two variables. Regression analyses, in contrast, are used to predict the value of the outcome, as well as to determine the relative contribution of each prognostic (risk) factor to this result. Both linear and logistic regression approaches may be used for evaluating predictors depending on whether the outcome is continuous or dichotomous, respectively.

Multiple logistic regression is implemented frequently because this technique produces odds ratios (ORs) for each factor retained in the equation. *Odds ratios* reflect the odds that an individual with a prognostic (risk) factor had an outcome of interest, as compared to the odds for an individual without the prognostic (risk) factor.[2,4] The odds are derived in consideration of all of the other independent variables in the regression equation.[11] ORs have the same values as likelihood ratios—that is, zero to infinity. Values that are less than 1 are recognized as decreased odds; values greater than 1 are recognized as increased odds. A value equal to 1 is a coin flip; in other words, the odds of developing the outcome of interest are no better than chance.

Table 12-3 provides results of a logistic regression analysis from a hypothetical study about predictors of re-injury upon return-to-work. The ORs are presented in the column with the heading "Exp (β)." Interpretation of ORs is similar to the interpretation of likelihood ratios. For example, the OR for body mass index in Table 12-3 is 2.398. This result would be interpreted to mean that subjects with a body mass index greater than 30 kg/m^2 had more than twice the odds of suffering re-injury compared to subjects with a lower body mass index. However, the OR for job satisfaction—0.790—indicates decreased odds for re-injury when job satisfaction is higher. This result is consistent with the negative sign in front of the β coefficient, which indicates an inverse relationship between the predictor (job satisfaction) and the outcome (reinjury).

ORs also can be calculated from a 2 × 2 table for an individual variable. **Figure 12-3** represents data from a hypothetical study of fall risk in relation to the presence or absence of peripheral neuropathy. The equation for calculating odds ratios from the table is:

$$OR = [a/b]/[c/d] \quad or \quad ad/bc$$

Using the data in the table produces an OR of 3.27; in other words, the odds that a subject with peripheral neuropathy fell more than once are three times the odds for a subject without neuropathy. This approach is useful when only one indicator is being evaluated; more than one factor or predictor requires a regression approach to isolate the effects of each predictor in the presence of the others.

Finally, investigators may report relative risks (RRs) and hazard ratios (HRs) for predictive factors for a particular outcome. *Relative risks* are the ratio of the risk of developing an outcome in patients with a prognostic (risk) factor compared to the risk in patients without the prognostic (risk) factor.[2,4]

TABLE 12-3   **Results from a Hypothetical Study Examining Predictors of Reinjury Following Return-to-Work**

Variable	Beta (β)	SE	*p* value	Exp (β): Odds Ratio	95% CI
Age (years)	0.181	0.049	0.102	1.198	0.98, 2.67
Body Mass Index (>30 kg/m²)	1.078	0.431	0.031	2.398	1.79, 3.56
Smoker (+)	0.389	0.084	0.070	1.475	0.93, 4.05
Prior Injury (+)	1.908	0.560	0.005	6.739	4.32, 7.23
Job Satisfaction (100 mm scale where 0 is completely unsatisfied and 100 is completely satisfied)	−0.986	0.341	0.022	0.790	0.69, 0.98
Constant	6.327	2.45	0.000		

Abbreviations:
(β) = Coefficient
SE = Standard error
Exp (β) = Exponent of the coefficient
CI = Confidence interval

FIGURE 12-3   **A 2 x 2 table for calculating the odds ratios from a hypothetical study about falls.**

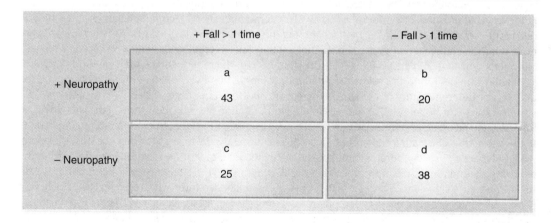

Hazard ratios commonly are reported in conjunction with survival curves. These values reflect relative risk for an outcome over time. As their names imply, these estimates are used in the context of adverse events. Conceptually, they are similar to ORs in that comparisons are made between the group that has the risk factor and the group that does not. Interpretation also is comparable: ratios greater than 1 indicate increased risk, ratios less than 1 indicate reduced risk, and ratios equal to 1 indicate that the risk of developing the outcome of interest is no better than chance.

RRs are different from ORs in that their calculation is based on the incidence of the outcome within the total group of subjects with (or without) the risk factor. This distinction is important because, by definition, RRs are used in longitudinal studies in which the incidence of an outcome of interest can be determined for individuals with, and without, the risk factor. They cannot be calculated in case-control designs in which the investigators define the number of subjects with and without the outcome and then identify risk factor distribution retrospectively.[4] RRs can be calculated from a 2 × 2 table using the following equation:

$$RR = [a/a + b]/[c/c + d]$$

Using the data from Figure 12-3, the relative risk of falls is 1.72, which means that subjects with neuropathy have more than 1.5 times the risk for falling as compared to subjects without neuropathy. RRs generally have lower values than ORs because the former value is a ratio of rates of events rather than a ratio of actual events. When the event rates are low, the RR and OR will approach each other. Readers must be cognizant of which estimate is used in order to interpret the study's results appropriately.

The Statistical Importance of Study Results

In addition to the correlation coefficients, odds ratios, relative risks, and hazard ratios reported in studies, investigators also provide information to determine the "meaningfulness"—or potential importance—of their results. The two primary ways to convey potential importance are via the *p* value and the confidence interval. A *p value* indicates the probability that the result obtained occurred due to chance. The smaller the *p* value (e.g., <0.05), the more important the result is statistically because the role of chance is so diminished, although not eliminated.

A *confidence interval* represents a range of scores within which the true score for a variable is estimated to lie within a specified probability (e.g., 90%, 95%, 99%).[3] An odds ratio, relative risk, or hazard ratio is meaningful if it lies within the confidence interval. As with any other estimate, a narrower confidence interval is preferred because it suggests that the ratio of interest is close to the "true" ratio according to the specified probability (e.g., 95%). Unfortunately, there are no criteria by which to judge whether a confidence interval is "too wide." Remember that if a confidence interval around an odds ratio, relative risk, or hazard ratio contains the value "1," then the odds, risks, or hazards are no better than chance, and the predictor is not useful.[9] Such a result also will be reported as statistically nonsignificant. Table 12-3 illustrates this situation for the prognostic factor "age" and "smoker."

Usually authors report the relevant confidence interval; however, readers also may calculate the interval for different estimates when they are not reported. Equations for confidence intervals for various ratios can be found elsewhere. Finally, authors choose what their threshold values will be for *p* values and confidence intervals. In the former case, the traditional threshold is alpha (α) $\leq$ 0.05. In the latter case, the traditional probability is 95%. Ultimately, these are arbitrary choices; therefore, evidence-based physical therapists must use their clinical judgment and expertise to determine the clinical meaningfulness or importance of a study's findings. This challenge will be apparent when results just miss significance (e.g., *p* = 0.07) or when confidence intervals are wide. Nevertheless, a study that minimizes bias and that demonstrates strong statistical significance with narrow confidence intervals should be taken seriously in terms of the information it provides.

Evidence and the Patient or Client

As with all evidence, a study about prognostic (risk) factors must be examined to determine if the subjects included resemble closely enough the patient or client to whom the results may be applied. The outcomes predicted in the study also should be relevant and meaningful to that individual.[7]

A more sensitive issue is the degree to which the evidence will influence what therapists will tell their patients or clients about their future, as well as how treatment planning will be influenced, if at all.[6] Predictions about the future can be complicated by expectations, fears, desires, and many other emotions that define the human experience and impact all stakeholders involved (including the therapist!). Although the evidence may be objective and unemotional, its implications may not be. This is where clinical judgment comes into play because therapists must decide whether their patient's or client's potential to experience an outcome is unique to him or her or matches the tendency of the group in the study. That conclusion, as well as the patient's or client's values, will provide guidance to therapists about how to use the prognostic information in the management process.

Evidence Appraisal Tools

Table 12-4 provides a checklist to guide the evaluation of evidence about prognostic (risk) factors for use in any practice setting.[8] Alternatively, the reader might consider accessing appraisal resources available online. A strategy worth considering is the creation of reference notebooks that contain completed checklists or worksheets along with their associated research articles. These compendia

TABLE 12-4	Evidence About Prognostic (Risk) Factors: Quality Appraisal Checklist
Research Validity of the Study	
Did the investigators operationally define the sample in their study?	___ Yes ___ No ___ Insufficient detail
Were the subjects representative of the population from which they were drawn?	___ Yes ___ No ___ Insufficient detail
Did all subjects enter the study at the same (preferably early) stage of their condition?	___ Yes ___ No ___ Insufficient detail
Was the study time frame long enough to capture the outcome(s) of interest?	___ Yes ___ No ___ Insufficient detail
Did the investigators collect outcome data from all of the subjects enrolled in the study?	___ Yes ___ No ___ Insufficient detail
Were outcome criteria operationally defined?	___ Yes ___ No ___ Insufficient detail

(continues)

TABLE 12-4	Evidence About Prognostic (Risk) Factors: Quality Appraisal Checklist (*Continued*)

Were the individuals collecting the outcome measures masked (or blinded) to the status of prognostic factors in each subject?	___ Yes ___ No ___ Insufficient detail
Did the sample include subgroups of individuals for whom prognostic estimates will differ?	___ Yes ___ No ___ Insufficient detail
If you answered "yes" to the previous question, did the investigators conduct separate subgroup analyses or statistically adjust for these different prognostic factors?	___ Yes ___ No ___ Insufficient detail
Did investigators confirm their findings with a new set of subjects?	___ Yes ___ No ___ Insufficient detail
Do you have enough confidence in the research validity of this paper to consider using this evidence with your patient or client?	___ Yes ___ Undecided ___ No

Relevant Study Findings

Results reported that are specific to your clinical question:

Correlation coefficient(s) _____

Coefficient(s) of determination _____

Odds ratio(s) _____

Relative risk ratio(s) _____

Hazard ratio(s) _____

Other _____

Statistical significance and/or precision of the relevant study results:

Obtained p values for each relevant statistic reported by the authors: _____

Obtained confidence intervals for each relevant statistic reported by the authors: _____

Application of the Evidence to Your Patient or Client

How likely are the outcomes over time (based on your experience or on the proportion of subjects in the study who achieved the outcome)? _____

Are there clinically meaningful differences between the subjects in the study and your patient or client?	___ Yes ___ No ___ Mixed results ___ Insufficient detail

TABLE 12-4	Evidence About Prognostic (Risk) Factors: Quality Appraisal Checklist (*Continued*)
Will sharing information from this study about prognostic indicators or risk factors help your patient or client given his or her expressed values and preferences?	___ Yes ___ No ___ Mixed results
Will you use this information with your patient or client?	___ Yes ___ No

These questions were adapted from the Oxford Centre for Evidence-Based Medicine and applied to physical therapist practice.

could facilitate the use of evidence regarding prognostic (risk) factors for all physical therapists in a particular setting (as long as there is a commitment to keeping them up to date).

Summary

Prognosis is the process of predicting a future outcome for a patient or client. Developing prognostic estimates from clinical practice alone is difficult because of the limited exposure physical therapists have to a representative group of individuals at risk for, or known to have, a particular problem or outcome. Evidence about prognostic (risk) factors for outcomes relevant to physical therapy should be evaluated when possible to improve the prognostic estimation process during patient/client management. Verification of the validity, importance, and relevance of the evidence about prognostic (risk) factors is central to the ability to use the information with patients or clients. Sensitivity to patient or client values and preferences is equally important considering the potential emotional impact of sharing information about unfavorable prognoses.

Exercises

1. Describe the three focus areas of prognosis in physical therapist patient/client management and give clinical examples of each.
2. Describe the three elements of a prognostic estimate and give a clinical example relevant to physical therapist practice that includes all of the relevant information.
3. Explain why clinical practice is insufficient for establishing precise prognostic estimates. Provide a clinical example relevant to physical therapist practice to illustrate your points.
4. Explain why it is important that subjects enter a study about prognostic (risk) factors at the same time in the course of their disease or disorder evolution or at the same level of health status. Provide a clinical example relevant to physical therapist practice to illustrate your points.
5. Explain why the length of time and completeness of follow-up is essential to the validity of studies about prognostic (risk) factors. Provide a clinical example relevant to physical therapist practice to illustrate your points.

6. Explain why adjustment for other factors is important when subgroups of subjects have different prognostic estimates for an outcome. Provide a clinical example relevant to physical therapist practice to illustrate your points.

7. Differentiate among odds ratios, relative risks, and hazard ratios. Use clinical examples relevant to physical therapist practice to illustrate interpretations for ratios that have values less than 1, equal to 1, and greater than 1.

8. Explain the usefulness of an odds ratio, a relative risk, or a hazard ratio when its associated confidence interval includes the value 1.

9. Use the following 2 × 2 table to calculate the odds ratio and relative risk for the hypothetical outcome:

	+ Outcome	− Outcome
+ Prognostic Factor	97	68
− Prognostic Factor	38	130

Interpret the results for each of the calculations. Why is the odds ratio different from the relative risk?

10. A study regarding the prognostic factor in question 9 provides the following confidence interval for the odds ratio: 95% CI (2.05, 22.8). What does this confidence interval indicate about the usefulness of this odds ratio?

References

1. Helewa A, Walker JM. *Critical Evaluation of Research in Physical Rehabilitation: Towards Evidence-Based Practice.* Philadelphia, PA: W.B. Saunders; 2000.

2. Guyatt G, Rennie D. *Users' Guides to the Medical Literature: A Manual for Evidence-Based Clinical Practice.* Chicago, IL: AMA Press; 2002.

3. Carter RE, Lubinsky J, Domholdt E. *Rehabilitation Research: Principles and Applications.* 4th ed. St. Louis, MO: Elsevier Saunders; 2011.

4. Straus SE, Richardson WS, Glaziou P, Haynes RB. *Evidence-Based Medicine: How to Practice and Teach EBM.* 3rd ed. Edinburgh, Scotland: Elsevier Churchill Livingstone; 2005.

5. American Physical Therapists Association. Guide to Physical Therapist Practice. 3.0. Available at: http://guidetoptpractice.apta.org. Accessed July 16, 2016.

6. Herbert R, Jamtvedt G, Hagen KB, Mead J. *Practical Evidence-Based Physiotherapy.* 2nd ed. Edinburgh, Scotland: Elsevier Butterworth-Heinemann; 2011.

7. Beattie PF, Nelson RM. Evaluating research studies that address prognosis for patients receiving physical therapy care: a clinical update. *Phys Ther.* 2007;87(11):1527–1535.

8. Centre for Evidence-Based Medicine–Oxford website. Critically Appraising the Evidence. Worksheets for Prognosis. Available at: www.cebm.net. Accessed October 1, 2016.

9. Altman DG. Systematic reviews of evaluations of prognostic variables. *BMJ.* 2001;323(7306):224–228.

10. Matsuzawa R, Matsunaga A, Wang G, et al. Relationship between lower extremity muscle strength and all-cause mortality in Japanese patients undergoing dialysis. *Phys Ther.* 2014;94(7):947–956.

11. Portney LG, Watkins MP. *Foundations of Clinical Research: Applications to Practice.* 3rd ed. Upper Saddle River, NJ: Pearson; 2009.

CHAPTER 13

APPRAISING EVIDENCE ABOUT INTERVENTIONS

OBJECTIVES

Upon completion of this chapter, the student/practitioner will be able to do the following:

1. Discuss the contribution of evidence to the decision making about interventions for patients or clients.

2. Critically evaluate evidence about interventions, including the

   a. Important questions to ask related to research validity; and

   b. Relative merits of experimental, quasi-experimental, and nonexperimental designs.

3. Interpret and apply information provided by the following calculations:

   a. Absolute benefit increase;

   b. Absolute risk reduction;

   c. Effect size;

   d. Intention to treat;

   e. Number needed to treat;

   f. Relative benefit increase; and

   g. Relative risk reduction.

4. Evaluate p values and confidence intervals to determine the potential importance of reported findings.

5. Discuss the role of the minimal clinically important difference in determining the potential usefulness of an intervention of interest.

6. Discuss considerations related to the application of evidence about interventions to individual patients or clients.

TERMS IN THIS CHAPTER

Absolute benefit increase (ABI): The absolute value of the difference in rates of positive outcomes between the intervention group and the control group (expressed as a percentage).[1]

Absolute risk reduction (ARR): The absolute value of the difference in rates of adverse outcomes between the intervention group and the control group (expressed as a percentage).[1]

Assignment (also referred to as *allocation*): The process by which subjects are placed into two or more groups in a study.

Attrition (also referred to as *dropout* or *mortality*): A term that refers to subjects who stop participation in a study for any reason; loss of subjects may threaten research validity (internal validity) by reducing the sample size and/or producing unequal groups.

Bias: Results or inferences that systematically deviate from the truth "or the processes leading to such deviation."[2(p.251)]

Biologic plausibility: The reasonable expectation that the human body could behave in the manner predicted.

Concealment: The methods by which investigators hide information about group assignment from individuals responsible for enrolling subjects.[3]

Confidence interval: A range of scores within which the true score for a variable is estimated to lie within a specified probability (e.g., 90%, 95%, 99%).[4]

Control group event rate (CER): The percentage of subjects who improved (or got worse) in the control group.

Effectiveness: The extent to which an intervention produces a desired outcome under usual clinical conditions.[2]

Effect size: The magnitude of the difference between two mean values; may be standardized by dividing this difference by the pooled standard deviation to compare effects measured by different scales.[5]

Efficacy: The extent to which an intervention produces a desired outcome under ideal conditions.[2]

Experimental design: A research design in which the behavior of randomly assigned groups of subjects is measured following the purposeful manipulation of an independent variable(s) in at least one of the groups; used to examine cause and effect relationships between an independent variable(s) and an outcome(s).[4,6]

Experimental group event rate (EER): The percentage of subjects who improved (or got worse) in the experimental group.

Imputation: A term referring to a collection of statistical methods used to estimate missing data.[7]

Intention-to-treat analysis: Statistical analysis of data from subjects according to the group to which they were assigned despite noncompliance with the study protocol.[3]

Intervention: "Physical therapists purposefully interact with the individual and, when appropriate, with other people involved in his or her care, using various" procedures or techniques "to produce changes in the condition."[8]

Masked (also referred to as *blinded*): (1) In diagnostic test and clinical measure papers, the lack of knowledge about previous test/measure results; (2) in prognostic factor papers, the lack of knowledge about exposure status; and (3) in intervention papers, the lack of knowledge about to which group a subject has been assigned.

Minimal clinically important difference (MCID): "The smallest treatment effect that would result in a change in patient management, given its side effects, costs, and inconveniences."[9(p.1197)]

Nonexperimental design (also referred to as an *observational study*): A study in which controlled manipulation of the subjects is lacking[4]; in addition, if groups are present, assignment is predetermined based on naturally occurring subject characteristics or activities.[1]

Number needed to treat (NNT): The number of subjects treated with an experimental intervention over the course of a study required to achieve one good outcome or prevent one bad outcome.[10]

Placebo: "An intervention without biologically active ingredients."[3(p.682)]

Power: The probability that a statistical test will detect, if it is present, a relationship between two or more variables (or scores) or a difference between two or more groups (or scores).[4,11]

***p* value**: The probability that a statistical finding occurred due to chance.

Quasi-experimental design: A research design in which there is only one subject group or in which randomization to more than one subject group is lacking; controlled manipulation of the subjects is preserved.[12]

Randomized clinical trial (also referred to as a *randomized controlled trial* and a *randomized controlled clinical trial* [RCT]): A clinical study that uses a randomization process to assign subjects to either an experimental group(s) or a control (or comparison) group. Subjects in the experimental group receive the intervention or preventive measure of interest and then are compared to the subjects in the control (or comparison) group who did not receive the experimental manipulation.[4]

Relative benefit increase (RBI): The absolute value of the rate of increase in positive outcomes for the intervention group relative to the control group (expressed as a percentage).[1]

Relative risk reduction (RRR): The absolute value of the rate of decrease in adverse outcomes for the intervention group relative to the control group (expressed as a percentage).[1]

CLINICAL SCENARIO

Which Physical Therapy Treatment Techniques Will Be Most Effective for My Elbow Pain?

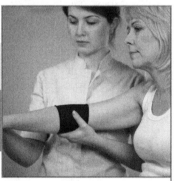

© Photographee.eu/Shutterstock

Anne knew she did not want medication (oral or injected) for her elbow pain, but she is not sure which physical therapy treatment techniques will be most helpful in her case. Ever curious, she has scoured Google Scholar and come across a study* comparing exercise with a form of manual therapy for treatment of elbow pain like hers. She brought you a copy of the publication and wants your opinion about its quality and the trustworthiness of its findings.

What will you tell her and how will you explain the results?

*Viswas R, Ramachandran R, Korde Anantkumar P. Comparison of effectiveness of supervised exercise program and Cyriax physiotherapy in patients with tennis elbow (lateral epicondylitis): a randomized clinical trial. *Scientific World Journal*. 2012;939645.

Introduction

Upon conclusion of the examination and evaluation process, physical therapists consider the *interventions* that are available to address identified patient or client needs. Several factors may influence decisions about which treatments to choose that are derived from both the therapist and the patient or client. For example, the physical therapist will (1) determine whether the signs and symptoms fit an established classification scheme; (2) consider the complexity of the case; (3) prioritize the problem list; (4) determine what resources are required, as well as their availability; (5) identify the patient or client's educational needs; and (6) make a judgment about enablers and barriers to adherence to the treatment plan. These issues will be evaluated in the context of past experiences with similar individuals, as well as within the ethical, legal, and socioeconomic parameters that inform practice.[8] The patient or client will offer his or her perspective on priorities, resources, educational needs, and adherence challenges in a manner that reflects his or her preferences and values about the usefulness of physical therapy, the effort required to recover or adapt function, and the opportunities lost as a result of spending time and money on rehabilitation, rather than on other activities or material pursuits.

As physical therapists and the individuals they manage review various treatment options, they also consider the trade-offs between the benefits and risks for each intervention. This deliberation may be illustrated by the following questions:

- If this intervention (versus another) is applied, will the condition improve, regress, remain unchanged, or will a new problem develop?
- If this intervention (versus another) is not applied, will the condition improve, regress, remain unchanged, or will a new problem develop?

Ideally, the answer to these questions will include details about the different responses possible, as well as estimations about the likelihood of their occurrence. Physical therapists may use previous experience with similar individuals, as well as theoretical premises based on *biologic plausibility*, to answer these questions. However, past experience is subject to bias and biologic plausibility may be refuted in unexpected ways. The incorporation of the best available evidence about the *efficacy* or *effectiveness* of different therapeutic approaches adds to this deliberative process by helping physical therapists and their patients or clients consider their options from an objectively tested point of view.

Table 13-1 provides some examples of studies about the effectiveness or efficacy interventions that physical therapists use in practice.

Study Credibility

Evidence pertaining to interventions physical therapists use first should be evaluated with an assessment of its research validity. Higher research validity provides greater confidence that a study's findings are reasonably free from *bias*. In other words, the results are believable. Appraisal of evidence about interventions starts with the questions itemized in **Table 13-2**. These questions are modeled after versions of the critical appraisal worksheets developed by the Centre for Evidence Based Medicine at the University of Oxford.[13] Their purpose is to help physical therapists determine whether there are problems with a study's design that may have biased the results.[1]

1. Did the investigators randomly assign (or allocate) subjects to groups?

Randomization of subjects to groups is the *assignment* method most likely to reduce bias by creating groups with equally distributed characteristics. Groups that are equivalent at the start of a study are necessary to isolate the impact, if any, of an experimental intervention. Investigators who used a randomized allocation process usually announce that fact in the title or abstract of the paper, making it easy for a reader to identify such studies. The importance of this *experimental design* feature is

TABLE 13-1	Examples of Studies About Interventions Relevant to Physical Therapist Practice

- Perez-Palomares S, et al. Contribution of dry needling to individualized physical therapy treatment of shoulder pain: a randomized controlled trial. *J Orthop Sports Phys Ther.* 2017;47(1):11-20.
- Sran M, et al. Physical therapy for urinary incontinence in postmenopausal women with osteoporosis or low bone density: a randomized trial. *Menopause.* 2016;23(3):286-293.
- Kalron A, et al. A personalized, intense physical rehabilitation program improves walking in people with multiple sclerosis presenting with different levels of disability: a retrospective cohort. *BMC Neurol.* 2015;15:21.
- Jang DH, et al. The influence of physical therapy and anti-botulinum toxin antibody on the efficacy of botulinum toxin-A injections in children with spastic cerebral palsy. *Dev Neurorehabil.* 2014;17(6):414-419.
- Sricharoenchai T, et al. Safety of physical therapy interventions in critically ill patients: a single-center prospective evaluation of 1110 intensive care unit admissions. *J Crit Care.* 2014;29(3):395-400.
- Sartor CD, et al. Effects of a combined strengthening, stretching and functional training program versus usual-care on gait biomechanics and foot function for diabetic neuropathy: a randomized controlled trial. *BMC Musculoskelet Disord.* 2012;13:36.

TABLE 13-2	Questions to Determine the Validity of Evidence About Interventions

1. Did the investigators randomly assign (or allocate) subjects to groups?
2. Was each subject's group assignment concealed from the people enrolling individuals in the study?
3. Did the groups have similar sociodemographic, clinical, and prognostic characteristics at the start of the study?
4. Were subjects masked (or blinded) to their group assignment?
5. Were clinicians and/or outcome assessors masked (or blinded) to the subjects' group assignment?
6. Were the instruments used to measure outcomes reliable and valid?
7. Did the clinicians and/or outcomes assessors have demonstrated competence applying the outcomes measures?
8. Did the investigators manage all of the groups in the same way except for the experimental intervention(s)?
9. Did the investigators apply the study protocol and collect follow-up data on all subjects over a time frame long enough for the outcomes of interest to occur?
10. Did subject attrition (e.g., withdrawal, loss to follow-up) occur over the course of the study?
11. If attrition occurred, did the investigators perform an intention-to-treat analysis?
12. Did the investigators confirm their findings with a new set of subjects?

emphasized by proponents of evidence-based practice who propose that research papers that do not include randomized subject assignment should be set aside in favor of a new literature search.[1,3,14] Unfortunately, many questions of interest to physical therapists are addressed by *quasi-experimental* and *nonexperimental designs* without randomized group assignment. The potential role of these designs is discussed later in this section.

2. Was each subject's group assignment concealed from the people enrolling individuals in the study?

The issue of *concealment* alludes to the possibility that study personnel may interfere with the randomization process such that bias is introduced into the study. This interference may be well intended. For example, investigators may feel compelled to respond to logistical challenges that make study participation difficult for the subjects, the research personnel, or the facilities. Prior knowledge of subject assignment during the enrollment period would allow the investigators to reassign subjects to resolve these problems.[3] In so doing, however, equal distribution of characteristics is undermined, resulting in the introduction of an alternative explanation for the study's results. Unfortunately, the concealment of group assignment during the enrollment period often is not addressed one way or the other in physical therapy research. Readers should not assume that concealment was performed unless explicitly stated.

3. Did the groups have similar sociodemographic, clinical, and prognostic characteristics at the start of the study?

Although randomized assignment methods are likely to result in equivalent groups at the start of the study, this result is not guaranteed. This question acknowledges this fact by asking whether the investigators confirmed group equality through statistical analysis of the relevant sociodemographic (e.g., age, gender, race/ethnicity), clinical (e.g., diagnosis, acuity/chronicity, medical management), and prognostic (e.g., prior experience, family support) characteristics. This information may be found in tables and text reported in the section describing subjects or in the results section of the paper, depending on journal formatting requirements. Ideally, investigators adjust for the imbalances in these factors in their statistical analyses. However, readers should note any statistically significant differences among the groups and consider whether, and in what ways, those differences may have played a role in the study's results.

4. Were subjects *masked* (or blinded) to their group assignment?

This question explores the possibility that subjects' behavior may have changed during the study due to knowledge about the group to which they were assigned. Subjects who know (or suspect) their group assignment may increase their efforts in the hopes of achieving the anticipated outcomes or decrease their efforts due to frustration that they are not in the experimental treatment group. As Herbert et al. note, it often is impractical to mask group assignment from the subjects in physical therapy research.[14] The one exception is the modification of electrotherapeutic modalities, such as ultrasound, to give the appearance of normal function without providing actual therapeutic effects. Creation of sham interventions for exercise and mobilization techniques often is not possible. Therefore, the potential for changes in subject behavior as a result of knowledge of their group assignment should be considered when evaluating the study's findings.

5. Were clinicians and/or outcome assessors masked (or blinded) to the subjects' group assignment?

This question explores the possibility that clinician or study personnel behavior may have changed during the study due to knowledge about the group to which subjects were assigned. Clinicians responsible for training subjects in the study may provide added encouragement to compensate for allocation to the control group. Outcomes assessors may unconsciously introduce bias into the measurement process because of expectations about how subjects in each group will respond over the course of the study. Authors usually indicate that clinicians and/or study personnel are masked by referring to their research as a "single-blind" design. When subjects also are masked, the label "double-blind" is used.

6. Were the instruments used to measure outcomes reliable and valid?

Clinicians and researchers alike need to have confidence that any treatment effect they are observing is "real." Using outcomes instruments that have established measurement reliability and validity is an essential step to ensure that an effect is captured appropriately and accurately. Researchers evaluating the effectiveness of an experimental intervention typically cite previously published literature to defend their choice of outcomes measures. They may report specific statistical findings related to reliability, validity, and responsiveness, but they are not required to do so. As a result, physical therapists may find themselves relying on their own knowledge of available instruments and their measurement properties to determine whether appropriate selections were made and the subsequent results are useful.

7. Did the clinicians and/or outcome assessors have demonstrated competence applying the outcomes measures?

Implementing reliable and valid instruments to measure study outcomes is the first step to ensure that a treatment effect can be captured. In addition, investigators should verify that the individuals implementing those instruments have the necessary knowledge and skills to apply the measures appropriately. Protocols may be designed and implemented in an effort to ensure that each individual is applying an instrument consistently. Instructions and any follow-up coaching of subjects should be delivered the same way so that any differences in performance can be attributed to the treatment itself and not differences in subject management. Investigators also may evaluate intrarater and/or interrater reliability and report the related correlation coefficients to demonstrate the necessary competence levels. Readers should not assume that either of these strategies has been implemented unless explicitly stated in the study.

8. Did the investigators manage all the groups in the same way except for the experimental intervention(s)?

This question clarifies the degree to which group equality was maintained when study personnel and/or clinicians interacted with subjects over the course of the project. Ideally, the only difference between or among the study groups will be the application of the experimental intervention(s). Other factors such as (1) the timing of treatment applications and outcomes measurement, (2) the environmental conditions in which these activities are performed, and (3) the methods for provision of instructions and application of treatments or measures should be comparable across groups so that the effect, if any, of the experimental intervention(s) may be isolated. Readers should note any differences in group management and consider whether, and in what ways, these differences may have influenced the study's results.

9. Did the investigators apply the study protocol and collect follow-up data on all subjects over a time frame long enough for the outcomes of interest to occur?

The issue regarding subject follow-up involves the time frame over which the study was conducted. Specifically, readers must determine whether the time allotted for application of the study protocol and the measurement of its effect was long enough for the outcome(s) of interest to occur. For example, a hypothetical study about an experimental strength training technique should include a training period of at least several weeks in order for changes in muscle fiber size and performance to develop.[15] In contrast, a study examining the comparative effects of once versus twice a day physical therapy on patients' functional status following orthopedic surgery will have a time frame defined by the length of the acute hospital stay. Depending on the research question, outcomes data also may be collected beyond the immediate conclusion of the intervention phase to determine over what length of time any treatment effects remain. In this scenario, the time frame(s) selected for follow-up are at the discretion of the investigators based on the purpose of the study. Readers should remember that long-term follow-up of treatment effects, although desirable, is not a requirement for intervention studies. The absence of such information is not a design flaw per se, but it does represent a limit to our understanding of an intervention's impact.

10. Did subject attrition (e.g., withdrawal, loss to follow-up) occur over the course of the study?

Readers must determine whether all subjects who were enrolled at the start of the study remained at the end of the study. The loss of subjects, or *attrition*, may create several problems. First, the distribution of subject characteristics among the groups may become unbalanced such that an alternative explanation for the study's results is generated. For example, groups that were previously equal in the proportion of male and female subjects now may be unequal in gender distribution. If there is an expectation that gender may influence the outcome of the study independent of the experimental intervention, then this imbalance is problematic. Second, statistical *power* may be undermined due to the decrease in sample size. In other words, the ability to detect a difference between groups at the end of the study, if present, may be lost. Third, the sample may be further compromised with respect to its representation of the population of interest for the study. Clinical research pertinent to physical therapist practice frequently relies on non-probabilistic methods for selecting subjects to study due to logistical constraints. The inability to randomly select individuals for participation introduces bias at the outset of the investigation that is likely to be exacerbated by subsequent dropout.

Attrition may occur for numerous reasons, including death, illness, subject loss of interest, or new circumstances making participation difficult. In addition, subjects may be dropped from the analyses when individual data points are missing from their cases. A variety of statistical methods are available for estimating missing data to avoid this reduction in sample size.[7] Details about these *imputation* methods are beyond the scope of this text. Readers should understand, however, that these methods provide estimates of the missing information that may introduce error to various degrees depending on the approach selected.[14,16] When imputation is not performed, then the reader must make a qualitative decision about whether bias likely has been introduced because of attrition. Several authors recommend that a data loss of 5% or less probably is inconsequential, whereas losses of 15% to 20% or more probably have undermined the research validity of the study.[1,14] Investigators may explicitly discuss the loss of subjects in the text of the paper or they may indicate attrition by noting the number (via the symbol "*n*") of subjects included in each of the analyses summarized in tables or figures.[14] Understandably, the longer a study is conducted, the greater the chance for attrition to occur.

11. If attrition occurred, did the investigators perform an intention-to-treat analysis?

This question pertains to situations in which some of the subjects are not compliant with the protocol for their assigned group. Noncompliance may occur because of factors outside of the subjects' control, such as illness, or because of purposeful decisions by the subjects not to participate according to plan. As noted earlier, the latter situation is likely to occur when subjects determine to which group they have been assigned and change their behavior as a result of this knowledge. If noncompliant subjects are still available for collection of follow-up data, then investigators may implement an *intention-to-treat analysis* in which the outcome data are analyzed according to group assignment.[16,17] In other words, statistical comparisons between the intervention and control groups are made as if every subject complied with the protocol for their group. The results likely will reflect a reduction in the effect size of the treatment; however, Herbert et al. point out that this reduction is what one should expect if subjects (or patients) are not compliant with the treatment.[14]

An intention-to-treat analysis is valued primarily because it preserves the randomized allocation process and, therefore, the baseline equality of group characteristics. In addition, sample size is maintained. There is some debate regarding the appropriateness of using imputed data from subjects lost to follow-up in these analyses because of the potential for error in the estimates. Sensitivity analyses provide an alternative approach to determine the impact on effect size of "best case" and "worst case" scenarios in which outcomes for missing subjects are assumed to be all favorable or all unfavorable, respectively. Authors should state clearly which, if any, analytic technique was used.

12. Did the investigators confirm their findings with a new set of subjects?
This question alludes to the possibility that the research findings regarding an intervention of interest occurred due to unique attributes of the sample. Repeating the study on a second group of subjects who match the inclusion and exclusion criteria outlined for the first group provides an opportunity to evaluate the consistency (or lack thereof) of an intervention's effect. Often this step is not included in a single research report due to insufficient numbers of subjects and/or lack of funds. As a result, evidence-based physical therapists may need to read several pieces of evidence about the same intervention if they wish to verify its usefulness to a greater degree.

Additional Considerations

The previous questions serve as an initial screening of the evidence to determine its potential usefulness—that is, its research validity. From an evaluative standpoint, a "no" answer to any of questions 1 through 11 may indicate a "fatal flaw" in the research design. Readers may use more latitude in their analysis with respect to question 12, given that researchers must conduct their studies within their resource limitations.

In addition to the 12 questions itemized above, concerns pertaining to research design in evidence about interventions include the presence or absence of a detailed description of the:

1. Setting in which the research was conducted;
2. Protocol for the intervention(s) used; and
3. Characteristics of the sample obtained.

This information allows evidence-based physical therapists to determine if the intervention of interest is applicable and feasible in their environment (1, 2) and if the subjects included resemble the patient or client about whom there is a question (3). Well-designed studies may have limited usefulness when these details are lacking.

Issues Related to Research Designs in Intervention Studies

Affirmative answers to most of the questions just listed are possible only in *randomized clinical trials*; however, the question of the validity of intervention papers is complicated by an ongoing debate regarding the relative merits of experimental, quasi-experimental, and nonexperimental (or observational) research designs. The evidence hierarchies promulgated by evidence-based practice sources consistently place experimental studies (e.g., randomized clinical trials) higher in ranking than the other two study types.[1,3,14] The rationale underlying this order is the ability of experimental designs to minimize bias by virtue of numerous controls directing subject assignment and management, study procedures, and study personnel knowledge and behavior. Studies suggesting that lower forms of evidence tend to overestimate treatment effects due to bias reinforce the value of experimental designs.[18,19]

   Unfortunately, randomized clinical trials are complex and expensive endeavors that may be logistically difficult to produce depending on the intervention in question. In addition, randomization to groups may be unethical if the necessary comparison is "no care" or a treatment alternative associated with high risk. Finally, experimental designs do not, by definition, resemble everyday clinical practice in which any number of factors may influence therapist and patient or client behavior, as well as outcomes from interventions. This latter point challenges the external validity of results from randomized clinical trials.

   In 1998, Britton et al. published a systematic review in response to this debate over study design.[18] These authors found that experimental designs are not inevitably better than quasi-experimental designs. For example, randomized clinical trials may produce a smaller effect size if they over-select subjects whose conditions are less severe, resulting in a smaller capacity to benefit from the experimental treatment. Such a scenario is reasonable to expect given the stringent exclusion criteria often used in experimental research designs. However, a treatment effect may be overestimated due to the potential influence of subject preferences in unmasked randomized trials. The authors also reported that quasi-experimental studies may produce comparable results to randomized clinical trials, if adjustment for group differences in important baseline prognostic factors is performed and that the same subject exclusion criteria are used. Anglemyer et al. drew similar conclusions in their 2014 systematic review comparing effects reported in randomized clinical trials to those reported in observational studies.[19] However, this more recent information does not provide a definitive resolution to the debate. For example, the authors noted that two previous reviews found that observational designs produced larger effect sizes, whereas a different review indicated these designs produced smaller effect sizes than randomized controlled trials. As a result, they recommended development of a standardized method to assess the potential for confounding influences when conducting systematic reviews of observational designs.

   Despite the emphasis on experimental designs, Straus et al. and Guyatt and Rennie do acknowledge that quasi-experimental and nonexperimental designs may be appropriate for determining the potential ineffectiveness or harm from an intervention of interest.[1,3] On a more practical level, physical therapists may find that the only research available to them to answer a question about interventions is not in the form of a randomized controlled trial. Rejecting this evidence because it is lower on the hierarchy would leave therapists without options beyond practice as it is currently conducted. Ultimately, evidence-based physical therapists will be required to use their clinical expertise and judgment regarding the potential usefulness of a quasi-experimental or nonexperimental study, keeping in mind that these research designs always are more vulnerable to bias.

Study Results

Studies about interventions may use descriptive statistics to elaborate on subject characteristics and to summarize baseline measures of performance. Whether an experimental treatment had an effect, as compared to an alternative or control, may be determined by "tests of differences"—those statistical tests that compare groups based on means, ranks, or frequencies. These tests come in parametric (e.g., t-test, ANOVA) and nonparametric (e.g., Kruskal-Wallis, chi square) forms depending on whether the outcome is a ratio, interval, ordinal, or nominal level measure. In addition, which test is used depends on whether the investigator is comparing only two groups or more than two groups. Finally, researchers need to decide if they are going to adjust for covariates (e.g., ANCOVA) and whether they are looking at only one outcome or multiple outcomes (e.g., MANOVA). Although these statistical tests indicate if a difference resulted from the experimental treatment, they do not provide information about the size of the treatment effect. This piece of information is vital to determine if the resulting outcome may be clinically meaningful for the physical therapist and the patient or client.

Treatment Magnitude: Continuous Data

One method for determining the magnitude of treatment impact is to calculate an effect size. This approach is appropriate for intervention studies in which the outcomes are continuous measures. An *effect size* identifies the magnitude of the difference between two group means.[5] In its simplest form, the absolute effect size is calculated by subtracting the mean outcome value for the control group from the mean outcome value for the experimental group at the conclusion of the study. In studies in which the comparison group is an alternative intervention rather than a true control (no intervention or *placebo*), then the "experimental group" may represent the larger mean score of the two groups.

For example, imagine a hypothetical study in which a customized ankle–foot orthosis (AFO) is compared to a molded arch support to determine if increased support of the foot and ankle improves the ambulatory ability of children with spastic hemiplegia. If the average walking distance in the AFO group was 250 feet further than in the arch support group at the conclusion of the study, then the effect size produced by the customized AFO is 250 feet.

A standardized version of the effect size is created when the variation in scores is included in the calculation (**Figure 13-1**). This approach evaluates the extent of overlap, if any, in the distribution of scores for each group (**Figure 13-2**). Standardized effect sizes often are used when investigators want to compare the magnitude of impact from the same intervention across different outcome measures within a study[20,21] or across numerous studies evaluated in a systematic review. Standardized effect sizes also are used in power calculations to determine the minimum sample size needed to detect a statistically significant difference or relationship, if it is present.

Standardized effect sizes often have a value between 0 and 1, although they may be less than 0 or greater than 1. The following guidelines have been recommended by some authors for interpreting standardized effect sizes[4,5]:

- 0.20   minimal effect size
- 0.50   moderate effect size
- 0.80   large effect size

However, an argument can be made that this scale has the potential to diminish the clinical relevance of smaller treatment effects when compared to other available alternatives.[22] In other words, interventions with small effect sizes may still be clinically meaningful to a physical therapist or a patient or client.

FIGURE 13-1   Calculation of standardized effect size.

$$\frac{\text{Mean Score of Group 1} - \text{Mean Score of Group 2}}{\text{Pooled Standard Deviation}}$$

$$\text{Pooled Standard Deviation} = \sqrt{\frac{(N_{exp} - 1)SD^2_{exp} + (N_{control} - 1)SD^2_{control}}{N_{exp} + (N_{control} - 2)}}$$

FIGURE 13-2   **Illustration of the influence of group variability on effect size.**

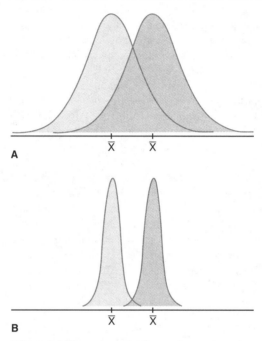

A

B

Effect of within-group variability on the overlap of sampling distributions.
A, High variability leads to overlap of sampling distributions.
B, Low variability leads to minimal overlap of sampling distributions.
$\overline{X}$ = mean.

This was published in Rehabilitation Research, Principles and Applications, 3rd edition, Elizabeth Domholdt, Page 294. Copyright 2005 by Elsevier. Reprinted with permission from Elsevier.

Treatment Magnitude: Dichotomous Data

An alternative method by which to demonstrate the magnitude of treatment impact is to calculate the change in the rate (expressed as a percentage) of developing the outcome of interest. This approach is useful when the outcome is captured using a dichotomous measure: either the outcome happened or it did not. The first step in this process is to determine whether the outcome of interest is beneficial or harmful to the subjects. Santos et al. considered a beneficial outcome when they investigated potential improvements in submaximal exercise capacity following an aerobic training program for overweight pregnant women.[23] In contrast, Emery et al. considered a harmful outcome when they studied whether a home balance training program prevented sports-related injuries in adolescent high school students.[24]

Changes in the rates of beneficial outcomes may be reflected by calculations of the increase in benefit achieved due to application of the experimental intervention. In the exercise study, the investigators wanted to know the extent to which aerobic training made a difference in submaximal cardiorespiratory capacity. Investigators can capture the impact of aerobic training by determining the absolute benefit increase and relative benefit increase. The *absolute benefit increase (ABI)* is calculated as follows:

$$ABI = |Experimental\ group\ event\ rate\ (EER) - Control\ group\ event\ rate\ (CER)|^1$$

These rates are the percentage of subjects who improved submaximal functional capacity in the exercise group and the control group, respectively. Santos et al. reported an EER of 26% and a CER of 5%[23]; therefore, the ABI achieved through aerobic exercise training was 21%. The ABI is useful for discriminating between large and small treatment effects.[1] Alternatively, the *relative benefit increase (RBI)* is calculated as follows:

$$RBI = \frac{|Experimental\ group\ event\ rate\,(EER) - Control\ group\ event\ rate\,(CER)|^1}{Control\ group\ event\ rate\,(CER)}$$

Using the same numbers from the prior calculation, the RBI in the exercise training study was 4.2, which should be interpreted to mean that aerobic exercise training increased submaximal functional capacity in the experimental group by 420% as compared to those who did not participate in the exercise program. Unlike the ABI, the RBI is insensitive to differences in magnitude of the treatment effect. For example, if 2.5% of the experimental group improved submaximal functional capacity versus 0.5% of the control group, the RBI would still be 420%. Yet the actual difference between the two groups is only 2.0%, which may have no clinical relevance depending on what other treatment techniques are available.

Changes in rates of adverse outcomes may be reflected by calculations of the reduction in risk achieved due to the experimental intervention. Risk reduction will be familiar to those with a background in public health epidemiology because prevention of adverse events is a central theme in this service area. In the balance training study, the risk pertains to the development of sports-related injury as a result of presumed proprioceptive deficiencies. An appropriate exercise program may reduce this risk by improving static and dynamic balance through proprioceptive training. Investigators can capture the impact of the balance training program by determining the absolute risk reduction and the relative risk reduction. The *absolute risk reduction (ARR)* is calculated as follows:

$$ARR = |Control\ group\ event\ rate\ (CER) - Experimental\ group\ event\ rate\ (EER)|^1$$

These rates are the percentage of subjects who developed a sports-related injury in the control group and the experimental group, respectively. Emery et al. reported a CER of 17% and an EER of 3%[24]; therefore, the ARR achieved by use of the balance training program was 14%. As with the ARI, the ARR is useful in distinguishing between small and large treatment effects. Alternatively, the *relative risk reduction (RRR)* is calculated as follows:

$$RRR = \frac{|Control\ group\ event\ rate\,(CER) - Experimental\ group\ event\ rate\,(EER)|^1}{Control\ group\ event\ rate\,(CER)}$$

Using the same numbers from the prior calculation, the RRR in the balance training study was 0.82. In other words, participation in the balance training program reduced the risk of developing a sports-related injury by 82% as compared to subjects who did not participate in the program. The RRR is limited in the same fashion as the RBI in that it is insensitive to small treatment effects.

Readers should note that the absolute and relative benefit and risk calculations can be derived from 2×2 tables if authors provide the data in their results. **Tables 13-3** and **13-4** illustrate this approach for both the Santos et al. and Emery et al. studies. However, results from hand calculations may vary slightly from those reported depending on whether the authors round values with decimal points up or down.

The Statistical Importance of Study Results

As is the case for evidence about diagnostic tests, clinical measures and prognostic (risk) factors, p values and confidence intervals may be employed in evidence about interventions to help determine the statistical importance of a study's results. A p value indicates the probability that the result obtained

---

TABLE 13-3   Results from a Study of Aerobic Exercise Training in Overweight Pregnant Women

	+ Improved $VO_2^\P$	− Improved VO_2
+ Aerobic Exercise Program	**a** 10	**b** 28
− Aerobic Exercise Program	**c** 2	**d** 36

$VO_2^\P$ = Oxygen consumption at anaerobic threshold in exercise test

$ABI = |a/(a + b) - c/(c + d)| = |10/38 - 2/38| = 0.21 \times 100\% = 21\%$

$RBI = \dfrac{|a/(a + b) - c/(c + b)|}{c/(c + d)} = \dfrac{|10/38 - 2/38|}{2/38} = 4.2 \times 100\% = 420\%$

TABLE 13-4   Results from a Study of Balance Training for Reducing Sports-Related Injuries

	+ Sports Injury	− Sports Injury
+ Balance Program	**a** 2	**b** 58
− Balance Program	**c** 10	**d** 50

$ARR = |c/(c + d) - a/(a + b)| = |10/60 - 2/60| = 0.14 \times 100\% = 14\%$

$RRR = \dfrac{|c/(c + d) - a/(a + b)|}{c/(c + d)} = \dfrac{|10/60 - 2/60|}{10/60} = 0.80 \times 100\% = 80\%$

occurred due to chance. Results become more convincing as the p value decreases (e.g., <0.05) because the role of chance is so diminished, although not eliminated. The p values usually are reported in conjunction with statistical tests of differences to determine whether an experimental intervention was more effective than a control or comparison intervention. As noted earlier, it is helpful to know that a difference in outcome occurred, but it is more helpful to know the magnitude of that difference. For this reason, a p value usually is not sufficient by itself to help determine the potential importance of findings in an intervention study.

Confidence intervals are more helpful in determining the potential meaningfulness of study findings because they establish the precision (or lack thereof) of effect sizes, as well as of absolute and relative benefit and risk calculations. A *confidence interval* represents a range of scores within which the true score for a variable is estimated to lie within a specified probability (e.g., 90%, 95%, 99%).[4] Usually, authors report the relevant confidence interval; however, readers may also calculate the interval for different estimates when they are not reported. Equations for confidence intervals for various outcomes are available in statistics textbooks.

There is an important difference between confidence intervals calculated around values for treatment magnitude and confidence intervals calculated around likelihood and odds ratios. Specifically, the lower bound of confidence intervals for likelihood and odds ratios is zero, whereas it is possible for the lower bound of confidence intervals for treatment effects to be a negative number. This difference is understandable if one considers what is being measured. Likelihood and odds ratios represent predictions about the probability of a specific outcome. As such, these ratios cannot have negative values in the mathematical sense. Put in practical terms, the statement "There is a –50% probability that a patient will have 'X' diagnosis or outcome" makes no sense. Either there is a probability of the diagnosis or outcome (however small or large) or there is not (the value zero). However, the evaluation of an experimental intervention in comparison to an alternative may produce one of three actual outcomes:

1. Subjects who receive the experimental intervention improve (or reduce their risk) compared to those who did not receive the intervention;
2. Subjects who receive the experimental intervention remain unchanged compared to those who did not receive the intervention; or
3. Subjects who receive the experimental intervention are worse off (or increase their risk).compared to those who did not receive the intervention.

As a result, it is possible to have negative values for both the measures of treatment magnitude (expressed as an effect size, ABI, RBI, ARR, or RRR), as well as for their confidence intervals.

Note that authors choose what their threshold values will be for p values and confidence intervals. In the case of p values, the traditional threshold is an alpha (α) ≤ 0.05. In the case of confidence intervals, the traditional parameter choice is 95% certainty. Ultimately, these are arbitrary choices; therefore, evidence-based physical therapists must use their clinical judgment and expertise to determine the clinical meaningfulness of a study's findings. This challenge will be apparent when results just miss significance (e.g., $p = 0.07$) or when confidence intervals are wide. Nevertheless, a study that minimizes bias and demonstrates strong statistical significance with narrow confidence intervals should be taken seriously in terms of the information it provides.

Evidence and the Patient or Client

Once the validity of a study about an intervention is established and the statistical importance of its results confirmed, the final step is to determine whether the evidence is appropriate for use with an individual patient or client. This is the point in the process during which physical therapists must add their clinical expertise and judgment, along with the patient or client's preferences and values, to the information gleaned from the research. Whether to use an intervention with an individual depends in part on the extent to which a study's results are clinically meaningful. Statistical significance does not equal clinical significance *per se*. However, physical therapists have tools with which to assess the relationship between these two judgments: the minimal clinically important difference and the number needed to treat.

Minimal Clinically Important Difference

The *minimal clinically important difference (MCID)* is defined as "the smallest treatment effect that would result in a change in patient management, given its side effects, costs, and inconveniences."[9(p.1197)] In other words, the MCID reflects the minimal level of change required in response to an intervention before the outcome would be considered worthwhile in terms of an individual's function or quality of life. An intervention that produces a statistically significant change in study subjects that does not cross this change threshold is likely to be disregarded as unimportant from a clinical standpoint. Ideally, investigators will evaluate their own findings in light of a predetermined MCID. This value often is stated as part of a power calculation to determine an appropriate sample size. However, Chan et al. reported that authors of randomized clinical trials inconsistently evaluate clinical importance.[9] As a result, evidence-based physical therapists must make their own determination based on their knowledge of other evidence and their clinical experience, as well as on input from the individual for whom the intervention is being considered.[14]

Number Needed to Treat

Interventions with large effects may still have limited usefulness if the associated outcomes are rare. Alternatively, interventions with modest effects may be more meaningful if the outcomes occur frequently. Investigators may estimate the number of subjects that must receive an intervention in order for one subject to increase his or her benefit (or reduce his or her risk).[10] This calculation is referred to as the *number needed to treat (NNT)* and is determined using one of the following equations:

$$\text{NNT} = 1/\text{ABI} \ or \ \text{NNT} = 1/\text{ARR}$$

In the aerobic training study, the NNT is 1/0.21, or 5. In the balance training study, the NNT is 1/0.14, or 7. In other words, investigators need to treat five overweight pregnant women or seven adolescent high school students to improve submaximal functional capacity in one woman or prevent one sports-related injury in one student, respectively. These values do not indicate which women or students will benefit—only that one of them is likely to do so within the parameters of this study.[10] The NNT also should be interpreted within the time lines of each study (12 weeks and 6 months, respectively). Understandably, a smaller NNT along with a shorter time line implies greater potential usefulness of the intervention. Physical therapists also may evaluate the precision of an NNT with confidence intervals reported or calculated for these values.

Readers may calculate the NNT if authors provide the necessary information about event rates in their results. However, hand-calculated results may vary from those reported depending on how values with decimals are handled. The tendency is to be conservative in estimating the NNT, as is illustrated in the study by Emery et al.[24] Although they rounded the event rates for calculation of the absolute risk reduction, they left these values intact for calculation of the NNT, thereby producing NNT = 8, rather than the 7 just calculated.

The NNT calculated from a study refers to the group of subjects, not to the individuals within it. To apply this value to an individual patient or client, physical therapists must consider the extent to which that person's probability of achieving the outcome of interest matches the probability of subjects in the study.[1] This determination is reached by considering the likelihood of achieving the desired outcome if the individual does not receive the intervention. As a result, the reference point used from the evidence is the probability for the control group (i.e., the control group event rate [CER]). Emery et al. reported a CER of 16.6%[24]; therefore, a therapist working with a high school athlete should consider whether that individual's risk is higher or lower than 16.6% given the degree to which this person's characteristics match those of the control group. This information may be used in combination with the relative risk reduction from the study to determine a number needed to treat for the individual athlete.

Fortunately, mathematical equations are not required for this purpose because a nomogram has been created to facilitate this evaluation of treatment effect for an individual (**Figure 13-3**).[25] The nomogram works in a similar fashion to the tool created for use with likelihood ratios. An individual's risk for the outcome of interest is identified on the line to the far left. A straight edge is applied from this point through the relative risk reduction from the study located on the center line to determine the NNT on the line to the far right. For example, the dark green line on the figure indicates that, for an athlete with a risk of injury of less than that of the control group (e.g., 10%), and a relative risk reduction from Emery et al. of 80%,[24] the NNT is approximately 12. Under these circumstances, the therapist might consider other interventions, especially in light of the compliance issues reported in the study. However, if the athlete's risk is estimated to be 35% (black line), then the NNT is reduced to approximately 3. Under these circumstances, the physical therapist and the high school athlete may decide to implement the balance training program.

Practical Considerations

In addition to the MCID and NNT, there are several practical considerations before putting the evidence about an intervention into practice. First, the intervention should be available, practical, and safe in the setting in which the physical therapist practices. Second, the intervention should have demonstrated performance on people that resemble the individual with whom the physical therapist is working. These commonalities may include age, gender, signs, symptoms, previous activity or functional levels, comorbidities, and so on. Important differences may indicate a need to discard the intervention in favor of another option. Alternatively, therapists may decide to adapt the intervention to accommodate to a patient or client's limitations. For example, a joint mobilization technique performed in a supine position in a study may be modified by having the patient sit in a semi-recumbent position to reduce the work of breathing associated with compromised cardiopulmonary function.

Physical therapists also must consider their patient or client's preferences and values with respect to their health status and its management. Areas of interest or concern for an individual may include, but are not limited to, the following[26]:

1. The potential risk of injury or pain involved with the intervention;
2. Whether sufficient benefit will occur to outweigh the risks;
3. Cost—including financial, as well as time away from work, school, or family;
4. Confidence in the physical therapist; and
5. Appreciation and belief in the value of scientific evidence.

Individual cultural and social norms will shape the direction of these issues for the patient or client, as well as for family members or other caregivers involved in the situation. Ideally, both the physical therapist and the patient or client will agree on the optimal course of action. However, the ethical principle of autonomy dictates that the person seeking physical therapist services must decide whether the intervention is worth the effort and risk to undergo the procedure.

FIGURE 13-3   Nomogram for determining numbers needed to treat an individual patient or client.

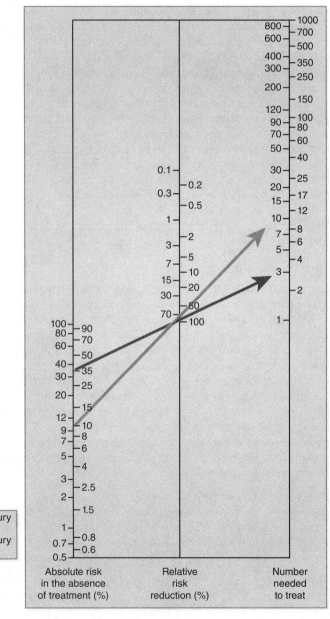

Adapted by permission from BMJ Publishing Group, Limited. The Number Needed to Treat: A Clinically Useful Nomogram in its Proper Context, Gilles Chatellier, Eric Zapletal, David Lemaitre et al. *BMJ*. 312. Copyright 1996.

Evidence Appraisal Tools

Table 13-5 provides a checklist to guide the evaluation of evidence about interventions for use in any practice setting.[13] Answers to these questions should be considered in the context of the debate about the relative merits of experimental, quasi-experimental, and nonexperimental studies. Alternatively, readers might consider accessing some of the appraisal resources available online. A strategy worth

TABLE 13-5	Evidence About Interventions: Quality Appraisal Checklist

Research Validity of the Study

Did the investigators randomly assign (or allocate) subjects to groups?	___ Yes ___ No ___ Insufficient detail
Was each subject's group assignment concealed from the people enrolling individuals in the study?	___ Yes ___ No ___ Insufficient detail
Did the groups have similar sociodemographic, clinical, and prognostic characteristics at the start of the study?	___ Yes ___ No ___ Insufficient detail
Were subjects masked (or blinded) to their group assignment?	___ Yes ___ No ___ Insufficient detail
Were clinicians and/or outcome assessors masked (or blinded) to the subjects' group assignment?	___ Yes ___ No ___ Insufficient detail
Did the investigators manage all of the groups in the same way except for the experimental intervention(s)?	___ Yes ___ No ___ Insufficient detail
Did the investigators apply the study protocol and collect follow-up data on all subjects over a time frame long enough for the outcomes of interest to occur?	___ Yes ___ No ___ Insufficient detail
Did subject attrition (e.g., withdrawal, loss to follow-up) occur over the course of the study?	___ Yes ___ No ___ Insufficient detail
If attrition occurred, did the investigators perform an intention-to-treat analysis?	___ Yes ___ No ___ Insufficient detail ___ Not applicable

(continues)

TABLE 13-5	Evidence About Interventions: Quality Appraisal Checklist (*Continued*)

Did the investigators confirm their findings with a new set of subjects?	___ Yes ___ No ___ Insufficient detail
Do you have enough confidence in the research validity of this paper to consider using this evidence with your patient or client?	___ Yes ___ Undecided ___ No

Relevant Study Findings

Results reported that are specific to your clinical question:

Test(s) of differences _____

Effect size(s) _____

Absolute benefit increase(s) _____

Relative benefit increase(s) _____

Absolute risk reduction(s) _____

Relative risk reduction(s) _____

Number needed to treat (harm) _____

Other _____

Statistical significance and/or precision of the relevant study results:

Obtained p values for each relevant statistic reported by the authors: _____

Obtained confidence intervals for each relevant statistic reported by the authors: _____

Do these findings exceed a minimal clinically important difference?	___ Yes ___ No ___ Insufficient detail

Application of the Evidence to Your Patient or Client

Are there clinically meaningful differences between the subjects in the study and your patient or client?	___ Yes ___ No ___ Mixed results ___ Insufficient detail
Can you perform the intervention of interest safely and appropriately in your clinical setting given your current knowledge and skill level and your current resources?	___ Yes ___ No ___ Insufficient description of the techniques used
Does the intervention of interest fit within the patient's or client's expressed values and preferences?	___ Yes ___ No ___ Mixed results

TABLE 13-5	Evidence About Interventions: Quality Appraisal Checklist (*Continued*)

Do the potential benefits outweigh the potential risks of using the intervention of interest with your patient or client?

___ Yes
___ No
___ Mixed results

Will you use the intervention of interest for this patient or client?

___ Yes
___ No

SAMPLE CALCULATIONS: BENEFIT INCREASE

	+ Outcome	− Outcome
+ Intervention	**a** 72	**b** 55
− Intervention	**c** 40	**d** 78

CER = control group event rate = c/(c + d) = 0.25 = 34%

EER = experimental group event rate = a/(a + b) = 0.57 = 57%

EER	CER	Relative Benefit Increase (RBI)	Absolute Benefitt Increase (ABI)	Number Needed to Treat (NNT)
		$\dfrac{EER - CER}{CER}$	EER − CER	1/ABI
57%	34%	56%	23%	4
		*95%CI →	10.9%−35.1%	3−9

*95% confidence interval (CI) on an NNT − 1/(limits on the CI of its ABI) =

$$\pm 1.96 \sqrt{\left[\frac{CER \times (1 - CER)}{\#Control\ Pts}\right] + \left[\frac{EER \times (1 - EER)}{\#\ Exper\ Pts}\right]} = \pm 1.96$$

$$= \sqrt{\left[\frac{0.34 \times 0.66}{118}\right] + \left[\frac{0.57 \times 0.43}{127}\right]} = \pm 12.1\%$$

SAMPLE CALCULATIONS: RISK REDUCTION

	+ Outcome	− Outcome
+ Intervention	**a** 10	**b** 50
− Intervention	**c** 26	**d** 34

CER = control group event rate = c/(c + d) = 0.43 = 43%

EER = experimental group event rate = a/(a + b) = 0.17 = 17%

(*continues*)

TABLE 13-5   Evidence About Interventions: Quality Appraisal Checklist (*Continued*)

CER	EER	Relative Risk Reduction (RRR)	Absolute Risk Reduction (ARR)	Number Needed to Treat (NNT)
CER	EER	$\dfrac{CER - EER}{CER}$	CER − EER	1/ARR
43%	17%	60%	26%	4
		*95%CI →	10.3%−41.7%	2−10

*95% confidence interval (CI) on an NNT − 1/(limits on the CI of its ARR) =

$$\pm 1.96 \sqrt{\left[\frac{CER \times (1 - CER)}{\# Control\ Pts}\right] + \left[\frac{EER \times (1 - EER)}{\#\ Exper\ Pts}\right]} = \pm 1.96$$

$$= \sqrt{\left[\frac{0.17 \times 0.83}{60}\right] + \left[\frac{0.43 \times 0.57}{60}\right]} = \pm 15.7\%$$

YOUR CALCULATIONS

	+ Outcome	− Outcome
+ Intervention	a	b
− Intervention	c	d

CER = control group event rate = c/(c + d) =

EER = experimental group event rate = a/(a + b) =

EER	CER	Relative Benefit Increase (RBI)	Absolute Benefit Increase (ABI)	Number Needed to Treat (NNT)
EER	CER	$\dfrac{EER - CER}{CER}$	EER − CER	1/ABI
		*95%CI →		

*95% confidence interval (CI) on an NNT − 1/(limits on the CI of its ABI) =

CER	EER	Relative Risk Reduction (RRR)	Absolute Risk Reduction (ARR)	Number Needed to Treat (NNT)
CER	EER	$\dfrac{CER - EER}{CER}$	CER − EER	1/ARR
		*95%CI →		

*95% confidence interval (CI) on an NNT − 1/(limits on the CI of its ARR) =

These questions were adapted from the Oxford Centre for Evidence-Based Medicine and applied to physical therapist practice.

considering is the creation of reference notebooks that contain completed checklists or worksheets along with their associated research articles. These compendia could facilitate the use of evidence regarding interventions for all physical therapists in a particular setting (as long as there is a commitment to keeping them up to date).

Summary

Physical therapists and the individuals they manage select interventions in consideration of a variety of objective and subjective factors. Evidence about interventions may inform the selection process if its design minimizes bias. The experimental research design has the greatest opportunity for control of bias; however, critics point out that the inherent restrictions in the design may limit the relevance of the evidence to "real-world" practice. Some published reports indicate that quasi-experimental and non-experimental (observational) studies may provide acceptable results if adjustment for important confounding factors is performed. Ultimately, evidence-based physical therapists must evaluate the evidence on its merits and use their clinical judgment to determine the strength of the research design.

In addition to design issues, physical therapists also should evaluate the magnitude of reported treatment effects and consider whether the response to the experimental intervention is clinically worthwhile. This determination may be made when findings are compared to the minimal clinically important difference identified by researchers, therapists, patients, or clients. In addition, therapists may use the number needed to treat to identify interventions that produce the desired outcome with an acceptable frequency.

Exercises

1. Discuss three factors that may influence the intervention selection process for physical therapists and their patients or clients. Provide clinical examples relevant to physical therapist practice to illustrate your points.
2. Discuss the different perspectives in the debate regarding the relative usefulness of experimental, quasi-experimental, and nonexperimental designs.
3. Explain why it is important to mask those responsible for allocating subjects to groups. Provide a clinical example relevant to physical therapist practice to illustrate your point.
4. It is often difficult to prevent subjects from knowing to which group they have been assigned in a study of interventions physical therapists may use. Describe this design limitation's potential impact on study results. Provide a clinical example relevant to physical therapist practice to illustrate your point.
5. Explain why it is important to mask the people responsible for measuring outcomes to group assignment. Provide a clinical example relevant to physical therapist practice to illustrate your point.
6. Discuss the potential consequences of subject attrition. What are the advantages and disadvantages of estimating the lost data? Provide a clinical example relevant to physical therapist practice to illustrate your point.
7. Explain the concept of an intention-to-treat analysis, including its purpose and benefits. Provide a clinical example relevant to physical therapist practice to illustrate your point.
8. Explain why the magnitude of treatment effect provides more useful information than the results of a statistical test of differences. Provide a clinical example relevant to physical therapist practice to illustrate your point.

9. Discuss the concept of effect size in both of its forms. Provide a clinical example relevant to physical therapist practice to illustrate your point.

10. Discuss the concept of the minimal clinically important difference and its contribution to determining the potential usefulness of an experimental intervention. Provide a clinical example relevant to physical therapist practice to illustrate your point.

11. Use the following 2 × 2 table to calculate the experimental group and control group event rates, the absolute and relative risk reductions, and the number needed to treat in this hypothetical study about an intervention to prevent pressure ulcers:

	+ Pressure Ulcer	− Pressure Ulcer
+ Intervention	6	38
− Intervention	17	32

12. Interpret the results for each of the calculations. The authors of the hypothetical study in question 11 report that a 95% confidence interval around the absolute risk reduction (ARR) is (14, 28). The minimal clinically important difference for the study is an ARR of 25%. Using this information, make an argument:
    a. In favor of using this intervention.
    b. Against using this intervention.

References

1. Straus SE, Richardson WS, Glaziou P, Haynes RB. *Evidence-Based Medicine: How to Practice and Teach EBM.* 3rd ed. Edinburgh, Scotland: Elsevier Churchill Livingstone; 2005.

2. Helewa A, Walker JM. *Critical Evaluation of Research in Physical Rehabilitation: Towards Evidence-Based Practice.* Philadelphia, PA: W.B. Saunders; 2000.

3. Guyatt G, Rennie D. *Users' Guides to the Medical Literature: A Manual for Evidence-Based Clinical Practice.* 3rd ed. Chicago, IL: AMA Press; 2014.

4. Carter RE, Lubinsky J, Domholdt E. *Rehabilitation Research: Principles and Applications.* 4th ed. St. Louis, MO: Elsevier Saunders; 2011.

5. Batavia M. *Clinical Research for Health Professionals: A User-Friendly Guide.* Boston, MA: Butterworth-Heinemann; 2001.

6. Campbell DT, Stanley JC. *Experimental and Quasi-Experimental Designs for Research.* Boston, MA: Houghton Mifflin; 1963.

7. Tabachnik BG, Fidell LS. *Using Multivariate Statistics.* 4th ed. Boston, MA: Allyn & Bacon; 2006.

8. American Physical Therapy Association, Guide to Physical Therapist Practice. *Practice 3.0.* Available at http://guidetoptpractice.apta.org. Accessed July 16, 2016.

9. Chan KBY, Man-Son-Hing M, Molnar FJ, Laupacis A. How well is the clinical importance of study results reported? An assessment of randomized controlled trials. *CMAJ.* 2001;165(9):1197-1202.

10. Dalton GW, Keating JL. Number needed to treat: a statistic relevant to physical therapists. *Phys Ther.* 2000;80(12):1214-1219.

11. Portney LG, Watkins MP. *Foundations of Clinical Research: Applications to Practice.* 3rd ed. Upper Saddle River, NJ: Pearson; 2009.

12. Cook TD, Campbell DT. *Quasi-Experimentation: Design and Analysis Issues for Field Settings.* Boston, MA: Houghton Mifflin; 1979.

13. Oxford Centre for Evidence-Based Medicine website. Available at: www.cebm.net. Accessed October 1, 2016.

14. Herbert R, Jamtvedt G, Hagen KB, Mead J. *Practical Evidence-Based Physiotherapy.* 2nd ed. Edinburgh, Scotland: Elsevier Butterworth-Heinemann; 2011.

15. Staron RS, Karapondo DL, Kraemer WJ, et al. Skeletal muscle adaptations during early phase of heavy-resistance training in men and women. *J Appl Physiol.* 1994;76(3):1247-1255.

16. Hollis S, Campbell F. What is meant by intention to treat analysis? Survey of published randomized controlled trials. *BMJ.* 1999;319(7211):670-674.

17. Montori VM, Guyatt GH. Intention-to-treat principle. *CMAJ.* 2001;165(10):1339-1341.

18. Britton A, McKee M, Black N, et al. Choosing between randomized and non-randomized studies: a systematic review. *Health Technol Assess.* 1998;2(13):i-iv, 1-124.

19. Anglemyer A, Horvath HT, Bero L. Healthcare outcomes assessed with observational study designs compared with those assessed in randomized trials. *Cochrane Database Syst Rev.* 2014;April 29;(4):MR000034.

20. Jette AM, Delitto A. Physical therapy treatment choices for musculoskeletal impairments. *Phys Ther.* 1997;77(2):145-154.

21. Jette DU, Jette AM. Physical therapy and health outcomes for patients with spinal impairments. *Phys Ther.* 1997;76(9):930-945.

22. What is an Effect Size: A Guide for Users. Centre for Evaluation and Monitoring website. Available at: http://www.cem.org/effect-size-resources. Accessed March 13, 2017.

23. Santos IA, Stein R, Fuchs SC, et al. Aerobic exercise and submaximal functional capacity in overweight pregnant women. *Obstet Gynecol.* 2005;106(2):243-249.

24. Emery CA, Cassidy JD, Klassen TP, et al. Effectiveness of a home-based balance-training program in reducing sports-related injuries among healthy adolescents: a cluster randomized controlled trial. *CMAJ.* 2005;172(6):749-754.

25. Chatellier G, Zapletal E, Lemaitre D, et al. The number needed to treat: a clinically useful nomogram in its proper context. *BMJ.* 1996;312(7028):426-429.

26. King M, Nazareth I, Lampe F, et al. Conceptual framework and systematic review of the effects of participants' and professionals' preferences in randomized controlled trials. *Health Technol Assess.* 2005;9(35):1-191.

CHAPTER 14

APPRAISING EVIDENCE ABOUT CLINICAL PREDICTION RULES

OBJECTIVES

Upon completion of this chapter, the student/practitioner will be able to do the following:
1. Discuss the contributions of clinical prediction rules to physical therapist patient/client management.
2. Critically appraise evidence about the development and accuracy of clinical prediction rules, including:
   a. Important questions to ask related to research validity; and
   b. Statistical approaches used.
3. Evaluate p values and confidence intervals to determine the potential importance of reported findings.
4. Discuss considerations related to the application of evidence about clinical prediction rules to individual patients or clients.

TERMS IN THIS CHAPTER

Bias: Results or inferences that systematically deviate from the truth "or the processes leading to such deviation."[1(p.251)]

Clinical prediction rule: A systematically derived and statistically tested combination of clinical findings that provides meaningful predictions about an outcome of interest.[2-4]

Confidence interval: A range of scores within which the true score for a variable is estimated to lie within a specified probability (e.g., 90%, 95%, 99%).[5]

Criterion validity: The degree to which a measure of interest relates to a measure with established validity ("criterion measure").[6]

Diagnosis: A process of "integrating and evaluating the data that are obtained during the examination to describe the individual condition in terms that will guide the physical therapist in determining the prognosis and developing a plan of care."[7]

Differential diagnosis: A process for distinguishing among "a set of diagnoses that can plausibly explain the patient or client's presentation."[8(p.673)]

Face validity: A subjective assessment of the degree to which an instrument appears to measure what it is designed to measure.[9]

"Gold standard" (also referred to as *reference standard*): A diagnostic test or clinical measure that provides a definitive diagnosis or measurement. A "best in class" criterion test or measure.[1]

Intervention: "Physical therapists purposefully interact with the individual and, when appropriate, with other people involved in his or her care, using various" procedures or techniques "to produce changes in the condition."[7]

Masked (also referred to as *blinded*): (1) In diagnostic test and clinical measure papers, the lack of knowledge about previous test/measure results; (2) in prognostic factor papers, the lack of knowledge about exposure status; and (3) in intervention papers, the lack of knowledge about to which group a subject has been assigned.

Minimal clinically important difference (MCID): "The smallest treatment effect that would result in a change in patient management, given its side effects, costs, and inconveniences."[10(p.1197)]

Negative likelihood ratio (LR–): The likelihood that a negative test result will be obtained in an individual with the condition of interest as compared to an individual without the condition of interest.[11]

Odds ratio (OR): The odds that an individual with a prognostic (risk) factor had an outcome of interest as compared to the odds for an individual without the prognostic (risk) factor.[8,12]

Positive likelihood ratio (LR+): The likelihood that a positive test result will be obtained in an individual with the condition of interest as compared to an individual without the condition of interest.[11]

Posttest probability: The odds (probability) that an individual has a condition based on the result of a diagnostic test.[12]

Power: The probability that a statistical test will detect, if it is present, a relationship between two or more variables or scores or a difference between two or more groups or scores.[5,9]

Predictive validity: A method of criterion validation that reflects the degree to which the score on a measure predicts a future criterion score.[6]

Pretest probability: The odds (probability) that an individual has a condition based on clinical presentation before a diagnostic test is conducted.[12]

Prognosis: "The determination of the predicted optimal level of improvement in function and the amount of time needed to reach that level and also may include a prediction of levels of improvement that may be reached at various intervals during the course of therapy."[7]

Prognostic factor: A sociodemographic, diagnostic, or comorbid characteristic of an individual that confers increased or decreased chances of positive or adverse outcomes from a disease/disorder or from interventions.[8,12]

***p* value**: The probability that a statistical finding occurred due to chance.

Sensitivity (Sn): The proportion of individuals with the condition of interest that have a positive test result. Also referred to as "true positives."[12]

Specificity (Sp): The proportion of individuals without the condition of interest who have a negative test result. Also referred to as "true negatives."[12]

Type II error: A result from a statistical test that indicates a significant relationship or difference does not exist when in fact one exists (i.e., a false negative).[9]

CLINICAL SCENARIO

What Does This Clinical Prediction Rule Mean About My Future?

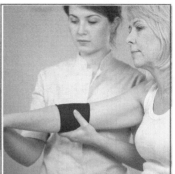

Anne discovered an article online about a clinical prediction rule aimed at identifying people with elbow pain like hers, who would respond to a combination of treatments.* She looked up the term "clinical prediction rule" and recognized that these algorithms are designed to expedite accurate clinical decision making. She wants to know whether this study will help you make decisions about how to manage her elbow pain.

What will you tell her and how will you explain the results?

*Vincenzo B, Smith D, Cleland J, Bisset L. Development of a clinical prediction rule to identify initial responders to mobilization with movement and exercise for lateral epicondylalgia. *Man Ther.* 2009;14(5):55-554.

Introduction

Physical therapists engage in a diagnostic process during the examination. Information is gathered via record review and interview as well as through systems review and application of diagnostic tests and clinical measures. The data obtained are used to:

- Identify and quantify the nature and extent of the individual's problem or concern (*diagnosis*);
- Predict future outcomes (*prognosis*); and
- Inform development of a plan of care (*intervention*).[5]

Throughout this endeavor physical therapists must make decisions about which pieces of information to gather and which methods to use to collect that data. They also must determine which information will confirm suspected causes or relationships, and which information will exclude other possibilities (*differential diagnosis*).[7, 8]

This iterative decision-making process may be facilitated when therapists know which pieces of information are most relevant as well as their relative contributions to the overall picture. The traditional practice paradigm relies on knowledge, experience, and intuition—often influenced by authority and tradition—to make these choices. However, the potential for inaccurate and/or costly misdirection exists in these circumstances because individual clinical practice is biased by exposure to patients or clients who may not be representative of the larger population for a given problem or concern.

Physical therapists can enhance the accuracy and efficiency of their decision making by using well-designed clinical prediction rules. *Clinical prediction rules* are systematically derived and statistically tested combinations of clinical findings that provide meaningful predictions about an outcome of interest. An outcome of interest may be a diagnostic category, a prognostic estimate, or a likely treatment response.[2-4] The potential utility of these algorithms is most pronounced in clinical situations that are complex and/or present with a significant degree of uncertainty. **Table 14-1** provides some examples of clinical prediction rules that are relevant to physical therapist practice.

TABLE 14-1	Examples of Studies About Clinical Prediction Rules Relevant to Physical Therapist Practice

- Wong CK, et al. Determining 1-year prosthetic use for mobility prognoses for community-dwelling adults lower-limb amputation: development of a clinical prediction rule. *Am J Phys Med Rehabil.* 2016;95(5):339-347.

- Wallenkamp MM, et al. The Amsterdam wrist rules: the multicenter prospective derivation and external validation of a clinical decision rule for the use of radiography in acute wrist trauma. *BMC Musculoskelet Disord.* 2015;16:389.

- Rabin A, et al. A clinical prediction rule to identify patients with low back pain who are likely to experience short-term success following lumbar stabilization exercises: a randomized controlled validation study. *J Orthop Sports Phys Ther.* 2014;44(1):6-13.

- Cleland JA, et al. Development of a clinical prediction rule for guiding treatment of a subgroup of patients with neck pain: use of thoracic spine manipulation, exercise, and patient education. *Phys Ther.* 2007;87(1):9-23.

- Kuijpers T, et al. Clinical prediction rules for the prognosis of shoulder pain in general practice. *Pain.* 2006;120(3):276-285.

- Stiell IG, et al. Decision rules for the use of radiography in acute ankle injuries. Refinement and prospective validation. *JAMA.* 1993;269(9):1127-1132.

Figure 14-1 is a schematic representation of the Ottawa Ankle Rules.[13] As the legend in the diagram illustrates, a combination of pain in a malleolar zone plus one of three possible other symptoms are the only pieces of information required to determine the need for radiographs in this rule.

These algorithms sometimes are referred to as "clinical decision rules," although there is some debate about the appropriateness of interchanging these labels.[14,15] In either case, physical therapists need to know for whom a prediction rule is intended, its performance characteristics, and the conditions under which it is appropriately applied. With that goal in mind, this chapter focuses on the evaluation of evidence that informs physical therapists' choices regarding clinical prediction rules.

Study Credibility

Evidence pertaining to clinical prediction rules may focus on derivation of the rule, validation of the rule, or both. **Table 14-2** itemizes the important questions to ask pertaining to the research validity of articles about rule development. **Table 14-3** provides the relevant assessment questions about studies pertaining to rule validation. These assessment criteria are drawn from a variety of authors,[2-4,14-16] and represent a blend of questions used for appraisal of evidence about diagnostic tests, *prognostic factors*, and interventions. Their purpose is to help physical therapists determine the extent to which research design elements may have introduced *bias* into a study.

Clinical Prediction Rule Derivation

1. Did the investigators operationally define the sample in their study?
Clearly articulated inclusion and exclusion criteria should be used to ensure that subjects fit the definition of individuals who have the potential to achieve the outcome of interest for the clinical prediction

FIGURE 14-1   Schematic representation of the Ottawa Ankle Rules.

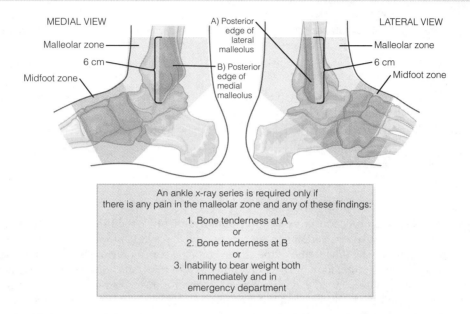

An ankle x-ray series is required only if
there is any pain in the malleolar zone and any of these findings:

1. Bone tenderness at A
or
2. Bone tenderness at B
or
3. Inability to bear weight both
immediately and in
emergency department

TABLE 14-2   Questions to Assess the Evidence About the Derivation of Clinical Prediction Rules

1. Did the investigators operationally define the sample in their study?
2. Were the subjects representative of the population from which they were drawn?
3. Did the investigators include all relevant predictive factors in the development process?
4. Were the predictive factors operationally defined?
5. Did the investigators include a large enough sample size to accommodate the number of predictive factors used to derive the clinical prediction rule?
6. Were the outcomes of interest operationally defined?
7. Were those responsible for measuring the outcomes masked to the status of the predictive factors (and vice versa)?
8. Did the investigators collect outcome data from all of the subjects enrolled in the study?

rule. For example, development of a hypothetical prediction rule to assist with identification of thoracic outlet syndrome should include subjects with identifiable and measurable anatomical (e.g., presence of a cervical rib) and behavioral (e.g., upper extremity positioning during sleep) characteristics that may predispose them to this condition rather than to adhesive capsulitis of the shoulder.

TABLE 14-3	Questions to Assess the Evidence About the Validation of Clinical Prediction Rules

1. Did the investigators compare results from the clinical prediction rule to results from an established criterion test or measure of the outcome of interest?
2. Were all subjects evaluated with the criterion test or measure of the outcome the rule is intended to predict?
3. Were the individuals interpreting the results of the clinical prediction rule unaware of the results of the criterion measure and vice versa?
4. Did the investigators confirm their findings with a new set of subjects?
5. Has the clinical prediction rule been validated on a population other than the one for which it originally was designed?

2. Were the subjects representative of the population from which they were drawn?

The issue of representativeness pertains to the degree to which investigators were able to capture all eligible subjects during the time frame of the study. Enrolling some individuals and not others may result in biased estimates that limit the accuracy and utility of the prediction rule. For the hypothetical thoracic outlet syndrome rule, this situation would occur if investigators only enrolled subjects with anatomic contributions to the condition and missed subjects with behavioral contributions to the problem. Of course, investigators cannot force all eligible patients to participate; however, they can perform statistical comparisons between participants and nonparticipants to determine whether the sample is representative of the population of interest. Statistically significant differences between the participants and nonparticipants suggest that biased prognostic estimates may have resulted.

3. Did the investigators include all relevant predictive factors in the development process?

Investigators have a variety of methods for developing a list of potential predictive factors, including patient interviews and focus groups, input from relevant health care providers and content experts, available evidence, and historical patient records. Physical therapists should consider whether the effort to build the list of possible predictors was exhaustive (i.e., were all possible contributors to thoracic outlet syndrome identified) as well as clinically sensible (i.e., the list has *face validity*). Ultimately, a larger list will be winnowed down to a narrower set of factors that have the most predictive value. This culling process should be performed statistically with pre-established criteria for maintaining and eliminating factors during each step of the analysis. Deviation from statistical approaches to selecting predictive factors should be supported by biologically plausible clinical theory.

4. Were the predictive factors operationally defined?

This question addresses the validity of the measures used to identify and quantify the predictive factors. A clear definition of these variables is necessary to correctly identify which subjects have these characteristics and to optimize the accuracy of the prediction rule. Investigators should articulate specific clinical and/or testing criteria prior to the start of data collection. They also should verify that individuals collecting the information are appropriately trained and that their measures are reliable. For the hypothetical thoracic outlet syndrome rule, investigators need to ensure they can accurately identify individuals with (versus without) a cervical rib or a predisposing sleep position, as well as any other potential predictive factors.

5. Did the investigators include a large enough sample size to accommodate the number of predictive factors used to derive the clinical prediction rule?

The issue of sample size is twofold. First, statistical modeling methods such as regression require adequate information to predict the value of an outcome.[17] Even when samples are homogeneous in composition, some individual subjects will not have all of the predictive characteristics of interest (i.e., some individuals will not have a cervical rib but still have symptoms of thoracic outlet syndrome). As a result, a limited amount of data may be available to represent these predictors in the model. Several consequences are possible in this situation including a *type II error* due to lack of *power* or an underspecified model that explains little of the variance in the outcome. Second, the precision of any estimate is improved with more information.[18] The most obvious example of this mathematical reality is a narrow confidence interval when sample sizes are large.

Investigators can anticipate these issues by performing a power analysis as part of the research design phase of the study. Alternatively, they can follow published recommendations regarding the number of cases needed for each predictive factor (e.g., prevalence of individuals with a cervical rib).[3,17] In either case, physical therapists should consider the potential impact of the actual sample size on the accuracy of the findings.

6. Were the outcomes of interest operationally defined?

This question addresses the validity of the measures used to capture the outcome(s) the rule is designed to predict. A clear definition of the outcome(s) is necessary to avoid misidentification—for example, classification of patients as positive for thoracic outlet syndrome when their true diagnosis is carpal tunnel syndrome. Investigators should articulate specific clinical and/or testing criteria prior to the start of data collection. They also should verify that individuals collecting the information are appropriately trained and that their measures are reliable.

7. Were those responsible for measuring the outcomes masked to the status of the predictive factors (and vice versa)?

Tester bias can occur when those responsible for collecting measures have knowledge of previous findings that could influence their interpretation. *Masking* those responsible for identifying and quantifying the predictive factors (e.g., presence or absence of a cervical rib) and those responsible for collecting the outcomes (e.g., presence or absence of thoracic outlet syndrome) reduces the opportunity for tester bias and should improve the prediction rule's accuracy.

When prediction rules are developed using historical patient data, then the clinicians who collected the information can be considered "masked" because they were conducting their usual patient management routines outside of a study framework. In other words, the clinicians had no way to know that future researchers would come along to develop a prediction rule for a specified outcome!

8. Did the investigators collect outcome data from all of the subjects enrolled in the study?

The ability to capture the outcomes from all subjects is important because attrition for any reason may provide a skewed representation of which outcomes occurred and when. Ideally, investigators will be able to determine what happened to subjects who left the study so that they can evaluate whether the outcomes were truly different than for those who remained. Differences between subjects who remained (e.g., individuals for whom sleep position was the primary contributor to thoracic outlet syndrome) and subjects who dropped out (e.g., individuals who developed thoracic outlet syndrome due to a cervical rib) indicate that bias likely has been introduced to the prognostic estimates. Straus et al. describe a "5 and 20 rule" in which the loss of 5% of subjects likely has little impact, whereas the loss of 20% (or more) of subjects will undermine study validity to a considerable extent.[12] Evidence-based physical therapists may then make their own decisions about whether the worst case scenario (i.e., >20% attrition) reflects bias that undermines the study's value.

Clinical Prediction Rule Validation

1. Did the investigators compare results from the clinical prediction rule to results from an established criterion test or measure of the outcome of interest?

This question addresses the need to confirm whether the outcome the rule is intended to predict actually occurred. This process is similar to confirming the validity of a diagnostic test. Ideally, the criterion test or measure will be the *gold standard*, or "best in class," instrument or method (e.g., the definitive method for determining the presence of thoracic outlet syndrome). However, the choice of a criterion is the researchers' prerogative. In any case, the criterion test or measure should have superior capability because of its technological features and/or its own track record of reliability and validity.

2. Were all subjects evaluated with the criterion test or measure of the outcome the rule is intended to predict?

This question clarifies the degree to which the investigators may have introduced bias into the study by administering the criterion test or measure only to subjects who achieved the outcome according to the clinical prediction rule (e.g., those individuals predicted to have thoracic outlet syndrome). As is the case with validation of diagnostic tests, selective comparisons can produce misleading results about the accuracy of the rule because there will be no information about the extent to which true and false negative results occurred when the clinical prediction rule was applied. Remember that the goal is to determine in an objective (i.e., statistical) fashion which pieces of information, in combination, enhance the prognostic estimate. Verification of the predictive model depends on the degree of congruence between the outcome identified by the prediction rule and the outcome captured by the criterion test or measure. Evidence-based physical therapists should be wary of prediction rules that were not evaluated using this design specification.

3. Were the individuals interpreting the results of the clinical prediction rule unaware of the results of the criterion measure and vice versa?

Ideally, the criterion test or measure will be applied by examiners who are masked to the results of the application of the clinical prediction rule for each subject (e.g., individuals who were predicted to have thoracic outlet syndrome versus individuals who were not). The concern for tester bias is the same as described previously.

4. Did the investigators confirm their findings with a new set of subjects?

This question alludes to the possibility that the research findings regarding the clinical prediction rule occurred due to unique attributes of the sample. Repeating the study on a second set of subjects who match the inclusion and exclusion criteria outlined for the first set provides an opportunity to evaluate whether the same combination of factors accurately predicts the outcome of interest. One strategy is to assemble a group of subjects and randomly select half of them to create the prognostic model, which then can be retested on the remaining half. Often, this step is not included in a single research report due to insufficient numbers of subjects (e.g., low prevalence of individuals with symptoms of thoracic outlet syndrome) and/or lack of funds. As a result, evidence-based physical therapists may have to read several pieces of evidence about the same clinical prediction rule if they wish to verify its usefulness to a greater degree.

5. Has the clinical prediction rule been validated on a population other than the one for which it originally was designed?

This question refers to efforts to expand the application of a clinical prediction rule to other patient populations. For example, a rule derived with an adult population might be tested for accuracy with a pediatric population presenting with a similar disorder or condition. The Ottawa Ankle Rules have undergone just such an evaluation.[19]

Additional Considerations

These questions serve as an initial screening of the evidence to determine its potential usefulness—that is, its research validity. From an evaluative standpoint, a "no" answer to any of the questions regarding derivation of the rule may indicate a "fatal flaw" in the research design. A "no" answer to questions 1 to 3 regarding validation of the rule may signal a similar concern. Readers may use more latitude in their analysis with respect to rule validation questions 4 and 5, given that researchers have the prerogative to frame a research question how they wish and to study it within their resource limitations.

Finally, there are additional concerns pertaining to research design in evidence about clinical prediction rules. Specifically, readers should note the presence or absence of a detailed description of the:

1. Setting in which the research was conducted;
2. Protocol for the test(s) and measure(s) used, including scoring methods; and
3. Characteristics of the sample obtained.

This information allows evidence-based physical therapists to determine if the clinical prediction rule of interest is applicable and feasible in their environment (1, 2) and if the subjects included resemble the patient or client about whom there is a question (3). Well-designed studies may have limited usefulness when these details are lacking.

Several authors have proposed a "levels of evidence" model to reflect the different phases of clinical prediction rule derivation and validation (**Figure 14-2**).[4,20] Rules that have been validated across broad populations are ranked more highly than rules limited to narrow populations within specific settings. Unfortunately, validation studies of prediction rules relevant to physical therapy continue to be in short supply.[21] Beneciuk et al. suggest that physical therapists give thoughtful consideration to well-designed derivation studies.[16]

FIGURE 14-2   Levels of evidence of clinical prediction rules.

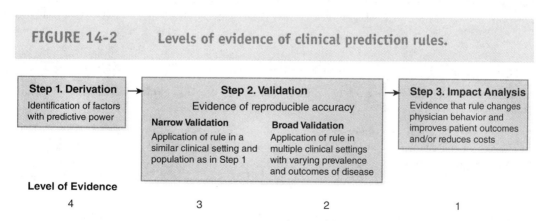

Reprinted from Childs JD, Cleland JA, Development and application of clinical prediction rules to improve decision making in physical therapist practice, *Phys Ther*. 2006;86:122-131, with permission from the American Physical Therapy Association. Copyright © 2006 American Physical Therapy Association.

Study Results

Statistical results from studies pertaining to clinical prediction rules vary depending on which phase of their evolution is being reported. Derivation studies typically use correlation and regression approaches to determine the smallest number of factors that have the most predictive ability for the outcome of interest. Validation studies also may use correlation coefficients to establish the *criterion* and/or *predictive validity* of the rules. In addition, these studies also may report values for sensitivity, specificity, likelihood ratios, and odds ratios. Receiver operating characteristic curves also may be displayed.

The interpretation of these findings is the same as that used for studies about diagnostic tests and prognostic factors. Clinical prediction rules with high *sensitivity* are good at detecting true positives (e.g., patients for whom an x-ray is needed), whereas those with high *specificity* are good at detecting true negatives (e.g., patients for whom an x-ray is not indicated). *Positive* and *negative likelihood ratios* indicate by how much a therapist's initial estimate (*pretest probability*) will change (*posttest probability*) based on which findings are obtained when the clinical prediction rule is applied. *Odds ratios* reflect the increase or decrease in probability of the outcome of interest occurring based on the results from implementation of the rule.

The Statistical Importance of Study Results

As with the other types of evidence, evaluation of the statistical importance or meaningfulness of the results about clinical prediction rules depends on the obtained *p values* and *confidence intervals*. A *p value* indicates the probability that the result obtained occurred due to chance. The smaller the *p* value (e.g., <0.05), the more important the result is statistically because the role of chance is very diminished, although not eliminated. Investigators will indicate their threshold for statistical significance; however, physical therapists should determine whether a *p* value is of sufficient magnitude to be convincing. A *confidence interval* represents a range of scores within which the true score for a variable is estimated to lie within a specified probability (e.g., "I am [90%, 95%, 99%] confident the true value for this variable lies within this range of values I have calculated from my data.").[5] Confidence intervals provide the information necessary to determine the precision of the result (e.g., a likelihood ratio, an odds ratio). Readers are reminded that if a confidence interval includes the value "1," the likelihood ratio or odds ratio is a coin flip (i.e., no better than chance) with respect to its ability to make a meaningful prediction.

Evidence and the Patient or Client

As always, the decision to use evidence during clinical decision making for an individual depends on the following factors:

- The extent to which the patient or client resembles the subjects in the study;
- The extent to which application of the clinical prediction rule is feasible in the physical therapist's setting; and
- The concordance between the options outlined in the study and the patient or client's preferences and values.

Some clinical prediction rules designed to guide treatment may be tied to outcomes that reflect a *minimal clinically important difference* (MCID), a concept that may have particular relevance to patients and clients.

At the individual level, well-designed and validated clinical prediction rules should enhance the efficiency and effectiveness of physical therapist patient/client management.[2,3] At the system and societal levels, rules should facilitate appropriate and judicious use of resources. Several authors have commented on the need for greater impact analysis to determine whether individual clinical prediction rules are living up to their potential to change practice while simultaneously improving patient outcomes.[15,22]

Evidence Appraisal Tools

Table 14-4 provides a checklist to guide the evaluation of evidence about clinical prediction rules. This checklist follows the same format as other appraisal worksheets adapted from the Oxford Centre for Evidence-Based Medicine.[23] The evaluative option "Separate study or studies cited" should be used when the evidence being reviewed focuses on validation of a previously established rule. Authors typically will reference prior work to establish what is known so far and will not repeat the derivation process. The absence of this information or a lack of clarity about the rigor of the derivation process should raise concerns about potential bias introduced during rule development.

TABLE 14-4	Evidence About Clinical Prediction Rules—Quality Appraisal Checklist

Research Validity of the Study

Clinical Prediction Rule Derivation

Did the investigators operationally define the sample in their study?	___ Yes ___ No ___ Insufficient detail ___ Separate study or studies cited
Were the subjects representative of the population from which they were drawn?	___ Yes ___ No ___ Insufficient detail ___ Separate study or studies cited
Did the investigators include all relevant predictive factors in the development process?	___ Yes ___ No ___ Insufficient detail ___ Separate study or studies cited
Were the predictive factors operationally defined?	___ Yes ___ No ___ Insufficient detail ___ Separate study or studies cited
Did the investigators include a large enough sample size to accommodate the number of predictive factors used to derive the clinical prediction rule?	___ Yes ___ No ___ Insufficient detail ___ Separate study or studies cited

(continues)

TABLE 14-4	Evidence About Clinical Prediction Rules—Quality Appraisal Checklist (*Continued*)
Were the outcomes of interest operationally defined?	___ Yes ___ No ___ Insufficient detail ___ Separate study or studies cited
Were those responsible for measuring the outcomes masked to the status of the predictive factors (and vice versa)?	___ Yes ___ No ___ Insufficient detail ___ Separate study or studies cited
Did the investigators collect outcome data from all of the subjects enrolled in the study?	___ Yes ___ No ___ Insufficient detail ___ Separate study or studies cited
Do you have enough confidence in the research validity of this paper to consider using this evidence with your patient or client even if the prediction rule has not been validated?	___ Yes ___ Undecided ___ No

Clinical Prediction Rule Validation

Did the investigators compare results from the clinical prediction rule to results from an established criterion test or measure of the outcome of interest?	___ Comparison to a gold standard test or measure was performed ___ Comparison to another test or measure was performed ___ Comparison was performed but the description is inadequate ___ No comparison was made
Were all subjects evaluated with the criterion test or measure of the outcome the rule is intended to predict?	___ Yes ___ No ___ Insufficient detail
Were the individuals interpreting the results of the clinical prediction rule unaware of the results of the criterion measure and vice versa?	___ Yes ___ No ___ Insufficient detail
Did the investigators confirm their findings with a new set of subjects?	___ Yes ___ No ___ Insufficient detail
Has the clinical prediction rule been validated on a population other than the one for which it originally was designed?	___ Yes ___ No ___ Insufficient detail ___ Not applicable
Do you have enough confidence in the research validity of this paper to consider using this evidence with your patient or client?	___ Yes ___ Undecided ___ No

TABLE 14-4	Evidence About Clinical Prediction Rules—Quality Appraisal Checklist (*Continued*)

Relevant Study Findings

Results reported that are specific to your clinical question:

Sensitivity _____

Specificity _____

+ Likelihood ratio(s) _____

– Likelihood ratio(s) _____

Odds ratio(s) _____

Correlation coefficients _____

Other _____

Statistical significance and/or precision of the relevant study results:

Obtained *p* values for each relevant statistic reported by the authors: _____

Obtained confidence intervals for each relevant statistic reported by the authors: _____

If this clinical prediction rule is specific to diagnostic options, does it have criterion validity?	___ Yes ___ No ___ Mixed results ___ Insufficient detail ___ Not applicable
If this clinical prediction rule is specific to prognostic estimates or plan of care options, does it have predictive validity?	___ Yes ___ No ___ Mixed results ___ Insufficient detail ___ Not applicable

Application of the Evidence to Your Patient or Client

Are there clinically meaningful differences between the subjects in the study and your patient or client?	___ Yes ___ No ___ Mixed results ___ Insufficient detail
Can you apply the clinical prediction rule safely and appropriately in your clinical setting given your current knowledge and skill level and your current resources?	___ Yes ___ No ___ Insufficient description of the techniques used
Does the clinical prediction rule fit within the patient's or client's expressed values and preferences?	___ Yes ___ No ___ Mixed results
Will you use the clinical prediction rule for this patient or client?	___ Yes ___ No

These questions were adapted from the Oxford Centre for Evidence-Based Medicine and applied to physical therapist practice.

Summary

Clinical prediction rules are systematically derived and statistically tested combinations of clinical findings that provide meaningful predictions about an outcome of interest. Use of these rules is intended to enhance physical therapist decision making during the examination process. Evidence about these rules may focus on their derivation, their validation, or both. The most useful clinical prediction rules are those that have (1) the most parsimonious, clinically sensible set of predictive factors; and (2) a demonstrated ability to make accurate predictions about the need for a specific diagnostic test, the odds of a specific prognosis, or the likely response to a specific intervention. In addition, rules whose accuracy has been tested successfully across a wide range of patient populations and clinical settings are considered the "best in class." Ultimately, their promise lies in their ability to effect change in practice habits that translate into improved patient or client outcomes at a lower cost to society.

Exercises

1. Describe the three focus areas of clinical prediction rules. Provide clinical examples relevant to physical therapist practice to illustrate your points.
2. Discuss the challenges of creating an accurate clinical prediction rule that can be readily adopted for use in clinical settings.
3. Discuss the potential sources of bias in the derivation of clinical prediction rules and describe strategies to minimize their influence. Provide clinical examples relevant to physical therapist practice to illustrate your points.
4. Discuss the potential sources of bias in the validation of clinical prediction rules and describe strategies to minimize their influence. Provide clinical examples relevant to physical therapist practice to illustrate your points.
5. Authors of a newly derived (hypothetical) clinical prediction rule for detecting thoracic outlet syndrome report an $R^2 = 32\%$ for the four retained predictive factors. Interpret these findings and discuss what they mean in terms of the rule's usefulness.
6. Differentiate between the sensitivity and specificity of a clinical prediction rule. Provide clinical examples relevant to physical therapist practice to illustrate your points.
7. The hypothetical clinical prediction rule for detecting thoracic outlet syndrome has a positive likelihood ratio of 4.5 and a negative likelihood ratio of 0.90. Interpret these values and discuss what they mean in terms of the rule's usefulness.

References

1. Helewa A, Walker JM. *Critical Evaluation of Research in Physical Rehabilitation: Towards Evidence-Based Practice.* Philadelphia, PA: W.B. Saunders; 2000.
2. Beattie P, Nelson N. Clinical prediction rules: what are they and what do they tell us? *Aust J Physiother.* 2006;52(3):157-163.

3. Childs JD, Cleland JA. Development and application of clinical prediction rules to improve decision-making in physical therapist practice. *Phys Ther.* 2006;86(1):122-131.

4. McGinn TG, Guyatt GH, Wyer PC, et al. Users' guides to the medical literature XXII: how to use articles about clinical decision rules. *JAMA.* 2000;284(1):79-84.

5. Carter RE, Lubinsky J, Domholdt E. *Rehabilitation Research: Principles and Applications.* 4th ed. St. Louis, MO: Elsevier Saunders; 2011.

6. Polit DF, Beck CT. *Nursing Research: Principles and Methods.* 7th ed. Philadelphia, PA: Lippincott Williams & Wilkins; 2003.

7. American Physical Therapy Association. *Guide to Physical Therapist Practice. 3.0.* Available at: http://guide toptpractice.apta.org. Accessed July 16, 2016.

8. Guyatt G, Rennie D. *Users' Guides to the Medical Literature: A Manual for Evidence-Based Clinical Practice.* Chicago, IL: AMA Press; 2002.

9. Portney LG, Watkins MP. *Foundations of Clinical Research: Applications to Practice.* 3rd ed. Upper Saddle River, NJ: Prentice Hall Health; 2009.

10. Chan KBY, Man-Son-Hing M, Molnar FJ, Laupacis A. How well is the clinical importance of study results reported? An assessment of randomized controlled trials. *CMAJ.* 2001;165(9):1197-1202.

11. Herbert R, Jamtvedt G, Hagen KB, Mead J. *Practical Evidence-Based Physiotherapy.* 2nd ed. Edinburgh, Scotland: Elsevier Butterworth-Heinemann; 2011.

12. Straus SE, Richardson WS, Glaziou P, Haynes RB. *Evidence-Based Medicine: How to Practice and Teach EBM.* 3rd ed. Edinburgh, Scotland: Elsevier Churchill Livingstone; 2005.

13. Stiell IG, Greenberg GH, McKnight RD, et al. Decision rules for the use of radiography in acute ankle injuries. Refinement and prospective validation. *JAMA.* 1993;269(9):1127-1132.

14. Laupacis A, Sekar N, Stiell IG. Clinical prediction rules. A review and suggested modifications for methodological standards. *JAMA.* 1997;277(12):488-494.

15. Reilly BM, Evans AT. Translating clinical research into clinical practice: impact of using prediction rules to make decisions. *Ann Intern Med.* 2006;144(3):201-209.

16. Beneciuk JM, Bishop MD, George SZ. Clinical prediction rules for physical therapy interventions: a systematic review. *Phys Ther.* 2009;89(2):114-124.

17. Tabachnik BG, Fidell LS. *Using Multivariate Statistics.* 4th ed. Boston, MA: Allyn & Bacon; 2006.

18. Sim J, Reid N. Statistical inference by confidence intervals: issues of interpretation and utilization. *Phys Ther.* 1999;79(2):186-195.

19. Dowling S, Spooner CH, Liang Y, et al. Accuracy of Ottawa Ankle Rules to exclude fractures of the ankle and midfoot in children: a meta-analysis. *Acad Emerg Med.* 2009;16(4):277-287.

20. Childs JD, Cleland JA. Development and application of clinical prediction rules to improve decision making in physical therapist practice. *Phys Ther.* 2006;86(1):122-131.

21. Stanton TR, Hancock MJ, Maher CG, Koes BW. Critical appraisal of clinical prediction rules that aim to optimize treatment selection for musculoskeletal conditions. *Phys Ther.* 2010;990(6):843-854.

22. Toll DB, Janssen KJM, Vergouwe Y, Moons KGM. Validation, updating and impact of clinical prediction rules: a review. *J Clin Epidemiol.* 2008;61(11):1085-1094

23. Oxford Centre for Evidence-Based Medicine Website. Available at: www.cebm.net. Accessed October 1, 2016.

CHAPTER 15

APPRAISING OUTCOMES RESEARCH

OBJECTIVES

Upon completion of this chapter, the student/practitioner will be able to do the following:

1. Discuss the purposes and potential benefits of outcomes research.

2. Critically evaluate outcomes research, including the

    a. Important questions to ask related to research validity; and

    b. Statistical approaches used.

3. Interpret and apply information provided by the statistical tests and calculations reported.

4. Evaluate p values and confidence intervals to determine the potential importance of reported findings.

5. Discuss considerations related to the application of outcomes research to individual patients or clients.

TERMS IN THIS CHAPTER

Bias: Results or inferences that systematically deviate from the truth "or the processes leading to such deviation."[1(p.251)]

Case-control design: A retrospective epidemiologic research design used to evaluate the relationship between a potential exposure (e.g., risk factor) and an outcome (e.g., disease, disorder); two groups of subjects—one of which has the outcome (i.e., the case) and one which does not (i.e., the control)—are compared to determine which group has a greater proportion of individuals with the exposure.[2]

Cohort design: A prospective epidemiologic research design used to evaluate the relationship between a potential exposure (e.g., risk factor) and an outcome (e.g., disease, disorder); two groups of subjects—one of which has the exposure and one of which does not—are monitored over time to determine who develops the outcome and who does not.[2]

Confidence interval: A range of scores within which the true score for a variable is estimated to lie within a specified probability (e.g., 90%, 95%, 99%).[3]

Confounding variable (also referred to as an *extraneous variable* or *extraneous factor*): A variable (factor) other than the independent variable that is said to influence, or confound, the dependent variable (outcome).[3]

Construct validity: The degree to which a measure matches the operational definition of the concept or construct it is said to represent.[4]

Cross-sectional study: A study that collects data about a phenomenon during a single point in time or once within a defined time interval.[5]

Effectiveness: The extent to which an intervention or service produces a desired outcome under usual clinical conditions.[1]

Effect size: The magnitude of the difference between two mean values; may be standardized by dividing this difference by the pooled standard deviation in order to compare effects measured by different scales.[6]

Efficacy: The extent to which an intervention or service produces a desired outcome under ideal conditions.[1]

Imputation: A term referring to a collection of statistical methods used to estimate missing data.[7]

Longitudinal study: A study that looks at a phenomenon occurring over time.[1]

Measurement reliability: The extent to which repeated measurements agree with one another. Also referred to as "stability," "consistency," and "reproducibility."[4]

Measurement validity: The ability of a test or measure to capture the phenomenon it is designed to capture.[4(p.77)]

Minimal clinically important difference (MCID): "The smallest treatment effect that would result in a change in patient management, given its side effects, costs, and inconveniences."[8(p.1197)]

Nonexperimental design (also referred to as an *observational study*): A study in which controlled manipulation of the subjects is lacking[3]; in addition, if groups are present, assignment is predetermined based on naturally occurring subject characteristics or activities.[5]

Number needed to treat (NNT): The number of subjects treated with an experimental intervention over the course of a study required to achieve one good outcome or prevent one bad outcome.[5]

Outcome: "The actual results of implementing the plan of care that indicate the impact on functioning;" may be measured by the physical therapist or determined by self-report from the patient or client.[9]

Outcomes research: The study of the impact of clinical practice as it occurs in the real world.[3,10,11]

Patient-centered care: Health care that "customizes treatment recommendations and decision making in response to patients' preferences and beliefs. . . . This partnership also is characterized by informed, shared decision making, development of patient knowledge, skills needed for self-management of illness, and preventive behaviors."[12(p.3)]

Prospective design: A research design that follows subjects forward over a specified period of time.

***p* value**: The probability that a statistical finding occurred due to chance.

Quasi-experimental design: A research design in which there is only one subject group or in which randomization to more than one subject group is lacking; controlled manipulation of the subjects is preserved.[13]

Randomized clinical trial (also referred to as a *randomized controlled trial* and a *randomized controlled clinical trial* [RCT])**: A clinical study that uses a randomization process to assign subjects to either an experimental group(s) or a control (or comparison) group. Subjects in the experimental group receive the intervention or preventive measure of interest and then are compared to the subjects in the control (or comparison) group who did not receive the experimental manipulation.[3]

Retrospective design: A study that uses previously collected information to answer a research question.

CLINICAL SCENARIO

Will I Be Able to Resume My Original Exercise Routine?

© Photographee.eu/Shutterstock

Anne has considered the possibility that she will remain susceptible to elbow pain and that she will have to modify her activities or self-care strategies as a result. You have searched the published literature and cannot find an outcomes study that addresses her question. However, you have managed other individuals with similar complaints and have documentation in your electronic medical record system that may provide a clue to her future.

How will you use that information in your discussions with her?

Introduction

The Guide to Physical Therapist Practice 3.0 describes *outcomes* as the "actual results of implementing the plan of care that indicate the impact on functioning."[9] Outcomes may be defined in terms of successful prevention of, remediation of, or adaptation to impairments in body structures and functions, activity limitations, and participation restrictions. The emphasis on *patient-centered care* and the processes of disablement have focused the discussion about outcomes on the latter two person-level concerns.[3,9,12] Physical therapists anticipate outcomes when they develop treatment goals with their patients or clients. They monitor progress toward these targets and adjust their plans of care in response to examination findings and to patient or client self-report. Finally, they document the extent to which patients or clients achieve the desired outcomes during, and at the conclusion of, the episode of care.

As with other elements of the patient/client management model, evidence may inform physical therapists about which person-level outcomes to expect. The available evidence, however, often uses *nonexperimental* research designs that generally are considered suspect because of their greater potential for *bias*.[1,2,5,14] This concern is fueled by research that indicates that *quasi-experimental* and *observational designs* tend to overestimate treatment effects.[15,16] In spite of these limitations, outcomes research has gained relevance in policy discussions pertaining to quality-of-care benchmarking and pay-for-performance initiatives.[17-19] Evidence-based physical therapists must be prepared to engage in these discussions to influence the selection of outcomes against which their practices will be judged. The purpose of this chapter is to provide information about the potential usefulness of nonexperimental studies about outcomes. In addition, considerations for the evaluation of outcomes research are discussed.

Outcomes Research

Outcomes research is the study of the impact of clinical practice as it occurs in the "real world."[3,10,11] By definition, these studies focus on the "end results" experienced by individuals following an episode of care, rather than on the relative *efficacy* or *effectiveness* of specific interventions.[10,20,21] The research designs used in outcomes studies are nonexperimental (or observational); therefore, investigators collect information about the phenomenon of interest without purposefully manipulating subjects.[3] These designs are comparable to those used in studies of prognostic (risk) factors.

Prospective outcome studies may be *cross-sectional* or *longitudinal*. In the former case, data are collected once during a single point in time or a limited time interval to describe the outcomes that occurred for the sample of interest. In the latter case, one or more groups, or cohorts, may be followed over an extended period of time to determine what outcomes occur and who develops them. Their appeal is the ability to establish a temporal sequence in which an intervention clearly precedes an outcome, an arrangement necessary to establish cause and effect. In addition, investigators are able to define the variables to be measured and to standardize data collection processes. Both design elements enhance the ability to answer the research question in a credible and useful manner. However, prospective studies may be logistically challenging in terms of subject identification and enrollment. Investigators must wait until potential subjects reveal themselves by virtue of admission to the clinical facility or service. Depending on referral or procedure volume, the time line for obtaining an adequate sample may be protracted considerably.

Retrospective outcomes studies also may be cross-sectional or longitudinal. The latter approach is preferred because it is the only opportunity to establish a temporal sequence of interventions and outcomes. Retrospective designs commonly are used to take advantage of a wealth of secondary data available in commercial and government health care–related databases.[3,10,21] Commercial databases refer to those developed for use by paying clients—such as Focus on Therapeutic Outcomes (FOTO), Inc.[22] and the Uniform Data System for Medical Rehabilitation—Functional Independence Measure (UDS-FIM)[23]—or to insurance company claims databases. Government sources may be federal or state level and include databases maintained by the National Center for Health Statistics, the Agency for Healthcare Research and Quality, and the Centers for Medicare and Medicaid Services.[24]

The primary advantage of using data from these sources is the large sample size that can be generated in comparison to prospective studies. Large sample sizes enhance the ability of statistical tests to detect a difference if one exists. In addition, estimates of treatment effect are more precise.[3] Depending on the database, it may be possible to make population-level estimates from the data it contains. A secondary benefit to using these databases is the variety of potential variables that may be accessed, including subject demographic characteristics, health service utilization and costs, and some diagnostic information. A third benefit is the opportunity to track subjects longitudinally, which may allow for causal inferences about the relationship between an intervention and an outcome.[21,24] The primary disadvantage of these databases is the lack of meaningful clinical information related to (1) impairments of body structures and function, activity limitations, and participation restrictions; (2) interventions provided; and (3) outcomes achieved.

Retrospective outcomes research also may be conducted using medical records. Assuming adequate documentation by the providers involved, these records can be sources of the clinical details missing in administratively oriented databases (e.g., insurance claims). Unfortunately, abstracting data about a large sample from individual medical records can be time consuming. In addition, the lack of standardization in terms of what and how clinicians document care may make it difficult for researchers to obtain consistent information within one record or across multiple records. These logistical problems can be addressed through the development of clinical data registries. A clinical data registry is "an organized system that uses observational study methods to collect uniform data (clinical and other) to evaluate specified outcomes for a population defined by a particular disease, condition, or exposure, and that serves one or more predetermined scientific, clinical, or policy purposes."[25(p.1)] These vast electronic databases contain a multitude of operationally defined variables that reflect sociodemographic, clinical, and administrative domains of interest to the registry developers. Individual providers, practices, organizations, and patients supply health care–encounter information that allows measurement of the variables in a standardized fashion. Participation usually is voluntary, but may require a fee depending on the services offered. Well-designed registries provide researchers with access to high volumes of standardized, "practice-based" data that provide a richer picture of "real-world" patient/client management and the resulting outcomes.

Table 15-1 provides a sample of outcomes research published in the journal *Physical Therapy* over the last 20 years. These citations reflect the variety of research designs readers will encounter when searching for outcomes studies. Regardless of the approach used, outcomes research should be evaluated in the same manner as evidence about diagnostic tests, prognostic (risk) factors, and interventions. Specifically, physical therapists should consider features of the design that may increase or reduce bias, the nature of the results provided, and their importance in statistical and clinical terms. Finally, findings from outcomes studies must be considered in light of patient or client preferences and values.

Study Credibility

Outcomes research first should be evaluated with the questions itemized in **Table 15-2**. These questions focus on the design elements that may enhance the research validity of observational studies.[26] Their purpose is to help physical therapists determine the extent to which the study's design may have produced biased results.

1. Was this a study with more than one group?

Outcomes studies provide the most information if they include at least two groups: one that received the interventions of interest and one that did not. These designs are analogous to *case-control* and *cohort designs* used in evidence about prognostic (risk) factors. Group comparisons may allow investigators to evaluate the impact of different therapeutic approaches on the outcomes achieved. Subjects are not randomly assigned to these groups; rather, their involvement is predetermined by the approach to their clinical management, which is out of the investigator's control.[5] Group comparisons in observational studies cannot eliminate bias because there may be inherent subject characteristics that influence the selection of the clinical management approach. Nevertheless, these study designs are preferable to single group designs when available.

2. Were the groups comparable at the start of the study?

As is the case with evidence about interventions, a primary concern is the equality of groups at the start of an outcomes study. Baseline equality enhances the researcher's ability to isolate the impact on outcomes, if any, of the interventions of interest. Unfortunately, the absence of random assignment may limit the degree to which subject characteristics may be distributed evenly between groups in

TABLE 15-1	Examples of Outcomes Research Relevant to Physical Therapist Practice

- Beck LA, et al. Functional outcomes and quality of life after tumor-related hemipelvectomy. *Phys Ther.* 2008;88(8):916-927.
- Cleland JA, et al. Predictors of short-term outcome in people with a clinical diagnosis of cervical radiculopathy. *Phys Ther.* 2007;7(12):1619-1632.
- DeJong G, et al. Physical therapy activities in stroke, knee arthroplasty, traumatic brain rehabilitation: their variation, similarities, and association with functional outcomes. *Phys Ther.* 2011;91(12):1826-1837.
- Fritz JM, et al. Utilization and clinical outcomes of outpatient physical therapy for Medicare beneficiaries with musculoskeletal conditions. *Phys Ther.* 2011;91(3):330-345.
- George SZ, et al. Depressive symptoms, anatomical region, and clinical outcomes for patients seeking outpatient physical therapy for musculoskeletal pain. *Phys Ther.* 2011;91(3): 358-372.
- Jewell DV, et al. Interventions associated with an increased or decreased likelihood of pain reduction and improved function in patients with adhesive capsulitis: a retrospective cohort study. *Phys Ther.* 2009;89(5):419-429.
- Magel J, et al. Outcomes of patients with acute low back pain stratified by the STarT Back screening tool: secondary analysis of a randomized trial. *Phys Ther.* 2017;20160298.
- Russell D, et al. Continuity in the provider of home-based physical therapy services and its implications for outcomes of patients. *Phys Ther.* 2012;92(2):227-235.
- Strenk ML, et al. Implementation of a quality improvement initiative improved congenital muscular torticollis outcomes in a large hospital setting. *Phys Ther.* 2017;pzx029.

TABLE 15-2	Questions to Determine the Validity of Outcomes Research

1. Was this a study with more than one group?
2. Were the groups comparable at the start of the study?
3. If the groups were not equal at the start of the study, was risk adjustment performed?
4. Were variables operationally defined and adequately measured by the data used for the study?
5. Were standardized person-level outcomes instruments used?
6. Were standardized data collection methods implemented?
7. Did the interventions of interest precede the outcomes?
8. Were other potentially confounding variables accounted for in the analysis?
9. Were missing data dealt with in an appropriate manner?
10. Did the investigators confirm their findings with a new set of subjects?

an observational study.[26] Investigators can develop and implement specific inclusion and exclusion criteria that may achieve some level of group equality; however, these criteria generally are less stringent than those imposed during *randomized controlled trials*. At a minimum, investigators should perform statistical comparisons to evaluate which, if any, characteristics were different and what these differences mean for their analytic approach and their results.

3. If the groups were not equal at the start of the study, was risk adjustment performed?
Risk adjustment is the process by which outcomes are modified to reflect differences in important subject characteristics. Factors of interest often include, but are not limited to, patient or client age, gender, race/ethnicity, baseline functional or health status, presence of comorbidities, and severity or acuity of the condition of interest. In addition, social and environmental factors, such as family support, household income, and accessible living arrangements, may be used.[27] The ability to adequately risk adjust depends on the availability of data about patient or client characteristics considered relevant to the outcomes of interest. Administrative databases may provide challenges in this regard due to their lack of detailed clinical and physiologic measures. Patient registries, in contrast, usually contain commonly encountered characteristics for which risk adjustment is necessary. A variety of methods for risk adjustment is available to outcomes researchers, the details of which are beyond the scope of this text. To learn more about these approaches, see *Risk Adjustment for Measuring Healthcare Outcomes, Fourth Edition*, by Lisa Iezzoni.[28]

4. Were variables operationally defined and adequately measured by the data used for the study?
The validity of any study is enhanced by the appropriate definition and adequate measurement of its variables. Variables may be concrete observable phenomena such as height, weight, blood pressure, and heart rate. Each of these physiologic parameters has one definition, although there may be multiple ways to measure them. Variables often are more abstract concepts or constructs, however, such as strength, endurance, level of dependence, or health status. Each of these terms has more than one interpretation; therefore, investigators have an obligation to provide their own operational definitions to avoid confusion regarding measurement and the interpretation of subsequent results.

The ability to measure variables adequately in a study depends in part on the *construct validity* of the measurement. This issue is particularly important for outcomes studies that use secondary data for their analyses. These data have been collected for purposes other than health care research. As a result, measures may be irrelevant or inadequately defined for the purposes of a particular study. Under these circumstances, "proxy measures" may be required as substitutes for preferred measures of the variables of interest.[21] A common example is the use of the billing procedure code "therapeutic exercise" as a measure for a physical therapy intervention variable. This code does not provide details pertaining to specific exercise method, intensity, or frequency, making it a blunt instrument at best for discerning the relationship between the treatment and the outcome. Secondary data also may be incomplete and/or inaccurate.[29] Accuracy problems often occur when conditions are labeled using diagnostic codes, in part because the codes are designed to support payment for services. The 2015 implementation of the International Statistical Classification of Diseases and Related Health Problems, 10th edition (ICD-10) should improve outcomes research that is dependent on diagnosis codes due to the expanded number of narrowly defined codes available.[30] However, the temptation to "up-code"—or assign additional diagnostic codes to enhance reimbursement—will continue to make it difficult to know whether these indicators of clinical status are valid.[27]

A related issue is the relative availability of clinical data meaningful to physical therapists. Commercial databases such as FOTO[22] and UDS-FIM[23] are designed to measure patient-level functional performance, such as the ability to transfer, ambulate, and climb stairs. The FIM instrument also provides information about the level of patient effort required to accomplish each functional task.[23] Institutional databases and registries also may be customized to include more detailed clinical measures that are relevant to their practices and market demands. Government and insurance databases, in contrast, often limit clinical detail to diagnostic and procedure codes or to mortality. These are undiscriminating measures that provide limited inferences about the impact of physical therapy on patient outcomes.[21,24,29]

Although the concerns discussed relate to secondary data, this question also should be addressed in prospective designs in which the investigators were able to create their variables and the methods with which they were measured. Important features include clearly articulated operational definitions, rationales for the measures collected, verification of the reliability of data recorders or those collecting measures, and data audits to ensure accuracy and completeness. Inadequacies here decrease the credibility of the evidence and should be noted.

5. Were standardized person-level outcomes instruments used?

One way investigators can enhance the validity of an observational design is to use standardized person-level outcomes tools with established *measurement reliability* and *validity*. An unstable instrument makes it difficult to determine whether the outcomes occurred in response to physical therapy interventions or because of problems with measurement variability. Outcomes measures may be performance based (e.g., balance tests, walk tests) or self-report tools (e.g., health status surveys). In both cases, the issue of "person-level" measures pertains to the focus on activity limitations, participation restrictions, and quality of life that distinguishes outcomes research.

6. Were standardized data collection methods implemented?

Standardized data collection is another method by which investigators may impose some level of control in observational studies. The most control is achieved in prospective designs because investigators can develop and implement their own procedures and forms for real-time data collection. They also may audit these processes to ensure their consistency and integrity. Problems with completeness or accuracy may be corrected as they occur. However, retrospective designs are limited to standardized data abstraction and maintenance procedures. The opportunity to influence the original data recording is, by definition, nonexistent in these studies. As a result, researchers using retrospective designs may find greater challenges with missing or inaccurate data elements.

7. Did the interventions precede the outcomes?

This question reflects an interest in potential causal connections between interventions and outcomes. Randomized clinical trials clearly are best suited to establishing cause and effect relationships because of the purposeful manipulation of the experimental intervention and because of the degree to which potential competing explanations may be managed. By definition, observational studies do not have these features. However, results from prospective and retrospective longitudinal designs may support causal inferences if the sequence of intervention and outcome can be established.[26] An investigator's ability to determine this temporal order depends on the nature and integrity of the data being used, as well as the nature of the phenomenon being studied. For example, a study of the effectiveness of physical therapy for the management of acute ankle sprains likely will be able to demonstrate that the injury preceded the intervention based on the dates on which the diagnosis was established and physical therapy was initiated, respectively. However, chronic conditions such as rheumatoid arthritis or multiple sclerosis, the symptoms of which ebb and flow in their own rhythm, may prove more challenging relative to determining whether the intervention was effective or the subjects experienced natural recovery.

8. Were other potentially confounding variables accounted for in the analysis?

Confounding (or *extraneous*) *variables* are factors that may influence the outcome independent of the interventions provided during an episode of care. By definition, subject characteristics (e.g., age, comorbidities, baseline functional level, etc.) may be confounding variables. However, if risk adjustment has been performed, then these factors have been accounted for. A key exception to this statement is the potential impact of underlying motivations individuals have for selecting one treatment option over another. Time also may influence outcomes due to the potential for natural recovery.

Other possible confounders in outcomes studies include characteristics of the health care providers and/or clinical facilities in which service occurs. For example, physical therapists may have varying professional degrees, specializations, amounts of experience, and so forth. If the study is large enough that the interventions of interest are provided by different therapists, then these factors may be important because they may influence how treatment is delivered. Similarly, clinical facilities may have different staff-to-patient ratios, skill mixes, payer mixes, and so on. Studies that use data from multiple sites also may require consideration of these factors because they may influence decision making regarding the frequency of service delivery and the time spent with the patient or client.

Investigators conducting outcomes research should identify potential confounding influences and account for them in their statistical analyses. Commonly used approaches are stratifying the analysis according to subgroups (e.g., different subject age groups or different levels of therapist experience) or by adding these factors as control variables in a multivariate statistical model.[26]

9. Were missing data dealt with in an appropriate manner?

As noted earlier, missing data is a common challenge with secondary databases. Investigators have several options for dealing with missing data. First, they may exclude cases with incomplete information from the analysis. This strategy is perhaps the most forthright, but it may introduce bias by creating a sample that is predisposed to a particular outcome. Sample sizes also are decreased when cases are excluded, a situation that may result in lack of statistical power to detect a difference in outcomes if it is present. Second, investigators may estimate missing values through statistical methods referred to as *imputation*.[7] These techniques may be as simple as averaging surrounding values and as complex as regression modeling. Error may be introduced in this process, but investigators may accept this consequence to preserve sample size and composition. At a minimum, researchers should report how much of the data were missing so that readers can make their own qualitative judgments about the nature and extent of the potential bias introduced and/or the potential impact on statistical power.

10. Did investigators confirm their findings with a new set of subjects?

This question alludes to the possibility that the research findings regarding outcomes occurred due to unique attributes of the sample. Repeating the study on a second set of subjects who match the inclusion and exclusion criteria outlined for the first set provides an opportunity to evaluate whether the same outcomes occurred to the same degree. One strategy is to assemble a group of subjects and randomly select half of them to evaluate the outcomes and then repeat the analysis on the remaining half. This approach is easiest to implement in retrospective designs using large databases with many patient cases. Otherwise, evidence-based physical therapists may have to read several pieces of evidence about the same outcomes if they wish to verify the results to a greater degree.

Additional Considerations

The previous questions serve as an initial screening of the evidence to determine its potential usefulness—that is, its research validity. From an evaluative standpoint, a "no" answer to any of questions 1 through 9 may indicate a "fatal flaw" in the research design. Readers may use more latitude in their analysis with respect to question 10, given that researchers must conduct their studies within their resource limitations.

In addition to the 10 questions just itemized, concerns pertaining to study design in outcomes research include the presence or absence of a detailed description of the:

1. Setting in which the research was conducted;
2. Protocol for the tests, measures, and intervention(s) used; and
3. Characteristics of the sample obtained.

This information allows evidence-based physical therapists to determine if the outcomes of interest are possible in their environment (1, 2) and if the subjects included resemble the patient or client about whom there is a question (3).

Study Results

Outcomes studies may use the variety of statistical analyses included in evidence about diagnostic tests, prognostic factors, or interventions. These techniques include tests of differences and tests of relationships as well as calculations of various ratios and *effect sizes*. Tests of differences are appropriate for both between-group and within-group (e.g., single group) designs. Tests of relationships usually are regression analyses used to predict the level of an outcome given the presence of an intervention or interventions. A common approach is to use multivariate models to control for possible confounding variables.[24] Statistical test results that indicate a dose–response relationship (e.g., an increased volume of exercise is associated with an increased functional performance level) are of particular interest. The presence of this association provides added support for a causal link between interventions and outcomes.[26] Finally, a calculation of ratios provides information about the magnitude of an effect or relationship.

The Statistical Importance of Study Results

Evaluation of the statistical importance or meaningfulness of the results from outcomes studies depends on the obtained *p values* and *confidence intervals*. Investigators indicate their threshold for statistical significance; however, physical therapists should determine whether a *p* value is of sufficient magnitude to be convincing. Confidence intervals provide the information necessary to determine the precision of the result within the specified probability.[3] Interpretation of confidence intervals for ratios is different than for measures of effect size. In the former case, an interval that includes the value "1" indicates that the result may be due to chance. In the latter case, an interval that includes the value "0" indicates that the true effect may be no change at all.

In addition to the statistical importance of the results, proponents of evidence-based medicine and practice acknowledge that "large" effects or "strong" relationships reported in observational studies should not be ignored, especially in cases where harmful outcomes are demonstrated.[5,14] There is no consensus about the minimum thresholds for "large" or "strong," so a commonsense judgment about the magnitude of the value in question is needed.

Evidence and the Patient or Client

As always, the decision to use evidence during clinical decision making for an individual depends on the following factors:

1. The extent to which the patients or clients resemble the subjects in the study;
2. The extent to which the interventions and outcomes of interest are feasible in the physical therapist's setting; and
3. The concordance between the options outlined in the study and the patient's or client's preferences and values.

Outcomes research may have an edge over other forms of evidence with respect to the first item because inclusion and exclusion criteria tend to be less stringent than those used in randomized controlled trials.[10,14,15,31] As a result, samples tend to be more representative of populations typically served in clinical settings. With respect to preferences and values, physical therapists may find it helpful to discuss a *minimal clinically important difference (MCID)* threshold with the patient or client to determine the acceptable amount of change. If outcome event rates are reported in the study, then it also may be possible to calculate the *number needed to treat (NNT)* to determine how much effort may be required to achieve the desired effect.

Ultimately, using evidence about outcomes requires physical therapists to integrate their critical-appraisal skills with their clinical judgment, perhaps more than would be the case when the evidence is a randomized clinical trial. Observational research designs are full of potential for bias that should not be ignored or overlooked. Nevertheless, the premise of this text is that these studies constitute evidence that may be more relevant to the circumstances in which patient/client management occurs. Careful evaluation of these studies' merits and thoughtful deliberation about their findings, are reasonable and appropriate strategies given that outcomes research is nonexperimental in form. Physical therapists should inform their patients or clients about the relative limitations of these studies so that truly informed decisions may occur.

Evidence Appraisal Tools

Table 15-3 provides a checklist to guide the evaluation of outcomes research. This form also may be used to critique studies using quasi-experimental designs. Answers to these questions should be considered in the context of the debate about the relative merits of experimental, quasi-experimental, and nonexperimental studies.

TABLE 15-3	Outcomes Research and Nonrandomized Trials: Quality Appraisal Checklist
Research Validity of the Study	
Was this a study with more than one group?	___ Yes
	___ No
	___ Insufficient detail
Were the groups comparable at the start of the study?	___ Yes
	___ No
	___ Insufficient detail
	___ Not applicable
If the groups were not equal at the start of the study, was risk adjustment performed?	___ Yes
	___ No
	___ Insufficient detail
	___ Not applicable
Were variables operationally defined and adequately measured by the data used for the study?	___ Yes
	___ No
	___ Insufficient detail

(continues)

TABLE 15-3   Outcomes Research and Nonrandomized Trials: Quality Appraisal Checklist (*Continued*)

Were standardized person-level outcomes instruments used?
___ Yes
___ No
___ Insufficient detail

Were standardized data collection methods implemented?
___ Yes
___ No
___ Insufficient detail

Research Validity of the Study

Did the interventions of interest precede the outcomes?
___ Yes
___ No
___ Insufficient detail

Were other potentially confounding variables accounted for in the analysis?
___ Yes
___ No
___ Insufficient detail

Were missing data dealt with in an appropriate manner?
___ Yes
___ No
___ Insufficient detail

Did the investigators confirm their findings with a new set of subjects?
___ Yes
___ No
___ Insufficient detail

Do you have enough confidence in the research validity of this paper to consider using this evidence with your patient or client?
___ Yes
___ Undecided
___ No

Relevant Study Findings

Results reported that are specific to your clinical question:

Test(s) of differences _____

Test(s) of relationships _____

Effect size(s) _____

Absolute benefit increase(s) _____

Relative benefit increase(s) _____

Absolute risk reduction(s) _____

Relative risk reduction(s) _____

Number needed to treat (harm) _____

Other _____

TABLE 15-3	Outcomes Research and Nonrandomized Trials: Quality Appraisal Checklist (*Continued*)

Statistical significance and/or precision of the relevant study results:

Obtained *p* values for each relevant statistic reported by the authors: _____

Obtained confidence intervals for each relevant statistic reported by the authors: _____

Do these findings exceed a minimal clinically important difference?	___ Yes
	___ No
	___ Insufficient detail
Application of the Evidence to Your Patient or Client	
Are there clinically meaningful differences between the subjects in the study and your patient or client?	___ Yes
	___ No
	___ Mixed results
	___ Insufficient detail
Can you perform the interventions of interest safely and appropriately in your clinical setting given your current knowledge and skill level and your current resources?	___ Yes
	___ No
	___ Insufficient description of the techniques used
Do the interventions of interest fit within your patient's or client's expressed values and preferences?	___ Yes
	___ No
	___ Mixed results
Do the outcomes fit within your patient's or client's expressed values and preferences?	___ Yes
	___ No
	___ Mixed results
Do the potential benefits outweigh the potential risks of using the interventions of interest with your patient or client?	___ Yes
	___ No
	___ Mixed results
Will you use the interventions of interest for this patient or client?	___ Yes
	___ No

These questions were adapted from the Oxford Centre for Evidence-Based Medicine and applied to physical therapist practice.[32]

Summary

Outcomes are the end results of physical therapy patient/client management. The focus on patient-centered care and the disablement process reinforces the need to understand treatment effectiveness in terms that are meaningful to the patient or client. Evidence in the form of outcomes research is challenging to use because of the vulnerability to bias inherent in its nonexperimental designs. Access to large samples from administrative databases and clinical data registries may overcome some of the concerns because of the volume of data involved and the potential for greater standardization of the information included. As a result, these studies constitute evidence worth considering, given their reflection of "real-world" physical therapist practice.

Exercises

1. Discuss the benefits and challenges of using nonexperimental research to evaluate outcomes of physical therapy interventions. Provide a clinical example relevant to physical therapist practice to illustrate your points.
2. Discuss the trade-off between prospective and retrospective design options in outcomes research. Provide a clinical example relevant to physical therapist practice to illustrate your points.
3. Discuss the benefits and challenges of using secondary data to conduct outcomes research. Provide a clinical example relevant to physical therapist practice to illustrate your points.
4. Define risk adjustment and the patient or client factors used in the adjustment process. Provide a clinical example relevant to physical therapist practice to illustrate your points.
5. Explain why risk adjustment is necessary when comparing outcomes. Provide a clinical example relevant to physical therapist practice to illustrate your points.
6. Discuss the philosophy behind the use of "person-level" measures in outcomes research. Provide a clinical example relevant to physical therapist practice to illustrate your points.
7. Describe the circumstances necessary to make causal inferences in outcomes research. Provide a clinical example relevant to physical therapist practice to illustrate your points.
8. Discuss the role confounding variables may play in outcomes research and the methods used to control them. Provide a clinical example relevant to physical therapist practice to illustrate your points.

References

1. Helewa A, Walker JM. *Critical Evaluation of Research in Physical Rehabilitation: Towards Evidence-Based Practice.* Philadelphia, PA: W.B. Saunders; 2000.
2. Guyatt G, Rennie D. *Users' Guides to the Medical Literature: A Manual for Evidence-Based Clinical Practice.* 3rd ed. Chicago, IL: AMA Press; 2014.
3. Carter RE, Lubinsky J, Domholdt E. *Rehabilitation Research: Principles and Applications.* 4th ed. St. Louis, MO: Elsevier Saunders; 2011.
4. Portney LG, Watkins MP. *Foundations of Clinical Research: Applications to Practice.* 3rd ed. Upper Saddle River, NJ: Prentice Hall Health; 2009.
5. Straus SE, Richardson WS, Glaziou P, Haynes RB. *Evidence-Based Medicine: How to Practice and Teach EBM.* 3rd ed. Edinburgh, Scotland: Elsevier Churchill Livingstone; 2005.
6. Batavia M. *Clinical Research for Health Professionals: A User-Friendly Guide.* Boston, MA: Butterworth-Heinemann; 2001.

7. Tabachnik BG, Fidell LS. *Using Multivariate Statistics.* 4th ed. Boston, MA: Allyn & Bacon; 2006.

8. Chan KBY, Man-Son-Hing M, Molnar FJ, Laupacis A. How well is the clinical importance of study results reported? An assessment of randomized controlled trials. *CMAJ.* 2001;165(9):1197-1202.

9. American Physical Therapy Association. *Guide to Physical Therapist Practice 3.0.* Available at: http://guidetoptpractice.apta.org. Accessed July 16, 2016.

10. Silverman SL. From randomized controlled trials to observational studies. *Am J Med.* 2009;122(2):115-120.

11. Matchar DB, Rudd AG. Health policy and outcomes research 2004. *Stroke.* 2005;36(2):225-227.

12. Greiner AC, Knebel E, eds. *Health Professions Education: A Bridge to Quality.* Institute of Medicine website. Available at: https://www.nap.edu/read/10681/chapter/1. Accessed March 1, 2017.

13. Cook TD, Campbell DT. *Quasi-Experimentation: Design and Analysis Issues for Field Settings.* Boston, MA: Houghton Mifflin; 1979.

14. Herbert R, Jamtvedt G, Hagen KB, Mead J. *Practical Evidence-Based Physiotherapy.* 2nd ed. Edinburgh, Scotland: Elsevier Butterworth-Heinemann; 2011.

15. Britton A, McKee M, Black N, et al. Choosing between randomized and non-randomized studies: a systematic review. *Health Technol Assess.* 1998;2(13):i-iv, 1-124.

16. MacLehose RR, Reeves BC, Harvey IM, et al. A systematic review of comparisons of effect sizes derived from randomized and nonrandomized studies. *Health Technol Assess.* 2000;4(34):1-154.

17. Measuring Performance. National Quality Forum website. Available at: www.qualityforum.org/Measuring_Performance/Measuring_Performance.aspx. Accessed March 1, 2017.

18. Medicare Hospital Value-Based Purchasing. Centers for Medicare and Medicaid website. Available at: www.cms.gov/Medicare/Quality-Initiatives-Patient-Assessment-Instruments/hospital-value-based-purchasing/index.html. Accessed March 1, 2017.

19. Jette AM. Outcomes research: shifting the dominant research paradigm in physical therapy. *Phys Ther.* 1995;75:965-970.

20. Dissemination of Patient-Centered Outcomes Research (PCOR). Agency for Healthcare Research and Quality website. Available at: https://www.ahrq.gov/pcor/dissemination-of-pcor/index.html. Accessed March 1, 2017.

21. Iezzoni LI. Using administrative data to study persons with disabilities. *Millbank Q.* 2002;80(2):347-379.

22. Focus on Therapeutic Outcomes, Incorporated. Available at: www.fotoinc.com. Accessed March 1, 2017.

23. Functional Independence Measure. Uniform Data System for Medical Rehabilitation website. Available at: www.udsmr.org. Accessed March 1, 2017.

24. Freburger JK, Konrad TR. The use of federal and state databases to conduct health services research related to physical and occupational therapy. *Arch Phys Med Rehabil.* 2002;83(6):837-845.

25. Gliklich RE, Dreyer NA, ed. *Registries for Evaluating Patient Outcomes.* 2nd ed. Rockville, MD: Agency for Healthcare Research and Quality; 2010.

26. Grimes DA, Schulz KF. Bias and causal associations in observational research. *Lancet.* 2002;359(9302):248-252.

27. Iezzoni LI. Risk adjusting rehabilitation outcomes. *Am J Phys Med Rehabil.* 2004;83(4):316-326.

28. Iezzoni LI, ed. *Risk Adjustment for Measuring Health Care Outcomes.* 4th ed. Chicago, IL: Health Administration Press; 2012.

29. Retchin SM, Ballard DJ. Commentary: establishing standards for the utility of administrative claims data. *Health Serv Res.* 1998;32(6):861-866.

30. ICD-10. Centers for Medicare and Medicaid Services website. Available at: https://www.cms.gov/Medicare/coding/ICD10/index.html. Accessed March 1, 2017.

31. Concato J. Observational versus experimental studies: what's the evidence for a hierarchy? *NeuroRx.* 2004;1(3):341-347.

32. Oxford Centre for Evidence-Based Medicine website. Available at: www.cebm.net. Accessed October 1, 2016.

CHAPTER 16

APPRAISING EVIDENCE ABOUT SELF-REPORT OUTCOMES MEASURES

OBJECTIVES

Upon completion of this chapter, the student/practitioner will be able to do the following:

1. Discuss the contributions of self-report outcomes measures to physical therapist patient/client management.

2. Critically appraise evidence about the development and measurement properties of self-report outcomes measures, including

   a. Important questions to ask related to research validity; and

   b. Statistical approaches used.

3. Interpret and apply information provided by the following calculations:

   a. Cronbach's alpha (α);

   b. Effect size;

   c. Factor analysis;

   d. Floor and ceiling effects;

   e. Intraclass correlation coefficient;

   f. Kappa (κ);

   g. Minimal detectable change;

   h. Minimal clinically important difference; and

   i. Standardized response mean.

4. Evaluate p values and confidence intervals to determine the potential importance of reported findings.

5. Discuss considerations related to the application of evidence about self-report outcomes measures to individual patients or clients.

TERMS IN THIS CHAPTER

Agreement: A form of measurement reliability that indicates how close repeated measures are to one another.[1]

Bias: Results or inferences that systematically deviate from the truth "or the processes leading to such deviation."[2(p.251)]

Ceiling effect: A limitation of a measure in which the instrument does not register a further increase in score for the highest scoring individuals.[3]

Clinimetric properties (also referred to as *psychometric properties*): The measurement characteristics of surveys or other indexes used in clinical practice to obtain patients' perspectives about an aspect (or aspects) of their condition or situation.

Confidence interval: A range of scores within which the true score for a variable is estimated to lie within a specified probability (e.g., 90%, 95%, 99%).[3]

Construct validity: The degree to which a measure matches the operational definition of the concept or construct it is said to represent.[4]

Content validity: The degree to which items in an instrument represent all of the facets of the variable being measured.[3]

Criterion validity: The degree to which a measure of interest relates to a measure with established validity ("criterion measure").[5]

Discriminant validity: A method of construct validation that reflects the degree to which an instrument can distinguish between or among different phenomena or characteristics.[5]

Effect size: The magnitude of the difference between two mean values; may be standardized by dividing this difference by the pooled standard deviation to compare effects measured by different scales.[6]

Factor analysis: A statistical method used to identify a concise set of variables, or factors, from a large volume of data.[3]

Floor effect: A limitation of a measure in which the instrument does not register a further decrease in score for the lowest scoring individuals.[3]

Internal consistency: The degree to which subsections of an instrument measure the same concept or construct.[5]

Measurement reliability: The extent to which repeated measurements agree with one another. Also referred to as "stability," "consistency," and "reproducibility."[4]

Measurement validity: The degree to which a measure captures what it is intended to measure.[4]

Minimal clinically important difference (MCID): "The smallest treatment effect that would result in a change in patient management, given its side effects, costs, and inconveniences."[7(p.1197)]

Minimal detectable change (MDC): The amount of change that just exceeds the standard error of measurement of an instrument.[4]

Nonexperimental design (also referred to as an *observational study*): A study in which controlled manipulation of the subjects is lacking[3]; in addition, if groups are present, assignment is predetermined based on naturally occurring subject characteristics or activities.[5]

Outcomes: "The actual results of implementing the plan of care that indicate the impact on functioning;" may be measured by the physical therapist or determined by self-report from the patient or client.[8]

***p* value**: The probability that a statistical finding occurred due to chance.

Reproducibility (also referred to as *test–retest reliability*): The stability of a measure as it is repeated over time.[3]

Responsiveness: The ability of a measure to detect change in the phenomenon of interest.[9]

Standard error of measurement (SEM): The extent to which observed scores are disbursed around the true score; "the standard deviation of measurement errors" obtained from repeated measures.[3(p.482)]

Standardized response mean (SRM): An indicator of responsiveness based on the difference between two scores (or the "change score") on an outcomes instrument.

CLINICAL SCENARIO

Does All That Paperwork Really Help You Manage My Elbow Pain?

That was Anne's question after completing several forms related to her medical history, her current problems, and her insurance during her initial visit with you. What she does not know is that you also want her to complete a standardized self-report instrument about the impact of her elbow pain on her daily function. You have selected the QuickDASH* for that purpose.

How will you explain your reasons for selecting this survey and the role her answers will play in your clinical decision making?

*About the QuickDASH. The Disabilities of the Arm, Shoulder, Hand (DASH) Outcome Measure website. Available at: http://www.dash.iwh.on.ca/about-quickdash. Accessed March 1, 2017.

© Photographee.eu/Shutterstock

Introduction

Physical therapists have a variety of motivations for measuring the *outcomes* of patient/client management. Assessment of outcomes may provide indications of progress over an episode of care for individual patients or clients. They also may be used to benchmark the quality of physical therapist services for specific conditions such as low back pain, dizziness, or frailty. Outcomes may be captured through a physical therapist's objective examination (i.e., performance-based measures) or through the patient's or client's perceptions about his or her status (i.e., self-report measures), or both (**Table 16-1**). Essential to this effort is the selection and application of instruments with established

TABLE 16-1	Examples of Outcomes Measures Used in Physical Therapist Practice	
Measure	**Type**	**Purpose**
Five times sit to stand test	Performance based	Tests functional strength of the lower extremities
Functional gait assessment	Performance based	Tests postural stability during a variety of walking tasks
Six-minute walk test	Performance based	Submaximal test of aerobic capacity/ endurance
Timed up & go	Performance based	Assesses mobility, balance, walking ability, and fall risk in older adults
Fear Avoidance Beliefs Questionnaire (FABQ)	Self-report (condition specific)	Measures fear of pain and resulting avoidance of physical activity
Lower Extremity Functional Scale (LEFS)	Self-report (body region specific)	Measures perceived impact of a condition on lower extremity function and mobility
Parkinson Disease Activities of Daily Living Scale (PADLS)	Self-report (condition specific)	Measures perceived impact of Parkinson's disease on performance of activities of daily living
Short Form 12 (v2) Health Survey (SF12v2)	Self-report (generic)	Measures health-related quality of life

Shirley Ryan AbilityLab

measurement reliability and *validity*. This challenge is the same demand that researchers face when determining the best way to measure the variables in their studies. Evidence may be used to assist decision making regarding the selection of outcomes measures for practice.

Studies pertaining to any type of measure have *nonexperimental designs* and often are referred to collectively as "methodologic research." Their goal is to document how an instrument was developed and/or to establish its measurement properties with subjects representing the population of patients or clients for whom it is intended. All measures have some degree of error with which they are associated (i.e., the *standard error of measurement*). If that error is not understood, then interpretation of the results is problematic because it is not possible to know if the result obtained is the "true" score. An instrument that has demonstrated reliability, validity, and responsiveness is useful to investigators and to clinicians because measurement error is defined and can be accounted for.

All measures physical therapists use may be evaluated for measurement reliability, validity, and responsiveness. The application of these concepts to patient self-report measures used to capture person-level outcomes is described here. The goal is to help physical therapists evaluate evidence about the development and implementation of these survey instruments so they may make informed decisions about which measures to use with their patients or clients.

Important Clinimetric Properties

Clinimetric properties is a term used to describe the measurement characteristics of surveys or other indexes used to obtain individuals' perspectives about an aspect (or aspects) of their condition or

TABLE 16-2	**Questions About Important Clinimetric Properties of Self-Report Outcomes Measures**

1. Did the investigators provide an adequate description of the survey development process, including identification of participants and methods for item development and selection?
2. Is the self-report instrument of interest easy to administer?
3. Is the self-report instrument of interest reliable?
4. Is the self-report instrument of interest valid?
5. Is the self-report instrument of interest responsive?
6. Can scores on the self-report instrument of interest be interpreted in a meaningful way?
7. If there is more than one method for administering the self-report instrument of interest, did the authors reexamine its measurement properties (questions 2–6) for each mode?
8. If the self-report instrument of interest is being considered for use in other cultures or languages, did the authors reexamine its measurement properties (questions 2–6) under these new conditions?

situation. Evidence about self-report measures (also referred to as "patient reported outcomes," or PROs) varies with respect to which clinimetric properties are evaluated based on the specific research questions posed. Some investigators create and assess brand new instruments; others test previously established instruments under new circumstances. As a result, the appraisal of evidence about self-report outcomes measures focuses on both instrument development and performance. Issues of potential bias relate to methods in both the development and testing phases. The evaluative criteria used in this text are those recommended by the Scientific Advisory Committee of the Medical Outcomes Trust in 2002 (**Table 16-2**).[10] Comparable appraisal guidelines developed using a qualitative research approach also have been published by Mokkink et al.[11]

1. Did the investigators provide an adequate description of the self-report instrument development process, including identification of participants and methods for item development and selection?

Evidence about the development of a new self-report instrument should include a description of the phenomenon to be captured. Disability, health status, and health-related quality of life are the person-level outcomes of interest most commonly addressed. These abstractions require operational definitions, preferably with a description of an underlying theoretical framework, if they are to be measured successfully. The instrument's scope also should be described. Surveys may be written generically so that they can be used for individuals with a variety of conditions. Alternatively, they may be designed to focus on a specific condition or body region.[12]

Once these features have been determined, then investigators start the item development process. The goal is to create an instrument that asks both the right type and the right number of questions to capture the phenomenon of interest. The use of focus groups of patients and/or providers is a common strategy to generate survey questions. This qualitative approach may be supplemented by the use of statistical methods to organize items into common themes. Investigators should describe both of these processes, including the characteristics of participants and criteria used to determine whether to keep or eliminate items. Readers should consider whether the methods are consistent with the research question, as well as the degree to which researchers controlled for *bias* in participant responses.

Additional features of the instrument, such as the style of questions (open versus closed ended) and the ease with which subjects can read and understand them, should be reported. The type and method for scoring individual items, subsets of items (subscales), and the entire instrument also should be described. Finally, investigators should make clear in which direction scores move as subjects improve or decline. A 0 to 100 scale in one instrument may have the anchors "0 = inability to function" and "100 = maximum function," respectively. Another instrument with the same numerical scale may be anchored in the opposite direction, or "0 = no disability" and "100 = maximum disability." Readers should carefully note this information to avoid confusion when interpreting results of a study or an individual's own self-report.

2. Is the self-report instrument of interest easy to administer?

Developers of self-report instruments must balance the need for adequate measurement of the phenomenon with the practical realities of the clinical environment. A survey with many questions may be a disincentive to patients or clients, and to physical therapists, because of the time required to complete it. Similarly, the comprehension level needed to understand the questions should be as accessible as possible to the widest range of individual cognitive abilities. The extent to which cultural context and preferred language will influence understanding and response also should be factored into the survey development process. An additional administrative challenge may be the resources required to score the instrument. The need for a computer or complex mathematical transformations may dissuade clinicians from adopting an otherwise useful outcome measure.[13] Investigators should provide information about all of these issues.

Physical therapists understandably want to see the self-report instrument while they are reading the evidence about it. If it is included, then clinicians have the opportunity to judge for themselves what administrative demands may be required. Unfortunately, instrument ownership issues often preclude full publication.

3. Is the self-report instrument of interest reliable?

The reliability of a self-report instrument may be established by testing for internal consistency, reproducibility, and agreement. *Internal consistency* reflects the degree to which subsections of a survey measure the same concept or construct.[5] In other words, questions within one domain (e.g., physical function, emotional function, social function) of the survey should be highly correlated with one another but not with items in other dimensions. *Reproducibility* reflects the stability of repeated scores from respondents presumed to be unchanged over a specified period of time.[3] *Agreement* indicates how close repeated measures are to one another.[1] By definition, demonstrating these latter forms of reliability requires at least two administrations of the survey. Ideally, investigators provide a detailed description of the methods used to establish reliability, as well as the characteristics of the subjects used and the conditions under which they were tested. Researchers conducting validation studies of established questionnaires may cite previously published articles to affirm the reliability of the instrument of interest.

4. Is the self-report instrument of interest valid?

Validity usually is examined on three fronts: content, construct, and criterion. *Content validity* is the degree to which items in an instrument represent all of the facets of the variable being measured.[3] In other words, if the survey is intended to measure the health-related quality of life of individuals with Parkinson's disease, then items should be phrased to reflect the experiences of individuals with this condition (e.g., stiffness interfering with movement or balance). The primary way in which content validity is established is by inviting content experts to help develop and/or comment on items the investigators hope to use. These experts may be clinicians, patients, caregivers, or some combination of members from these groups.

Construct validity is the degree to which a measure matches the operational definition of the concept or construct it is said to represent.[3] This approach to validity is theory driven. For example, investigators may hypothesize that individuals with Parkinson's disease have restrictions in physical and social function due to the symptoms of their condition. If this is the case, then the survey should contain questions that capture the constructs "physical function" and "social function." A form of construct validity known as *discriminant validity* may be demonstrated if individuals with higher severity levels consistently report lower functioning on these subscales, as compared to individuals with milder forms of the disease.

Criterion validity reflects the degree to which a measure of interest relates to an external criterion measure.[5] This is the same form of validity that is examined when diagnostic tests or clinical measures of impairment or function are compared to "gold standard" or "reference standard" tests. The challenge is to find the best-in-class self-report instrument against which to judge the self-report measure of interest. The most commonly used criterion measure is the Medical Outcomes Study Short Form-36 because of its demonstrated reliability and validity in a variety of patient populations around the world. The survey also has been norm referenced on healthy subjects.[14]

As with reliability, investigators should describe the methods by which they examined instrument validity, including the characteristics of the subjects they used and the conditions under which they were tested.

5. Is the self-report instrument of interest responsive?

Responsiveness is the ability of a measure to detect change in the phenomenon of interest. "Change" may be defined simply as the smallest amount of difference the instrument can detect.[4,9] A responsive instrument registers change beyond measurement error (i.e., the *minimal detectable change*). In addition, the degree to which an instrument can be responsive depends in part on the scale that is used to measure the phenomenon. The more values on the scale of the instrument, the greater the opportunity to detect change when it occurs. Survey developers should provide a rationale for the range of their response scale (i.e., 0 to 3 versus 0 to 10). *Floor* and *ceiling effects* occur when the scale of the measure does not register a further decrease or increase in scores for the lowest or highest scoring individuals, respectively.[3] Investigators should report which survey questions demonstrated floor and ceiling effects, along with the criteria used to maintain or eliminate problematic items.

6. Can scores on the self-report instrument of interest be interpreted in a meaningful way?

Interpretability is defined as "the degree to which one can assign qualitative meaning—that is, clinical or commonly understood connotations—to an instrument's quantitative scores or change in scores."[15] From a qualitative perspective, the interpretation of scores starts with an analysis of the data's distribution in the context of various influences the subjects experience, such as the initiation of treatment, the exacerbation of symptoms, the start of a new activity, and so on. Comparisons also may be made across subgroups of condition severity level or functional status. In both cases, the scores should reflect the meaning of the event or influence.[10] In other words, health-related quality of life would be anticipated to improve if an intervention is effective and to worsen if symptoms flare up. Comparisons with results from other studies using similar subjects and circumstances also may aid in the interpretation process.

From a quantitative perspective, investigators may identify the minimal amount of change in the measure that is required to be meaningful.[16] "Meaningfulness" is reflected by the concept of a *minimal clinically important difference (MCID)*. The MCID is defined as "the smallest treatment effect that would result in a change in patient management, given its side effects, costs, and inconveniences."[7(p.1197)] The MCID may be defined in an objective or subjective way. For example, investigators may compare a change in survey score to a change in a performance-based measure, such as a walk test or balance test. Patients or clients also may express their own values with respect to the meaning of survey scores over time, in which case the minimal amount of change required to be clinically relevant may be different. Investigators should report how this minimal threshold for change was determined and which meaning they are using.

Other Circumstances

Questions 7 and 8 in Table 16-2 reflect the need to repeat assessments of clinimetric properties when the self-report instrument will be used under conditions different from those under which it was originally developed. These new circumstances may include translation into a different language, administration in a different format (such as oral rather than written), or administration to a different population. All of the same evaluative criteria apply in these situations.

A related issue is whether investigators confirmed their findings with a new set of subjects. This question alludes to the possibility that the research findings regarding a self-report instrument are reflective only of the subjects in the study. Repeating the study on a second group of individuals who match the inclusion and exclusion criteria outlined for the first group provides an opportunity to evaluate the consistency (or lack thereof) of the measure's performance. If the authors have a large enough sample, then they might split it into two groups, evaluate the self-report instrument on one group, and then repeat the evaluation using the second group. If not, then evidence-based physical therapists may have to read several pieces of evidence about the same outcome measure if they wish to verify its usefulness to a greater degree.

Study Results

Results of an evaluation of a self-report instrument's clinimetric properties may be presented in both qualitative and quantitative form. In both cases, physical therapists will find it easier to draw their own conclusions if more detail, rather than less, is provided.

Initial Survey Development

The statistical approach commonly implemented in survey development is *factor analysis*. The goal of the process is to determine whether items on a survey group together to form independent subsets or factors.[17] These factors should be theoretically and intuitively meaningful based on the content of the questions with which they are associated. For example, questions that address walking, running, climbing, and performing physical activities in the home likely reflect a factor that could be defined as "physical functioning." In contrast, questions that address mood and emotional state may cluster together to form a subset regarding "psychological functioning."

Numerous factor analytic methods are available. Investigators using these techniques often report which items are grouped together, as well as the strength of the association between each item and the factor. This association is represented by a "factor loading score," which is interpreted in the same manner as a correlation coefficient. Scores close to one (1) indicate a strong association between the item and the factor. Threshold values usually are established below which items may be eliminated from the survey, thereby providing empirical support for the contents of the final instrument.

Reliability

Internal consistency usually is determined using Cronbach's alpha (α). This statistic evaluates the correlation among items within each dimension of the survey.[3] The standard identified by the Medical

Outcomes Trust Scientific Advisory Committee is a correlation coefficient between 0.70 and 0.90 to 0.95.[10] Similarly, the intraclass correlation coefficient (ICC) is commonly used to assess reproducibility. Portney and Watkins suggest the following score interpretations for ICC statistics:[4(p.595)]

- >0.90   reliability sufficient to "ensure reasonable validity"
- >0.75   "good reliability"
- <0.75   "poor to moderate reliability"

Finally, the kappa (κ) statistic, along with the standard error of measurement, is often used to evaluate agreement among repeated scores. Recommended standards for κ are as follows:[18]

- 0.81–1.0   "almost perfect agreement"
- 0.61–0.80   "substantial agreement"
- 0.41–0.60   "moderate agreement"
- 0.21–0.40   "fair agreement"
- 0.01–0.20   "slight agreement"
- <0.00   "poor agreement"

Validity

Content validity is not tested statistically. Instead, investigators may describe the degree of consensus among content experts who review the survey. Construct validity also may be described qualitatively, or it may be assessed via testing of hypothesized relationships among items or scale dimensions. Criterion validity, in contrast, may be evaluated based on the relationship between scores on the self-report instrument of interest and scores on a gold standard or reference standard instrument. A high correlation coefficient suggests that the survey measures a comparable phenomenon. The challenge for investigators is to find an appropriate criterion against which to judge their instrument. Shorter versions of previously established surveys may be compared to their longer "parent" instrument.

Responsiveness

Responsiveness may be demonstrated through the calculation of an effect size or a standardized response mean, or both. The *effect size* may be the simple difference between the scores on the first and second administration of the self-report instrument. Alternatively, the calculation may include the standard deviation (SD) of the initial survey scores to capture the variability within the effect. The following guidelines have been recommended for interpreting this standardized effect size[4]:

- 0.80   large effect size
- 0.50   moderate effect size
- 0.20   minimal effect size

The *standardized response mean* (SRM) is similar in concept to the standardized effect size; however, the variability included in the calculation is the standard deviation of the change scores rather than the standard deviation of the initial scores. An SRM of 1.0 is a commonly stated threshold criterion for establishing responsiveness. **Figure 16-1** provides the calculations for these indicators of responsiveness.

The limitations to responsiveness reflected by floor and ceiling effects may be detected when most of the answers to the questions on the survey are scored at the low end or the high end of the scale, respectively. If items demonstrating these effects are maintained, then investigators should describe the characteristics of individuals for whom the survey is not responsive.

FIGURE 16-1   Calculations for indicators of responsiveness.

Effect Size	$Mean_{test1} - Mean_{test2}$
Standardized Effect Size	$(Mean_{test2} - Mean_{test2})/SD_{test1}$
Standardized Response Mean	$(Mean_{test2} - Mean_{test2})/SD_{difference}$

Interpretability

As noted earlier, the interpretation of the meaning of survey scores may be achieved descriptively by evaluating patterns of responses in subsets of respondents defined by different characteristics or different circumstances. However, the minimal change needed to make a meaningful impact may be identified via opinion gathering, estimates using the standard error of measurement, or predictive modeling using receiver operating characteristic (ROC) curves.[4] Fortunately, this minimal clinically important difference is reported in the units of the self-report instrument (e.g., 12 points).

The Statistical Importance of Study Results

The statistical importance of the quantitative assessments of clinimetric properties is determined with *p values* and *confidence intervals*. In both instances, researchers must choose a threshold that indicates at what point they will consider the results to be "significant," rather than a chance occurrence. It goes without saying that an instrument with clearly established reliability and validity is worth considering to measure outcomes of physical therapy interventions from the individual's point of view.

Evidence and the Patient or Client

All self-report instruments are developed and tested with a group of individuals that may be defined by the nature of their condition, as well as other characteristics, such as age, gender, race/ethnicity, cognitive status, native language, and so forth. If the patient or client for whom the instrument is being considered is described by these attributes, then the survey may be an appropriate selection. Remember that the measurement properties of an instrument designed for one purpose should not be assumed to hold true when the survey is used under different circumstances. The extent of the administrative burden also may influence a decision to use the instrument.

Another consideration is a growing understanding that the amount of change needed for meaningful improvement in an individual's status often is more than the amount of change needed when comparing groups of subjects.[19] Physical therapists should keep this point in mind as they engage patients or clients in discussions about their expectations for outcomes of physical therapist services delivery.

Evidence Appraisal Tools

At the time of this publication, a generally accepted worksheet for appraisal of evidence about outcome measures does not exist. **Table 16-3** provides a checklist to guide the evaluation

TABLE 16-3	Evidence About Patient Self-Report Instruments: Quality Appraisal Checklist

Research Validity of the Study

Instrument Development and Application

Did the investigators provide an adequate description of the self-report instrument development process, including identification of participants and methods for item development and selection?	___ Yes ___ No ___ Insufficient detail ___ Separate study or studies cited
Is the self-report instrument of interest understandable (readable) by all populations for whom it is intended?	___ Yes ___ No ___ Insufficient detail ___ Separate study or studies cited
Does the self-report instrument of interest take a reasonable amount of time to administer?	___ Yes ___ No ___ Insufficient detail ___ Separate study or studies cited
Is the self-report instrument of interest easy to score and interpret?	___ Yes ___ No ___ Insufficient detail ___ Separate study or studies cited

Instrument Reliability

Did the investigators evaluate the internal consistency of the self-report instrument of interest?	___ Adequate design and method; factor analysis used; $\alpha = 0.70\text{–}0.90$ ___ Inadequate description of methods used ___ Inadequate internal consistency ($\alpha < 0.70$) ___ Separate study or studies cited ___ No information found on internal consistency
Did the investigators evaluate the reproducibility (test–retest reliability) of the self-report measure of interest?	___ Adequate design, method, and ICC > 0.70 ___ Inadequate description of methods use ___ Inadequate reliability (ICC ≤ 0.70) ___ Separate study or studies cited ___ No information found on test–retest reliability

(continues)

TABLE 16-3	**Evidence About Patient Self-Report Instruments: Quality Appraisal Checklist (*Continued*)**
Did the investigators evaluate the limits of agreement of the self-report measure of interest?	___ Adequate design, method, and result (κ and/or SEM) ___ Inadequate description of methods used ___ Inadequate agreement ___ Separate study or studies cited ___ No information found on agreement
Instrument Validity	
Did the investigators evaluate the content validity of the self-report measure of interest?	___ Patients (or clients) and investigators (or experts) involved in assessment ___ Only patients (or clients) involved in assessment ___ No patients (or clients) involved in assessment ___ Inadequate description of methods used ___ Separate study or studies cited ___ No information found on content validity
Did the investigators evaluate the construct validity of the self-report measure of interest?	___ Adequate design, method, and result ___ Inadequate description of methods used ___ Inadequate construct validity ___ Separate study or studies cited ___ No information found on construct validity
Did the investigators evaluate the criterion validity of the self-report measure of interest?	___ Adequate design, method, and result ___ Inadequate description of methods used ___ Inadequate criterion validity ___ Separate study or studies cited ___ No information found on criterion validity
Did the investigators evaluate the self-report instrument of interest on a population other than the one for which it originally was designed?	___ Adequate design, method, and result ___ Inadequate description of methods used ___ Separate study or studies cited ___ Not applicable
Instrument Responsiveness and Interpretability	
Did the investigators evaluate the responsiveness of the self-report instrument of interest?	___ Adequate design, method, and result (effect size and/or standardized response mean) ___ Inadequate description of methods used ___ Inadequate responsiveness ___ Separate study or studies cited ___ No information found on responsiveness

TABLE 16-3   Evidence About Patient Self-Report Instruments: Quality Appraisal Checklist (*Continued*)

Instrument Responsiveness and Interpretability

Did the investigators evaluate the floor and ceiling effects of the self-report instrument of interest?

___ No floor or ceiling effects identified

___ Floor and/or ceiling effects exceed 15% of instrument

___ Separate study or studies cited

___ No information found on floor and/or ceiling effects

Did the investigators evaluate the interpretability of the self-report instrument of interest?

___ Two or more types of information provided (including standard deviations)

___ Inadequate description of methods used

___ Separate study or studies cited

___ No information found on interpretation

Did the investigators evaluate the minimal clinically important difference (MCID) of the self-report instrument of interest?

___ MCID calculated

___ Inadequate MCID

___ Separate study or studies cited

___ No information found on MCID

Do you have enough confidence in the research validity of this paper to consider using this evidence with your patient or client?

___ Yes

___ Undecided

___ No

Relevant Study Findings

Results reported that are specific to your clinical question:

Cronbach's α: _____

Correlation coefficient(s): _____

Effect size(s): _____

Standardized response mean(s): _____

Other: _____

Statistical significance and/or precision of the relevant study results:

Obtained p values for each relevant statistic reported by the authors: _____

Obtained confidence intervals for each relevant statistic reported by the authors: _____

(continues)

TABLE 16-3	Evidence About Patient Self-Report Instruments: Quality Appraisal Checklist (*Continued*)

Application of the Evidence to Your Patient or Client

Are there clinically meaningful differences between the subjects in the study and your patient or client?	___ Yes
	___ No
	___ Mixed results
	___ Insufficient detail
Can you administer the self-report instrument of interest appropriately in your clinical setting with your current resources?	___ Yes
	___ No
	___ Insufficient description of the techniques used
Does the self-report instrument of interest fit within the patient's or client's expressed values and preferences?	___ Yes
	___ No
	___ Mixed results
Will you use the self-report instrument of interest for this patient or client?	___ Yes
	___ No

These questions were adapted from the Oxford Centre for Evidence-Based Medicine and applied to physical therapist practice.

of evidence about self-report outcomes instruments. This checklist follows the same format as the appraisal worksheets developed by the Oxford Centre for Evidence Based Medicine.[20] The content reflects the criteria proposed by the Medical Outcomes Trust Scientific Advisory Committee,[10] as well as those used by Bot et al. as part of their systematic review of shoulder disability questionnaires.[21] A strategy worth considering is the creation of reference notebooks that contain completed checklists or worksheets along with their associated research articles. These compendia could facilitate the use of evidence regarding self-report outcomes instruments for all physical therapists in a particular setting (as long as there is a commitment to keeping them up to date).

Summary

Outcomes are the end result of physical therapist patient/client management. Measuring person-level outcomes from the patient's or client's point of view represents a holistic approach to care. Disability, health status, and health-related quality of life are the person-level outcomes of interest most commonly addressed via self-report instruments. Clinimetric properties are the measurement characteristics of these tools. Evidence about self-report instruments may focus on their development, their validation, or both. Instruments with demonstrated reliability, validity, and responsiveness are preferred when available.

Exercises

1. Discuss the challenges of creating a meaningful self-report instrument that can be readily adopted for use in clinical settings.
2. Compare and contrast the clinimetric properties of reproducibility and agreement with respect to self-report instruments. Provide a clinical example relevant to physical therapist practice to illustrate your points.
3. Creators of a hypothetical self-report instrument report a Cronbach's α of 0.54 for the psychosocial functioning subscale. Interpret this value and discuss what it means in terms of the reliability of this survey.
4. Investigators report a κ of 0.68 when they evaluated the agreement of a hypothetical self-report instrument. Interpret this value and discuss what it means in terms of the reliability of this survey.
5. Compare and contrast content validity, construct validity, and criterion validity with respect to self-report instruments. Provide a clinical example relevant to physical therapist practice to illustrate your points.
6. Differentiate between floor and ceiling effects and discuss their implications for the use of a survey instrument. Provide a clinical example relevant to physical therapist practice to illustrate your points.
7. Differentiate between the standardized effect size and the standardized response mean. Provide a clinical example relevant to physical therapist practice to illustrate your points.
8. Compare and contrast the minimal detectable change and the minimal clinically important difference. Discuss why a change in score may be interpreted differently by a physical therapist and a patient or client.
9. Explain why it is necessary to reevaluate the clinimetric properties of a self-report instrument when it is going to be used with a population different from that originally used to create the instrument. Provide a clinical example relevant to physical therapist practice to illustrate your points.
10. Access and read the article by Jette et al.,[13] and discuss the implications of its findings for evidence-based physical therapist practice.

References

1. de Vet HCW, Terwee CB, Knol DL, Bouter LM. When to use agreement versus reliability measures. *J Clin Epidemiol.* 2006;59(10):1033-1039.
2. Helewa A, Walker JM. *Critical Evaluation of Research in Physical Rehabilitation: Towards Evidence-Based Practice.* Philadelphia, PA: W.B. Saunders; 2000.
3. Carter RE, Lubinsky J, Domholdt E. *Rehabilitation Research: Principles and Applications.* 4th ed. St. Louis, MO: Elsevier Saunders; 2011.
4. Portney LG, Watkins MP. *Foundations of Clinical Research: Applications to Practice.* 3rd ed. Upper Saddle River, NJ: Prentice Hall Health; 2009.
5. Polit DF, Beck CT. *Nursing Research: Principles and Methods.* 7th ed. Philadelphia, PA: Lippincott Williams & Wilkins; 2003.
6. Batavia M. *Clinical Research for Health Professionals: A User-Friendly Guide.* Boston, MA: Butterworth-Heinemann; 2001.
7. Chan KBY, Man-Son-Hing M, Molnar FJ, Laupacis A. How well is the clinical importance of study results reported? An assessment of randomized controlled trials. *CMAJ.* 2001;165(9):1197-1202.

8. American Physical Therapy Association. *Guide to Physical Therapist Practice 3.0.* Available at: http://guidetoptpractice.apta.org. Accessed July 16, 2016.

9. Beaton DE, Bombardier C, Katz JN, Wright JG. A taxonomy of responsiveness. *J Clin Epidemiol.* 2001;54(12):1204-1217.

10. Scientific Advisory Committee of the Medical Outcomes Trust. Assessing health status and quality-of-life instruments: attributes and review criteria. *Qual Life Res.* 2002;11(3):193-205.

11. Mokkink LB, Terwee CB, Patrick DL, et al. The COSMIN checklist for assessing the methodological quality of studies on measurement properties of health status measurement instruments: an international Delphi study. *Qual Life Res.* 2010;19(4):539-549.

12. Law M, MacDermid J, eds. *Evidence-Based Rehabilitation. A Guide to Practice.* 2nd ed. Thorofare, NJ: SLACK Inc.; 2008.

13. Jette DU, Halbert J, Iverson C, et al. Use of standardized outcome measures in physical therapist practice: perceptions and applications. *Phys Ther.* 2009;89(2):125-135.

14. Short Form-36. Medical Outcomes Study. Available at: www.rand.org/health/surveys_tools/mos/mos_core_36item.html. Accessed March 1, 2017.

15. Mokkink LB, Terwee CB, Patrick DL, et al. The COSMIN study reached international consensus on taxonomy, terminology, and definitions of measurement properties for health-related patient-reported outcomes. *J Clin Epidemiol.* 2010;63(7):737-745.

16. Beaton DE, Boers M, Wells GA. Many faces of the minimal clinically important difference (MCID): a literature review and directions for future research. *Curr Opin Rheumatol.* 2002;14(2):109-114.

17. Tabachnik BG, Fidell LS. *Using Multivariate Statistics.* 4th ed. Boston, MA: Allyn & Bacon; 2006.

18. Simm J, Wright CC. The kappa statistic in reliability studies: use, interpretation and sample size requirements. *Phys Ther.* 2005;85(3):257-268.

19. Riddle D, Stratford P. *Is This Change Real?* Philadelphia, PA: F.A. Davis Company; 2013.

20. Oxford Centre for Evidence-Based Medicine Web site. Available at: www.cebm.net. Accessed October 1, 2016.

21. Bot SDM, Terwee CB, van der Windt DAWM, et al. Clinimetric evaluation of shoulder disability questionnaires: a systematic review of the literature. *Ann Rheum Dis.* 2004;63(4):335-341.

APPRAISING COLLECTIONS OF EVIDENCE: SYSTEMATIC REVIEWS

OBJECTIVES

Upon completion of this chapter, the student/practitioner will be able to do the following:

1. Discuss the purposes and potential benefits of systematic reviews.

2. Critically evaluate systematic reviews, including the

   a. Important questions to ask related to research validity; and

   b. The relevance of these products to physical therapist practice.

3. Apply the following concepts during the evaluation of systematic reviews:

   a. Effect size;

   b. Heterogeneity;

   c. Homogeneity;

   d. Meta-analysis;

   e. Publication bias;

   f. Relative risk;

   g. Selection bias;

   h. Subgroup analysis; and

   i. Vote counting.

4. Interpret relative risks for beneficial and adverse outcomes.

5. Interpret forest plots and evaluate confidence intervals to determine the potential importance of reported findings in systematic reviews.

6. Discuss the potential benefits of using individual subject versus aggregate data in meta-analyses.

7. Discuss considerations related to the application of systematic reviews to individual patients or clients.

TERMS IN THIS CHAPTER

Assignment (also referred to as *allocation*): The process by which subjects are placed into two or more groups in a study; inadequate assignment procedures may threaten research validity (internal validity) by producing groups that are different from one another at the start of the study.

Attrition (also referred to as *dropout* or *mortality*): A term that refers to subjects who stop participation in a study for any reason; loss of subjects may threaten research validity (internal validity) by reducing the sample size and/or producing unequal groups.

Bias: Results or inferences that systematically deviate from the truth "or the processes leading to such deviation."[1(p.251)]

Compensatory equalization of treatments: A threat to research validity (internal validity) characterized by the purposeful or inadvertent provision of additional encouragement or practice to subjects in the control (comparison) group in recognition that they are not receiving the experimental intervention.

Confidence interval: A range of scores within which the true score for a variable is estimated to lie within a specified probability (e.g., 90%, 95%, 99%).[2]

Effect size: The magnitude of the difference (or the relationship) between two mean values; may be standardized by dividing this difference by the pooled standard deviation to compare effects measured by different scales.[3]

Fixed effects model: A statistical method that assumes that differences in results among studies in a meta-analysis are due to chance; in other words, the results are assumed to be similar.[4]

Heterogeneity: In systematic reviews, differences in the results of individual studies that are more than a chance occurrence.

Homogeneity: The consistency of results of individual studies included in systematic reviews.

Likelihood ratio (LR): The likelihood that a test result will be obtained in a patient or client with the condition of interest as compared to a patient or client without the condition of interest.[5]

Meta-analysis: A statistical method used to pool data from individual studies included in a systematic review.[5]

Nonexperimental design (also referred to as an *observational study*): A study in which controlled manipulation of the subjects is lacking[2]; in addition, if groups are present, assignment is predetermined based on naturally occurring subject characteristics or activities.[6]

Number needed to treat (NNT): The number of subjects treated with an experimental intervention over the course of a study required to achieve one good outcome or prevent one bad outcome.[7]

Odds ratio (OR): The odds that an individual with a prognostic (risk) factor had an outcome of interest as compared to the odds for an individual without the prognostic (risk) factor.[6,8]

Power: The probability that a statistical test will detect, if it is present, a relationship between two or more variables or a difference between two or more groups.[2,9]

Publication bias: The tendency of health sciences and health policy journal editors to publish studies based on the direction and statistical significance of the outcomes.[8]

***p* value**: The probability that a statistical finding occurred due to chance.

Quasi-experimental design: A research design in which there is only one subject group or in which randomization to more than one subject group is lacking; controlled manipulation of the subjects is preserved.[10]

Random effects model: A statistical method that assumes studies in a meta-analysis are measuring different effects.[4]

Randomized clinical trial (also referred to as a *randomized controlled trial* and a *randomized controlled clinical trial* [RCT]): A clinical study that uses a randomization process to assign subjects to either an experimental group(s) or a control (or comparison) group. Subjects in the experimental group receive the intervention or preventive measure of interest and then are compared to the subjects in the control (or comparison) group who did not receive the experimental manipulation.[2]

Relative risk (RR): In clinical trials, a ratio of the risk of the outcome in the experimental (intervention) group relative to the risk of the outcome in the control group.[8]

Research validity: "The degree to which a study appropriately answers the question being asked."[8(p.225)]

Selection bias: Error that occurs as a result of systematic differences between individual studies included in, and those excluded from, a systematic review.[1]

Systematic review: A method by which a collection of individual research studies is gathered and critically appraised in an effort to reach an unbiased conclusion about the cumulative weight of the evidence on a particular topic[4]; also referred to as a "synthesis."[11]

Testing: A threat to research validity (internal validity) characterized by a subject's change in performance due to growing familiarity with the testing or measurement procedure or to inconsistent implementation of the procedures by study personnel.

Vote counting: A method for generating a summary statement about the weight of evidence in a systematic review; for reviews about interventions, effectiveness is determined by the number of trials with positive results.[4]

Introduction

This chapter focuses on collections of evidence that have been systematically preappraised and synthesized into single research reports. These secondary analyses—referred to as systematic reviews—potentially provide physical therapists with a broader view of the evidence than any single study may accomplish. Their availability also may enhance the efficiency with which busy clinicians access scientific information. As a result, they often are recommended as the first place to look for answers to clinical questions. However, just like individual studies, systematic reviews may be flawed in terms of their design and execution. Results from these lower quality products may be less trustworthy as a result. This chapter discusses the nature and potential benefits of syntheses of preappraised evidence and provides methods by which they may be evaluated for their quality, meaningfulness, and usefulness.

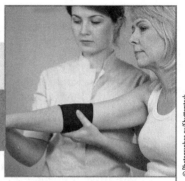

CLINICAL SCENARIO

How Do You Keep Up With All of the Studies That Are Published?

Anne's internet search for information about how to manage her elbow pain revealed hundreds of citations from all types of sources.

She was aware that medical professionals, including physical therapists, needed to stay current with the evidence and recognized how much time that could take. You also checked the scientific literature and found a recent systematic review specific to physical therapist management of lateral epicondylitis.*

How will you describe the purpose of systematic reviews and the potential usefulness of the information in this publication?

*Weber C, Thai V, Neuheuser K, Groover K, Christ O. Efficacy of physical therapy for the treatment of lateral epicondylitis: a meta-analysis. *BMC Musculoskelet Disord.* 2015;16:223.

Systematic Reviews

A *systematic review*, or "synthesis," is a secondary analysis of original individual studies. Most commonly these analyses are performed using research about interventions, although systematic reviews of evidence about other components of the physical therapist patient/client management model have been published.[12-16] The goal of conducting a review is to draw a conclusion based on the cumulative weight of the evidence about the management element of interest.

Systematic reviews possess research designs with specifically outlined (1) methods for identifying and selecting individual studies for evaluation, (2) review criteria and procedures to determine individual study quality, and (3) processes for drawing conclusions from the body of evidence. A formal results section also is included that may provide qualitative and/or statistical conclusions about the utility of the patient/client management element based on the studies included in the review.

Qualitative judgments may be determined through *vote counting*, a process in which each individual study included in the review receives one vote. For example, a summary conclusion about evidence for an intervention's effectiveness may be made based on the number of votes that represent a positive treatment effect.[4] Qualitative judgments derived from vote counting are limited, in part, because they reduce the question of utility down to a "yes/no" answer. There is no ability to assess the magnitude of the cumulative effect generated by gathering numerous studies. Alternatively, authors may qualify their judgments about the usefulness of a patient/client management element by indicating the level of evidence, as determined by a specified hierarchy, used to support their statements. A levels-of-evidence approach is challenged because of the inconsistencies among evidence hierarchies. The extent to which a judgment is supported may vary depending on which hierarchy is applied. For these reasons, a quantitative analysis is preferred when available.

Systematic reviews that use a quantitative method for drawing conclusions are referred to as *meta-analyses*. Meta-analyses pool data from individual studies, thereby creating larger sample sizes. For intervention studies, larger sample sizes have greater *power* to detect differences in treatment effect, if they exist, between the group that received the experimental intervention and the group that did not. In addition, the larger sample improves the estimate of the effect size as indicated by narrower confidence intervals. The same benefits may be achieved for reviews of prognostic indicators in the sense that larger sample sizes increase the power to detect relationships between predictive factors and outcomes, if they exist. Similarly, meta-analyses of diagnostic tests have larger samples with which to examine the test's ability to correctly classify individuals with and without a condition of interest. Regardless of the focus of the review, meta-analytic techniques require that the patient/client management techniques and outcomes of interest in individual studies be similar. Meta-analyses may be performed using aggregate data or using individual subject data from the studies reviewed.[6] The latter is preferable to obtain the most information from the data.

The most prolific source of systematic reviews is the Cochrane Collaboration.[17] This international organization has assembled multiple review groups (53 as of this publication) whose mission is to conduct systematic reviews of studies relevant to their category (**Table 17-1**). As the titles suggest, the products from many of these clinical topic groups are relevant to evidence-based physical therapists. Additional groups exist for the purpose of establishing methods for conducting systematic reviews. Of note are groups dedicated to the development of methods related to reviews of individual studies about diagnostic tests and clinical measures, nonrandomized trials, qualitative studies, and patient-reported outcomes.[18] These studies potentially have more opportunities for *bias*; therefore, different approaches to synthesizing and drawing conclusions from their data are warranted. The Cochrane Library houses the completed systematic reviews, which may be accessed online for a subscription fee. Updates are scheduled and performed regularly to incorporate new evidence as appropriate.

TABLE 17-1	Cochrane Review Groups
Acute Respiratory Infections Group	
Airways Group	
Anaesthesia, Critical and Emergency Care Group	
Back and Neck Group	
Bone, Joint and Muscle Trauma Group	
Breast Cancer Group	
Childhood Cancer Group	
Colorectal Cancer Group	
Common Mental Disorders Group	
Consumers and Communication Group	
Cystic Fibrosis and Genetic Disorders Group	
Dementia and Cognitive Improvement Group	
Developmental, Psychosocial, and Learning Problems Group	
Drugs and Alcohol Group	
Effective Practice and Organisation of Care Group	

(continues)

TABLE 17-1 Cochrane Review Groups *(Continued)*
ENT Group
Epilepsy Group
Eyes and Vision Group
Fertility Regulation Group
Gynaecological, Neuro-Oncology and Orphan Cancer Group
Gynaecology and Fertility Group
Haematological Malignancies Group
Heart Group
Hepato-Biliary Group
HIV/AIDS Group
Hypertension Group
IBD Group
Incontinence Group
Infectious Diseases Group
Injuries Group
Kidney and Transplant Group
Lung Cancer Group
Menstrual Disorders and Subfertility Group
Metabolic and Endocrine Disorders Group
Methodology Review Group
Movement Disorders Group
Multiple Sclerosis and Rare Diseases of the CNS Group
Musculoskeletal Group
Neonatal Group
Neuromuscular Group
Oral Health Group
Pain, Palliative and Supportive Care Group
Pregnancy and Childbirth Group
Public Health Group
Schizophrenia Group
Skin Group
STI Group
Stroke Group
Tobacco Addiction Group
Upper GI and Pancreatic Diseases Group
Urology Group
Vascular Group
Work Group
Wounds Group

Systematic reviews also are conducted independently from the Cochrane Collaboration and published in numerous health sciences and health policy journals. Format and required content are established by each journal, a situation that poses a challenge to readers when appraising the review. Important questions related to the quality of the review may not be answered simply because of reporting differences in the various publications. In an effort to remedy this situation, Moher et al. developed a checklist and flow diagram, originally referred to as the "Quality of Reporting of Meta-Analyses" (QUOROM) statement, for reporting meta-analyses conducted using clinical randomized controlled trials.[19] These authors expressed particular concern regarding the inclusion of information pertaining to:

- The evidence appraisal criteria;
- The quality of studies included in the meta-analysis, as judged by the appraisal criteria;
- The assessment of publication bias;
- The inclusion of unpublished studies or abstracts;
- The use of language restrictions as criteria for identification and selection of individual studies; and
- The relationship between the findings from the meta-analysis and other results reported from similar reviews.

In addition, the statement included recommendations for report formats to standardize the look, along with the content, for easier reading and appraisal. The PRISMA, or "Preferred Reporting Items of Systematic Reviews and Meta-Analyses," statement provides expanded and updated guidance in this area.[20,21] Stroup et al. produced a similar statement—the "Meta-Analysis of Observational Studies in Epidemiology" (MOOSE)—addressing reporting issues for meta-analyses of studies using nonexperimental research designs.[22] These are the studies used to evaluate the usefulness of diagnostic tests, prognostic indicators, and patient or client outcomes. The degree to which journal editors have adopted either or both the PRISMA and MOOSE statements is not clear. The bottom line for readers, however, is that appraisal of systematic reviews will be more accurate and thorough if authors provide more details about the review's methods and results.

Hierarchies developed for evidence-based medicine and practice generally rank systematic reviews at the top because their conclusions are based on a synthesis of several (sometimes many) studies rather than a single trial. This ranking assumes that the review in question is high quality in its own right, a fact that must be determined by the reader rather than taken for granted. The potential for low quality exists both due to the manner in which the review is conducted and how the raw materials (i.e., the individual studies) were synthesized. For example, Jadad et al. compared the quality of reviews produced by the Cochrane Collaboration with reviews published in health sciences journals.[23] These authors found that Cochrane reviews appeared to be more methodologically sound based on their descriptions of processes used to identify, select, and appraise individual studies. However, reviews published in other health sciences journals were noted to contain a higher number of individual studies and larger sample sizes.

As stated previously, Cochrane reviews are updated regularly, a fact that was supported to some extent by the results of Jadad et al. Fifty percent of the Cochrane reviews were updated compared to only 2.5% of the reviews published in other journals. Shea et al. conducted a similar study but appraised the included meta-analyses using an established checklist and scale.[24] These authors reported that the quality of reviews from both sources was low, as demonstrated by the lack of a statistically significant difference in quality scale scores for the two groups of reviews. Both Jadad et al.'s and Shea et al.'s findings reinforce the need for evidence-based physical therapists to perform their own appraisal of systematic reviews rather than accepting them at face value.

Study Credibility

Evidence pertaining to systematic reviews that physical therapists use should first be evaluated with the questions itemized in **Table 17-2**. These questions are adapted from the critical appraisal worksheets developed by the Oxford Centre for Evidence-Based Medicine.[25] Their purpose is to help physical therapists determine whether there are problems with a review's design and execution that may have biased the results.[6]

1. Did the investigators limit the review to high-quality studies?

This question reflects the importance of using study designs in which bias is minimized. Different designs are best suited for different types of research questions. Systematic reviews about patient/client management elements other than intervention appropriately use *nonexperimental* or *quasi-experimental designs*. Studies about interventions, in contrast, are most likely to have bias reduced through experimental research designs. The assumption is that *randomized clinical trials (RCTs)* are better than quasi-experimental and nonexperimental designs because of the methods available to control extraneous influences. However, there is considerable debate about the usefulness of studies that lack randomization. In addition, many of the interventions available to physical therapists have yet to be studied using RCTs or may not be eligible for an experimental design because of ethical considerations. If review authors include studies about interventions with different types of designs, then they should make that point clear in their report. They also should provide a rationale for that decision and should describe methods for handling information from each type of design included.

2. Did the investigators implement a comprehensive search and study selection process?

Systematic reviews may be limited by selection of a non-representative sample just like individual research projects. The difference is that the "subjects" in the review are studies, whereas the subjects in an individual clinical study are people. To reduce the chances of committing *selection bias*, review authors should describe a process whereby all relevant electronic and print databases and collections are searched. Commonly cited sources include Medline (PubMed),[26] EMBASE,[27] the Cochrane Controlled Trials Register,[17] and CINAHL.[28] Databases also are available for identifying dissertations and unpublished studies.[5] Citation lists in the articles initially located also may be searched, along with Web sites of professional associations whose meetings include presentation of scientific reports. Thorough searches require both electronic and manual efforts to be successful.

TABLE 17-2   Questions to Determine the Validity of Systematic Reviews

1. Did the investigators limit the review to high-quality studies?
2. Did the investigators implement a comprehensive search and study selection process?
3. Did the investigators assess the quality of individual studies with standardized processes and/or tools?
4. Did the investigators provide details about the research validity (or quality) of studies included in the review?
5. Did the investigators address publication bias?
6. If this is a meta-analysis, did the investigators use individual subject data in the analysis?

A related issue is the inclusion of studies published in languages other than English. Concerns have been expressed about the contribution to selection bias that language restrictions might create. Moher et al. compared meta-analyses that included non-English-language studies to those that excluded them and found no difference in effect size between these groups.[29] Juni et al. reported a similar result.[30] These authors also indicated that the non-English-language studies included in the meta-analyses studied had smaller sample sizes and lower methodological quality. In addition, these trials were more likely to demonstrate statistically significant results. However, they noted that individual meta-analyses might be differentially affected by the exclusion of non-English-language works. Both Moher et al. and Juni et al. acknowledged the improved precision of effect size estimates that occurred when foreign language studies were included in meta-analyses.[29,30] More recently, Morrison et al. "found no evidence of a systematic bias from the use of language restrictions in systematic review-based meta-analyses in conventional medicine."[31] Ideally, authors of meta-analyses will make clear in their reports whether a language restriction was implemented so that readers may determine whether, and to what extent, bias may have been introduced into the review.

In addition, review authors should indicate whether they included both published and unpublished materials. This point refers to the editorial tendency to publish studies with statistically significant positive results rather than studies that demonstrate no difference or relationship.[30] McAuley et al. investigated the impact of including unpublished material in 41 meta-analyses published between 1966 and 1995.[32] These authors found that, on average, reviews that excluded unpublished works produced a 15% larger estimate of effect as compared to reviews that included them. One approach to counteracting publication bias is to include "gray literature," such as unpublished studies, dissertations, theses, proceedings from meetings, and abstracts, in systematic reviews. Unfortunately, unpublished works are more time intensive to locate and retrieve, a situation that likely deters some authors from pursuing this type of material. In addition, Egger et al. found that many unpublished works were of lower quality and cautioned that the extra effort put into searching for this material may not be fruitful.[33]

Once again, authors should make clear whether they included unpublished works and, if not, why they were omitted. Potential candidates for review should be identified using predetermined inclusion and exclusion criteria that are consistent with the purpose of the review. Criteria may refer to the study design, the type of patient/client management element(s) investigated, the characteristics of subjects included in the individual studies, and the types of outcomes and the methods for their measurement. Ideally, authors will itemize studies that were excluded, as well as those that were included, so that readers can make their own judgments about the appropriateness of article selection.

3. Did the investigators assess the quality of individual studies with standardized processes and/or tools?

The quality of individual studies is an essential ingredient for a successful systematic review. The phrase "garbage in, garbage out" illustrates the point. Individual trials that have weak *research validity* will only produce more misleading results when synthesized for the purposes of a review. Juni et al. argue that four types of threats to research validity in clinical trials of interventions are particularly concerning:[34]

- Bias that occurs when subject allocation to groups is manipulated by the researcher(s);
- Bias that occurs when groups are managed differently apart from the experimental treatment;
- Bias that occurs when outcome measures are collected by unmasked investigators; and
- Bias that occurs when the loss of subjects produces systematic imbalances in group characteristics and/or when methods used to deal with this loss are inappropriate.

These sources of bias contribute to the research validity threats referred to as *assignment*, *compensatory equalization of treatment*, *testing*, and *attrition*. Threats to research validity may introduce competing explanations for a study's results. Juni et al. along with several others, demonstrated that the inclusion of lower quality trials suffering from one or more types of bias produced overestimates of beneficial treatment effects in meta-analyses.[34-36]

The challenge for review authors is to determine the method by which the quality of individual studies will be assessed. In 1995, Moher et al. published an annotated bibliography of tools available to assess the quality of clinical trials.[37] These instruments were categorized either as checklists that itemized what design elements should be included in a trial or scales that produced quality scores. Only 1 of the 25 scales identified at that time was thoroughly tested for its reliability and validity, whereas several others had information about components of reliability or validity.

Olivo et al. conducted a systematic review of scales used to assess the quality of RCTs.[38] Twenty-one scales were identified in this report; however, the scale with the strongest evidence of reliability and validity has not been tested on evidence specific to physical therapy. This lack of methodological appraisal means that different scales may produce different quality ratings of the same clinical trial. In fact, Colle et al. investigated the impact of choice of scale on quality scores for studies included in a systematic review of exercise for the treatment of low back pain.[39] These authors reported that the quality scale implemented influenced conclusions regarding the effectiveness of exercise therapy. In addition, correlation among the different scale scores and interrater reliability was low. In a subsequent study, Moher et al. reported that masked quality appraisal provided higher quality scores using a validated scale, as compared to unmasked appraisals.[35]

Until a methodologically sound and useful scale is developed, Juni et al. suggested that review authors assess the quality of individual trials using a descriptive component method that identifies the presence or absence of important elements of the review, such as allocation concealment, masking of investigators collecting outcome measures, and so forth.[34] The bottom line for evidence-based physical therapists is that authors of a systematic review should clearly describe the method and instruments used to perform a quality assessment of individual studies. Ideally, they will have selected a validated instrument to perform the appraisal and will have masked those conducting the quality assessments so that individual conclusions are not influenced by knowledge of other reviewers' findings.

4. Did the investigators provide details about the research validity (or quality) of studies included in the review?

Appraising the quality of individual studies is not sufficient by itself; something should be done with the information acquired from the assessment. At a minimum, authors should report the level of quality for each article reviewed. If a threshold quality score was required for study inclusion, then it should be stated along with a rationale for its selection. Moher et al. suggested incorporating quality scores into the meta-analysis calculation to reduce the overestimate of effect size.[35] In contrast, Juni et al. discouraged this practice due to the variability in scales. Instead, these authors recommended conducting sensitivity analyses by performing the meta-analysis both with, and without, the lower quality individual trials.[34] Either way, a systematic review is likely to be more useful if the quality of individual studies is reported and results are interpreted in light of these appraisals.

5. Did the investigators address publication bias?

Publication bias reflects the tendency of health sciences and health policy journal editors to publish studies based on the direction and statistical significance of the outcomes.[8] Specifically, preference is given to studies that have found statistically significant beneficial treatment effects (i.e., subjects improved or subjects' risk was reduced). The PRISMA statement recommends that review authors address explicitly the potential for publication bias by stating whether they included gray literature and/or non-English-language publications.[21] Sterne et al. state that publication bias also may be detected by graphing effect sizes used in the meta-analysis.[40] A nonbiased review results in a plot that looks like an inverted funnel with a wide base and narrow top. Bias will be suggested if pieces of the funnel are missing; that is, if effect sizes from studies that do not show treatment effects are not included in the plot. However, these authors also note that publication bias may be only one of several reasons for this result. Ultimately, readers must make a qualitative judgment about the potential role publication bias may have played in a review's findings.

6. If this is a meta-analysis, did the investigators use individual subject data in the analysis?
As noted earlier, meta-analyses may be conducted using aggregate data—that is, summary scores for effect size—or individual subject data. Which data are selected depends entirely on their availability. Review authors start with the information that is included in written study reports. When possible, they also may contact investigators from the individual studies to request access to any data that have been maintained over time. Individual subject data are preferred because they provide more detail than summary scores. Of interest is the potential to create subgroups of subjects based on different prognostic indicators or other baseline characteristics.[6] Analysis with subgroups allows investigators to examine whether an intervention(s) has differential effectiveness. For example, a technique used to facilitate ventilator weaning in patients with tetraplegia may perform differently if some of these individuals were smokers and others were not. Subgroup analysis using individual subject data would permit exploration of this hypothesized difference. Similar opportunities exist when subgroup analysis is possible for reviews about diagnostic tests, clinical measures, prognostic factors, outcomes research, and self-report outcomes measures. Unfortunately, logistical impediments may prevent review authors from obtaining this level of information. From a validity standpoint, this is not a fatal flaw in the review but rather a lost opportunity. Resulting limitations in the interpretation of findings from a meta-analysis should be acknowledged.

Study Results

One of the motivations to conduct a systematic review is to try to resolve conflicting results from individual studies. For this resolution to be meaningful, studies must not be extraordinarily divergent in their findings. Extreme differences in results suggest that these contradictory findings are more than a chance occurrence, which makes drawing conclusions about the utility of the patient/client management element, or lack of it, problematic. Review authors and readers may get a sense of the *homogeneity* of individual study findings by examining a plot of the individual estimates (e.g., ratios, effect sizes) and associated confidence intervals. Overlapping confidence intervals indicate a more homogeneous collection of results.[40]

Review authors also may perform statistical tests to determine the consistency of findings. In this case, a *p value* below a specified threshold (e.g., $\alpha = 0.05$) indicates that *heterogeneity* of results is present more than chance alone would explain. Under these circumstances, review authors should offer their insights as to possible reasons for the divergence of study findings. Differences in sample composition, patient or client management protocol, or outcomes measured are some of the commonly identified sources of heterogeneity. Depending on possible reasons for the differences in results, review authors may either make statistical adjustments or conduct separate meta-analyses for identified subgroups to deal with heterogeneity. In situations where these adjustments are inappropriate, meta-analyses are skipped altogether.[4]

Qualitative judgments about the strength of the evidence may be all that review authors can provide when individual studies have different methods for addressing the research question or when results are sufficiently heterogeneous that pooling data is not feasible. Under these circumstances, the findings from each study usually are reported along with details about the relative strength of their designs.

When meta-analyses are possible, review authors must decide which statistical methods to use to obtain a pooled estimate. The details of these approaches are beyond the scope of this text. In general, investigators must first determine whether the differences in results of individual studies are due to chance variation. If the differences are thought to be random occurrences, authors conduct a meta-analysis using a *fixed effects model* (also known as a Mantel-Haenszel test). A fixed effects model assumes that the results among the included studies are similar. If the differences in results among individual studies are thought to be meaningful but cannot be explained, review authors describe the use of a *random effects model*.[4]

Next, authors pool the data by weighting each study based on the precision of the ratio or effect that is being estimated. Studies with large sample sizes usually produce more precise estimates, as reflected by narrower confidence intervals. Therefore, greater weights are assigned to studies that reflect these properties. Once the analysis is conducted, the final product reported may be:

- *Likelihood ratios;*
- *Odds ratios;*
- *Relative risks;*
- A mean difference in outcomes between the groups (the *effect size*); or
- The standardized mean difference in outcomes (the standardized effect size).

The first three options are used with dichotomous data (e.g., present/absent, yes/no); the remaining options are used with continuous data (e.g., degrees, seconds, meters).[5]

Reporting Formats

Review authors may present information from individual trials in a variety of formats. Descriptive details and qualitative assessments usually are summarized in tables. **Table 17-3** is an example of descriptive information about each study included in a systematic review of the use of whole-body vibration as treatment for individuals with Parkinson's disease.[41] These details provide readers with a quick way to identify the subjects included, the study design and the level of evidence in which the systematic review authors classified the individual studies.

Table 17-4 elaborates on the qualitative assessment of the individual studies using the rating scale developed by PEDro, the Australian physiotherapy evidence database.[42] Note that this scale looks for the presence of key design components necessary to optimize the research validity of a clinical trial. Readers of this review must make their own determination about whether a minimum threshold score is needed before the individual trial will be considered trustworthy. Cochrane reviews generally have the most comprehensive collection of descriptive and qualitative tables; however, access to this information generally means there are many pages to print!

Quantitative results from individual studies may be presented in table or in graph format. **Table 17-5** illustrates a tabular summary of trials included in a systematic review of interventions for idiopathic scoliosis in adolescents.[43] Where possible, Lenssinck et al. calculated the relative risk for individual trials. The *relative risk (RR)* is a ratio of the risk of the outcome in the experimental (intervention) group relative to the risk of the outcome in the control group.[8] A ratio less than 1 indicates that the outcome is less likely to occur in the experimental group versus the control group. A ratio greater than 1 indicates that the outcome is more likely to occur in the experimental group versus the control group. A ratio equal to 1 indicates no difference between the experimental group and the control group. In Table 17-5 the outcomes measured primarily are adverse events—surgery or progression of the spinal curvature. If the interventions studied are effective, then the relative risk should be less

TABLE 17-3   Study Design and Characteristics of Study Participants[a]

Study	Level of Evidence[b]	Study Design	Characteristics of Participants[c] Sample Size (n)	Age (y)[d]	Sex	Severity of Pretest UPDRS Motor Score[d]
Turbanski et al.[46]	2b	Nonrandomized controlled trial	52 (26 in WBV and 26 in CON)	69.1 (8.9)	14 women and 38 men	40.0 (11.2)
Haas et al.[47]	1b	Randomized controlled trial with crossover	68	65.0 (7.8)	15 women and 53 men	29.9 (11.9)
Haas et al.[48]	2b	Nonrandomized controlled trial	28 (19 in WBV and 9 in CON)	63.1 (7.3)	NR	NR
Ebersbach et al.[49]	2b	Randomized controlled trial	21 (10 in WBV and 11 in CON)	WBV: 72.5 (6.0) CON: 75.0 (6.8)	14 women and 7 men	WBV: 23.0 (4.9) CON: 25.9 (8.1)
Arias et al.[50]	2b	Nonrandomized controlled trial	21 (10 in WBV and 11 in CON)	WBV: 66.9 (11.1) CON: 66.6 (5.6)	9 women and 12 men	WBV: 24.8 (7.1) CON: 30.5 (7.1)
King et al.[51]	2b	Randomized controlled trial with crossover	40	65.4 (9.9)	15 women and 25 men	NR

[a] UPDRS=Unified Parkinson Disease Rating Scale, WBV=whole-body vibration group, CON=control group, NR=not reported.
[b] Based on the PEDro scores and guidelines set by the Centre for Evidence-Based Medicine (level 1b indicated a good-quality randomized controlled trial, and level 2b indicated a poor-quality randomized controlled trial).
[c] Participants in all of the studies were patients with idiopathic Parkinson's disease.
[d] Reported as mean (standard deviation).

Note: The references cited within the table are relevant to the originally published source from which this table has been picked up.
Reproduced from Lau RWK, Teo T, Yu F, Chung RCK, Pang MYC. Effects of whole-body vibration on sensorimotor performance in people with Parkinson disease: a systematic review. *Phys Ther.* 2011;91(2):198-209, by permission of Oxford University Press.

TABLE 17-4   Methodological Quality Determined with the Physiotherapy Evidence Database (PEDro) Scale[a]

Criterion	Turbanski et al.[46]	Haas et al.[47]	Haas et al.[48]	Ebersbach et al.[49]	Arias et al.[50]	King et al.[51]
Eligibility criteria	No	No	No	No	Yes	No
Random allocation	0	1	0	1	0	1
Concealed allocation	0	0	0	0	0	0
Baseline comparability	0	1	1	1	1	0
Masking of patients	0	0	0	0	1	0
Masking of therapists	0	0	0	0	0	0
Masking of assessors	0	1	0	1	1	0
Adequate followup	1	1	1	0	1	1
Intention-to-treat analysis	0	0	0	0	0	0
Between-group comparisons	1	1	1	1	0	1
Point estimates and variability	0	1	1	1	1	1
Total	2	6	4	5	5	4

[a] Numeric values are scores.
*PEDro score calculated by the authors of this review.
Note: The references cited within the table are relevant to the originally published source from which this table has been picked up.
Reproduced from Lau RWK, Teo T, Yu F, Chung RCK, Pang MYC. Effects of whole-body vibration on sensorimotor performance in people with Parkinson disease: a systematic review. *Phys Ther.* 2011;91(2):198-209, by permission of Oxford University Press.

than 1. Note that calculations were conducted only for individual trials; data could not be pooled to perform a meta-analysis because of the variety of manual therapeutic approaches investigated.

Results from systematic reviews also may be presented graphically using forest plots. These visual displays usually are designed to indicate treatment effect size, along with associated confidence intervals, for individual studies reviewed. If a meta-analysis was performed, then the cumulative effect size will be presented as well.[44] These same displays can be used to summarize likelihood ratios, odds ratios, and relative risks. **Figure 17-1** is a forest plot from a systematic review examining the effects of high-intensity resistance exercise on bone loss in postmenopausal women.[45] The plot summarizes results from each trial for the comparison between an exercise intervention group and a non-exercise control group.

The outcome of interest is change in bone mineral density in the lumbar spine. The midline of the graph represents "no difference" in bone mineral density between groups at the conclusion of the studies. The negative values to the left of the midline indicate that the non-exercise control groups maintained their bone mineral density more than the experimental treatment groups ("favors control"). The positive values to the right of the midline indicate high-intensity resistance exercise

TABLE 17-5	Quantitative Results from Individual Trials in a Systematic Review of Interventions for Scoliosis		
Study	**Intervention**	**Results**	**RR as Calculated by the Reviewers**
Athanasopoulos et al.[27]	I: Boston brace + training, $n = 20$ C: Boston brace, $n = 20$	I: increased ability to perform aerobic work, 48.1% C: decreased ability to perform aerobic work, 9.2%	
el-Sayyad and Conine[33]	I: exercise + Milwaukee brace, $n = 8$ C1: exercise, $n = 10$ C2: exercise + electrical stimulation, $n = 8$	I change: −4.05° C1 change: −2.93% C2 change: −3.76°	
den Boer et al.[29]	I: side shift therapy, $n = 44$ C: brace therapy, $n = 120$	I change: +2.6°, failure = 34.1% C change: −1.5°, failure = 31.7%	Failure I versus C: RR = 1.08 (0.66–1.75), meaning no differences in failure rate between I and C
Birbaumer et al.[28]	I: behaviorally posture-oriented training, $n = 15$ C: noncompliers, $n = 4$	I change: −6.14° C change: +8.20°	
Carman et al.[30]	I: Milwaukee brace + exercises, $n = 21$ C: Milwaukee brace, $n = 16$	I ($n = 12$) change: −3.7° C ($n = 12$) change: −3.4°	Surgery I versus C: RR = 1.52 (0.45–5.18), meaning no difference in surgery rate between I and C
Gepstein et al.[35]	I: Charleston bending brace, $n = 85$ C: thoraco-lumbo-sacral orthosis, $n = 37$	Success: I = 80%, C = 81% Surgery: I = 12.3%, C = 11.8% Failure: I = 7.4%, C = 5.4%	Surgery I versus C: RR = 1.09 (0.36–3.25), meaning no difference in surgery rate between I and C Failure I versus C: RR = 1.31 (0.28–6.17), meaning no difference in failure between I and C

(continues)

TABLE 17-5	Quantitative Results from Individual Trials in a Systematic Review of Interventions for Scoliosis (*Continued*)		
Study	**Intervention**	**Results**	**RR as Calculated by the Reviewers**
Nachemson and Peterson[38]	I: underarm plastic brace, $n = 111$ C1: night time electrical surface stimulation, $n = 46$ C2: no treatment, $n = 129$	Failure: I = 15%, C1 = 48%, C2 = 45%	Failure I versus C1: RR = 0.3 (0.16–0.56), meaning failure rate in I significantly lower compared with C1 Failure I versus C2: RR = 0.28 (0.16–0.48), meaning failure rate in I significantly lower compared with C2 Failure C1 versus C2: RR = 0.93 (0.62–1.41), meaning no difference in failure rate between both control groups
Dickson and Leatherman[32]	I: traction, $n = ?$ C: exercises, $n = ?$	I change: standing curve in cast +3°, curve on lateral bending +1° C change: standing curve in cast +1°, curve on lateral bending –4°	
von Deimling et al.[31]	I: Chêneau corset, $n = 21$ C: Milwaukee brace, $n = 26$	I change: +1.2°, 19% success C change: +2.9°, 3.8% success	Success I versus C: RR = 0.84 (0.67–1.05), meaning no difference in success rate between I and C
Fiore et al.[34]	I: 3-valve orthosis, $n = 15$ C: Boston brace, $n = 15$	I angle change: –6° C angle change: –3°	
Mulcahy et al.[37]	I: Milwaukee brace, throat mold design, $n = 7$ C: conventional Milwaukee brace, $n = 30$	I: 42.85% remain in brace, 14.3% surgery C: 36.7% remain in brace, 16.7% surgery	Surgery I versus C: RR = 0.86 (0.12–6.23), meaning no difference in surgery rate between I and C

			RR as Calculated
Study	**Intervention**	**Results**	**by the Reviewers**
Schlenzka et al.[39]	I: lateral electrical surface stimulation, $n = 20$	I ($n = 6$) change: posttreatment +5°, follow-up (2.3 y) +8°	
	C: Boston brace, $n = 20$	C change: posttreatment −6°, follow-up (2.7 y) −2°	
Minami[36]	I: Milwaukee brace C: thoraco-lumbo-sacral orthosis, Boston-Milwaukee brace	No information about results of different treatment groups; results in curve and age groups	

TABLE 17-5   Quantitative Results from Individual Trials in a Systematic Review of Interventions for Scoliosis (*Continued*)

[a]Degrees with "−" sign indicate a decrease of the spinal curvature; degrees with "+" sign indicate an increase of the spinal curvature. Failure is >5 degrees progression of spinal curvature. RR = relative risk (95% confidence interval); RR <1 means effect in favor of first-mentioned comparison. I = intervention, C = control.
Note: The references cited within the table are relevant to the originally published source from which this table has been picked up. Reprinted from Lenssinck MLB, Frijlink AC, Berger MY, et al. Effect of bracing and other conservative interventions in the treatment of idiopathic scoliosis in adolescents: a systematic review of clinical trials. *Phys Ther.* 2005;85(12):1329-1339; Table 3 with permission from the American Physical Therapy Association. Copyright © 2005. American Physical Therapy Association.

groups maintained or increased their bone mineral density more than the non-exercise control groups ("favors treatment"). The effect size, calculated as a weighted mean difference (WMD) between the groups, is measured in grams/centimeter^2 (g/cm^2) and is represented by a vertical hash mark on the plot. The boxes on each hash mark indicate the weight assigned to each trial and coincide with the values in the second column from the right (weight %). A bigger box reflects the sample size of the trial and the extent to which subjects in the experimental group achieved the outcome of interest. Finally, the large diamond at the bottom of the plot represents the pooled estimate of the effect size, which, based on the values in the far right column, is an increase in bone mineral density of 0.00637 g/cm^2. Note that information regarding the test for heterogeneity also is printed on the plot; in this case, the high p value indicates homogeneity of the trials.

Readers should examine all details of a forest plot to ensure accurate interpretation. Specifically, it is important to note what outcome is being reported as well as the measure used. In Figure 17-1, the outcome of interest is a change in bone mineral density of the lumbar spine (an effect size measure). Studies demonstrating beneficial effects of the experimental intervention will have point estimates to the right of the midline (i.e., increased bone mineral density). In contrast, **Figure 17-2** is a forest plot from a different systematic review that examined the association between physical activity and osteoporotic fractures.[46] The outcome in this instance is a change in the fracture rate. The plot displays results that are risk ratios rather than effect sizes, so the midline represents "1," or a 50–50 chance of the outcome occurring. As a result, studies that demonstrate a beneficial association with physical activity will have point estimates to the left of the midline that reflect a decreased risk of a fracture occurring.

FIGURE 17-1 Forest plot of study results evaluating the effect of high-intensity resistance training on postmenopausal bone mineral density loss.

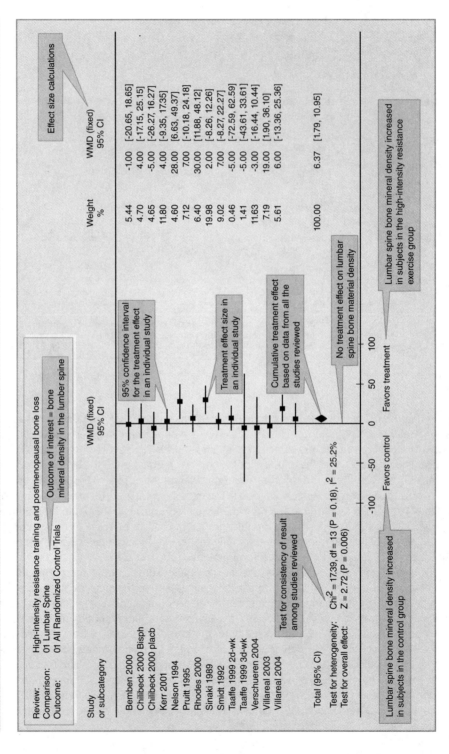

Reproduced from Osteoporosis International, High-intensity resistance training and postmenopausal bone loss: a meta-analysis, 17(8), 2006, 1225–1240, M. Martyn-St James, Copyright © 2006, International Osteoporosis Foundation and National Osteoporosis Foundation, with permission of Springer.

FIGURE 17-2   Forest plot of the association between physical activity and hip fracture.

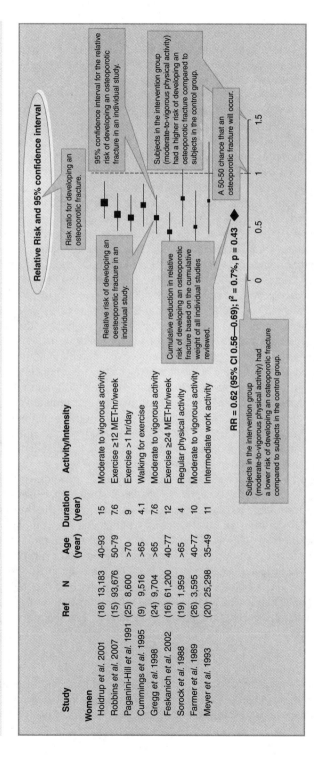

Reprinted from *Annals of Epidemiology*, 18(11), Moayyeri, A., The association between physical activity and osteoporotic fractures: a review of the evidence and implications for future research, 827–835, Copyright 2008, with permission from Elsevier.

The Meaning of Study Results

When meta-analyses cannot be performed, the "importance" of the findings is inferred from the extent to which individual studies report similar results. This determination is influenced by the quality of each trial, as well as by the statistical importance of their results as indicated by *p* values, confidence intervals, or magnitude of the effect. Review authors tell you what they think by creating summary statements about the weight of the evidence. For example, a treatment effect is considered likely if a collection of studies reports beneficial outcomes from the intervention of interest.

Calculation of a cumulative likelihood ratio, odds ratio, effect size, or relative risk is the first step in deciding about the weight of the evidence in a meta-analysis. These values are point estimates derived from the pooled sample; however, their statistical importance is determined based on the level of certainty that the result represents the "true value," if it could be measured. The most useful way to demonstrate statistical importance in meta-analyses is to calculate confidence intervals. The *confidence interval* provides a range within which the true score is estimated to lie within a specified probability.[2] Most often the probability selected is 95%. Interpretation of the confidence interval depends on the summary statistic used. For effect sizes, the confidence interval must exclude the value "0," because that represents "no change." For likelihood ratios, odds ratios, and relative risks, the confidence interval must exclude the value "1," because that represents equal likelihoods, odds, or risks between the two groups of subjects studied.

Confidence intervals may be reported in text and/or graphic form. In forest plots, confidence intervals calculated for the individual trials are indicated by straight lines through the point estimates. In Figure 17-1, eleven of the studies have 95% confidence intervals that cross the midline of the plot, indicating that the intervals include "0" or "no change." The remaining three studies have confidence intervals that do not cross the midline of the plot, so a positive treatment effect is acknowledged. Note that the confidence intervals overlap to a considerable degree, a situation that is consistent with the results of the heterogeneity test. The confidence interval for the cumulative effect size is represented by a diamond, a shape that reflects the increased precision of the estimate due to the increased sample size. Again in Figure 17-1, this confidence interval does not include zero. This result would be interpreted to mean that, based on the weight of the evidence included, high-intensity resistance training increases bone mineral density in the lumbar spine.

Another method by which to determine the importance of findings from a meta-analysis is to calculate the *number needed to treat (NNT)* based on studies that use odds ratios. Fortunately, reference tables are available to make these conversions.[6] What the therapist must determine is the rate with which his or her patients or clients will achieve the outcome of interest if provided with the experimental intervention. This value is a percentage expressed in decimal form and is referred to with the acronym "PEER" (patient's expected event rate). This step is comparable to determining a patient or client's pretest probability for a diagnostic test. Once the PEER has been identified on the *y*-axis of the table, then the odds ratio from the review can be identified on the *x*-axis. The number needed to treat is found at the intersection of the PEER row and the OR column. Not surprisingly, the lower the number needed to treat, the more useful the experimental intervention may be.

Clinical Importance

As always, statistical importance should not be considered synonymous with clinical importance. This point is exemplified in Figures 17-1 and 17-2. Both figures indicate that a statistically significant benefit was achieved because the confidence intervals around the pooled estimates do not cross the midline. However, the actual amount of change that occurred may be viewed by some as clinically unimportant because it is so small. An increase of 0.006 g/cm² may not translate into meaningful protection from fracture risk in the lumbar spine. However, a 38% decrease in risk of osteoporotic fracture in postmenopausal women may provide sufficient support for an exercise prescription that increases the dose of physical activity. As always, clinical judgment along with patient or client preferences and values must be used to determine whether this evidence is convincing enough to support the additional cost, discomfort, and effort required to provide the interventions described in the meta-analyses.

Evidence and the Patient or Client

The following considerations apply here with respect to using evidence from systematic reviews with a patient or client:

- The diagnostic test, clinical measure, prognostic indicator, intervention, clinical prediction rule, or self-report outcomes measure is appropriate and feasible in the physical therapist's practice setting;
- The subjects in the review resemble the patient or client to whom the evidence may be applied; and
- The diagnostic test, clinical measure, prognostic indicator, intervention, clinical prediction rule or self-report outcomes measure must be compatible with the patient or client's preferences and values.

Evidence Appraisal Tools

Table 17-6 provides a checklist to guide the evaluation of systematic reviews for use in any practice setting. Answers to these questions should be considered in the context of the debate about the relative merits of experimental, quasi-experimental, and nonexperimental studies and their inclusion in systematic reviews.[24]

Readers should also consider the following questions pertaining to subgroup analysis in systematic reviews[25]:

1. "Do the qualitative differences in treatment effectiveness really make biologic and clinical sense?"
2. "Is the qualitative difference both clinically (beneficial for some, but useless or harmful for others) and statistically significant?"
3. "Was this difference hypothesized before the study began (rather than the product of dredging the data), and has it been confirmed in other independent studies?"
4. "Was this one of just a few subgroup analyses carried out in this study?"

These points challenge physical therapists to consider the extent to which meaningful subgroups are likely to exist among a population of patients or clients with a particular disorder or condition. Answers to these questions depend on a physical therapist's knowledge and understanding of the disorder or condition of interest, as well as possible prognostic and risk factors with which it is associated. The potential for different responses to a diagnostic test, clinical measure, or experimental intervention must also be considered from a clinical and statistical perspective. Finally, differential effects that result from data dredging may be artifact and, therefore, clinically meaningless. Straus et al. argue that subgroup analysis should only be taken seriously if a reader can answer "yes" to all four questions.[6]

TABLE 17-6   Systematic Reviews: Quality Appraisal Checklist

Research Validity of the Study

Did the investigators limit the review to high-quality studies?	___ Yes ___ No ___ Insufficient detail
Did the investigators implement a comprehensive search and study selection process?	___ Yes ___ No ___ Insufficient detail
Did the investigators assess the quality of individual studies with standardized processes and/or tools?	___ Yes ___ No ___ Insufficient detail
Did the investigators provide details about the research validity (or quality) of studies included in the review?	___ Yes ___ No ___ Insufficient detail
Did the investigators address publication bias?	___ Yes ___ No ___ Insufficient detail
If this article includes a meta-analysis, did the investigators use individual subject data in the analysis?	___ Yes ___ No ___ Insufficient detail ___ Not applicable
How confident are you in the research validity of this paper?	___ Yes ___ Undecided ___ No

Relevant Study Findings

Were the results consistent from study to study (e.g., homogeneous)?	___ Yes ___ No

Results reported that are specific to your clinical question:

Likelihood ratios: _____

Odds ratios: _____

Effect size: _____

Relative risks: _____

Other: _____

Relevant Study Findings

Statistical significance and/or precision of the relevant study results:

Obtained *p* values for each relevant statistic reported by the authors: _____

Obtained confidence intervals for each relevant statistic reported by the authors: _____

TABLE 17-6 Systematic Reviews: Quality Appraisal Checklist (*Continued*)

If this paper is not a meta-analysis, is there a substantive conclusion that can be drawn about the cumulative weight of the evidence?	___ Yes ___ No ___ Insufficient detail ___ Not applicable
Application of the Evidence to Your Patient or Client	
Are there clinically meaningful differences between the subjects in the study and your patient or client?	___ Yes ___ No ___ Mixed results ___ Insufficient detail
If this review is about a diagnostic test, clinical measure, intervention, or clinical prediction rule can you perform this technique safely and appropriately in your clinical setting given your current knowledge and skill level and your current resources?	___ Yes ___ No ___ Insufficient description of the techniques used ___ Not applicable
If this review is about prognostic factors, can you modify them or provide information/education about them in your clinical setting given your current knowledge and skill level and your current resources?	___ Yes ___ No ___ Not applicable
Does the technique (or information about the prognostic factors) fit within the patient's or client's expressed values and preferences?	___ Yes ___ No ___ Mixed results
Will you use this technique (modify or provide information about the prognostic factors) for this patient or client?	___ Yes ___ No

These questions were adapted from the Oxford Centre for Evidence-Based Medicine and applied to physical therapist practice.

Summary

Systematic reviews synthesize information from individual studies to arrive at a conclusion based on the cumulative weight of the evidence. Conclusions may be qualitative or quantitative. Meta-analyses are a form of systematic review in which data are pooled to draw quantitative conclusions. These statistical assessments are possible when the types of subjects, procedures, and outcomes are consistent among the individual projects. Most systematic reviews relevant to physical therapist practice focus on therapeutic interventions; however, some reviews about diagnostic tests, clinical measures, prognostic indicators, clinical prediction rules, and self-report outcomes measures have been published. Systematic reviews are vulnerable to bias both due to the methods with which they are conducted, as well as the quality of the individual studies reviewed. Evidence-based physical therapists should evaluate systematic reviews carefully before accepting them at face value because of their high ranking on evidence hierarchies.

Exercises

1. Discuss the potential benefits of using systematic reviews to inform clinical decision making. Provide a clinical example relevant to physical therapist practice to illustrate your points.
2. Discuss the potential sources of bias in systematic reviews and strategies to minimize their influence. Provide a clinical example relevant to physical therapist practice to illustrate your points.
3. Describe the conditions under which a meta-analysis is appropriate to conduct. Provide a clinical example relevant to physical therapist practice to illustrate your points.
4. Forest plots may be used to illustrate likelihood ratios, odds ratios, effect sizes, and relative risks. Identify what the midline of the graph represents for each of these summary statistics. Provide a clinical example relevant to physical therapist practice to illustrate your points.
5. Interpret the meaning of a confidence interval that crosses the midline of a forest plot for likelihood ratios, odds ratios, effect sizes, and relative risks. Provide a clinical example relevant to physical therapist practice to illustrate your points.

References

1. Helewa A, Walker JM. *Critical Evaluation of Research in Physical Rehabilitation: Towards Evidence-Based Practice.* Philadelphia, PA: W.B. Saunders; 2000.
2. Carter RE., Lubinsky J, Domholdt E. *Rehabilitation Research: Principles and Applications.* 4th ed. St. Louis, MO: Elsevier Saunders; 2011.
3. Batavia M. *Clinical Research for Health Professionals: A User-Friendly Guide.* Boston, MA: Butterworth-Heinemann; 2001.
4. Higgins JPT, Green S, eds. Cochrane Handbook for Systematic Reviews of Interventions, version 5.1.0 [updated March 2011]. The Cochrane Collaboration, 2011. Available at: http://training.cochrane.org/handbook. Accessed March 1, 2017.
5. Herbert R, Jamtvedt G, Hagen KB, Mead J. *Practical Evidence-Based Physiotherapy.* 2nd ed. Edinburgh, Scotland: Elsevier Butterworth-Heinemann; 2011.
6. Straus SE, Richardson WS, Glaziou P, Haynes RB. *Evidence-Based Medicine: How to Practice and Teach EBM.* 3rd ed. Edinburgh, Scotland: Elsevier Churchill Livingstone; 2005.
7. Dalton GW, Keating JL. Number needed to treat: a statistic relevant to physical therapists. *Phys Ther.* 2000;80(12):1214-1219.
8. Guyatt G, Rennie D. *Users' Guides to the Medical Literature: A Manual for Evidence-Based Clinical Practice.* Chicago, IL: AMA Press; 2002.
9. Portney LG, Watkins MP. *Foundations of Clinical Research: Applications to Practice.* 3rd ed. Upper Saddle River, NJ: Prentice Hall Health; 2009.
10. Cook TD, Campbell DT. *Quasi-Experimentation: Design and Analysis Issues for Field Settings.* Boston, MA: Houghton Mifflin; 1979.
11. DiCenso A, Bayley L, Haynes RB. Accessing pre-appraised evidence: fine-tuning the 5S model into a 6S model. *Evid Based Nurs.* 2009;12(4):99-101.
12. Moreau NG, Bodkin AW, Bjornson K, et al. Effectiveness of rehabilitation interventions to improve gait speed in children with cerebral palsy: systematic review and meta-analysis. *Phys Ther.* 2016;96(12):1938-1954.

13. Hidding JT, Viehoff PB, Beurskens CHG, et al. Measurement properties of instruments for measuring of lymph-edema: systematic review. *Phys Ther.* 2016;96(12):1965-1981.

14. Hutting N, Scholten-Peeters GGM, Vijverman V, Keesenberg MDM, Verhagen AP. Diagnostic accuracy of upper cervical spine instability tests: a systematic review. *Phys Ther.* 2013;93(12):1686-1695.

15. Verkerk K, Luijsterburg PAJ, Miedema HS, Pool-Goudzwaard A, Koes BS. Prognostic factors for recovery in chronic nonspecific low back pain: a systematic review. *Phys Ther.* 2012;92(9):1093-1108.

16. Beneciuk JM, Bishop MD, George SZ. Clinical prediction rules for physical therapy interventions: a systematic review. *Phys Ther.* 2009;89(2):114-124.

17. The Cochrane Collaboration website. Available at: www.cochrane.org. Accessed March 1, 2017.

18. Methodology Review Group. Cochrane Collaboration website. Available at: http://methodology.cochrane.org. Accessed March 1, 2017.

19. Moher D, Cook DJ, Eastwood S, et al. Improving the quality of reports of meta-analyses of randomised controlled trials: the QUOROM statement. *Lancet.* 1999;354(9193):1896-1900.

20. Moher D, Liberatti A, Tetzlaff J, et al. Preferred reporting items for systematic reviews and meta-analyses: the PRISMA statement. *BMJ.* 2009;339:b2535.

21. PRISMA. Transparent Reporting of Systematic Reviews and Meta-Analyses. Available at: http://www.prisma-statement.org. Accessed March 1, 2017.

22. Stroup DF, Berlin JA, Morton SC, et al. Meta-analysis of observational studies in epidemiology. *JAMA.* 2000;283(15):2008-2012.

23. Jadad AR, Cook DJ, Jones A, et al. Methodology and reports of systematic reviews and meta-analyses. *JAMA.* 1998;280(3):278-280.

24. Shea B, Moher D, Graham I, et al. A comparison of the quality of Cochrane reviews and systematic reviews published in paper-based journals. *Eval Health Prof.* 2002;25(1):116-129.

25. Oxford Centre for Evidence-Based Medicine website. Available at: www.cebm.net. Accessed October 1, 2016.

26. PubMed. National Library of Medicine website. Available at: https://www.ncbi.nlm.nih.gov/pubmed. Accessed September 1, 2016.

27. EMBASE. Elsevier. Available at: https://www.elsevier.com/solutions/embase-biomedical-research. Accessed March 1, 2017.

28. Cumulative Index of Nursing and Allied Health Literature. Available via Ovid website at: https://health.ebsco.com/products/cinahl-complete. Accessed September 1, 2016.

29. Moher D, Pham B, Klassen TP, et al. What contributions do languages other than English make on the results of meta-analyses? *J Clin Epidemiol.* 2000;53(9):964-972.

30. Jüni P, Holenstein F, Stern J, et al. Direction and impact of language bias in meta-analyses of controlled trials: empirical study. *Int J Epidemiol.* 2002;31(1):115-123.

31. Morrison A, Polisena J, Husereau D, et al. The effect of English-language restriction on systematic review-based meta-analyses: a systematic review of empirical studies. *Int J Technol Assess Health Care.* 2012;28(2):138-144.

32. McAuley L, Pham B, Tugwell P, Moher D. Does the inclusion of grey literature influence estimates of intervention effectiveness in meta-analyses? *Lancet.* 2000;356(9237):1228-1231.

33. Egger M, Juni P, Bartlett C, et al. How important are comprehensive literature searches and the assessment of trial quality in systematic reviews? Empirical study. *Health Technol Assess.* 2003;7(1):1-82.

34. Juni P, Altman DG, Egger M. Systematic reviews in health care: assessing the quality of controlled clinical trials. *BMJ.* 2001;323(7303):42-46.

35. Moher D, Pham B, Jones A, et al. Does quality of reports of randomised trials affect estimates of intervention efficacy reported in meta-analyses? *Lancet.* 1998;352(9128):609-613.

36. Moher D, Cook DJ, Jadad AR, et al. Assessing the quality of reports of randomised trials: implications for the conduct of meta-analyses. *Health Technol Assess.* 1999;3(12):i-iv,1-98.

37. Moher D, Jadad AR, Nichol G, et al. Assessing the quality of randomized controlled trials: an annotated bibliography of scales and checklists. *Control Clin Trials.* 1995;16(1):62-73.

38. Olivo SA, Macedo LG, Gadotti IC, et al. Scales to assess the quality of randomized controlled trials: a systematic review. *Phys Ther.* 2008;88(2):156-175.

39. Colle F, Rannou F, Revel M, et al. Impact of quality scales on levels of evidence inferred from a systematic review of exercise therapy and low back pain. *Arch Phys Med Rehabil.* 2002;83(12):1745-1752.

40. Sterne JAC, Egger M, Smith GD. Systematic reviews in health care: investigating and dealing with publication and other biases in meta-analysis. *BMJ.* 2001;323(7304):101-105.

41. Lau RWK, Teo T, Yu F, Chung RCK, Pang MYC. Effects of whole-body vibration on sensorimotor performance in people with Parkinson disease: a systematic review. *Phys Ther.* 2011;91(2):198-209.

42. Physiotherapy Evidence Database. Centre for Evidence-Based Physiotherapy. Available at: www.pedro.org. au. Accessed September 1, 2016.

43. Lenssinck MLB, Frijlink AC, Berger MY, et al. Effect of bracing and other conservative interventions in the treatment of idiopathic scoliosis in adolescents: a systematic review of clinical trials. *Phys Ther.* 2005;85(12):1329-1339.

44. Lewis S, Clarke M. Forest plots: trying to see the wood and the trees. *BMJ.* 2001;322(7300):1479-1480.

45. Martyn-St. James M, Carroll S. High-intensity resistance training and postmenopausal bone loss: a meta-analysis. *Osteoporos Int.* 2006;17(8):1225-1240.

46. Moayyeri A. The association between physical activity and osteoporotic fractures: a review of the evidence and implications for future research. *Ann Epidemiol.* 2008;18(11):827-835.

APPRAISING COLLECTIONS OF EVIDENCE: CLINICAL PRACTICE GUIDELINES

OBJECTIVES

Upon completion of this chapter, the student/practitioner will be able to do the following:

1. Discuss the purposes and potential benefits of clinical practice guidelines (CPGs).

2. Critically evaluate CPGs, including the

    a. Important questions to ask related to research validity; and

    b. The relevance of these products to physical therapist practice.

3. Discuss the challenges of creating and updating CPGs.

4. Discuss considerations related to the application of CPGs to individual patients or clients.

TERMS IN THIS CHAPTER

Bias: Results or inferences that systematically deviate from the truth "or the processes leading to such deviation."[1(p.251)]

Clinical practice guideline: ". . . statements that include recommendations intended to optimize patient care. They are informed by a systematic review of evidence and an assessment of the benefits and harms of alternative care options."[2] Also referred to as summaries.[3]

Meta-analysis: A statistical method used to pool data from individual studies included in a systematic review.[4]

Nonexperimental design (also referred to as an *observational study*): A study in which controlled manipulation of the subjects is lacking[5]; in addition, if groups are present, assignment is predetermined based on naturally occurring subject characteristics or activities.[6]

Quasi-experimental design: A research design in which there is only one subject group or in which randomization to more than one subject group is lacking; controlled manipulation of the subjects is preserved.[7]

Randomized clinical trial (also referred to as a *randomized controlled trial* and a *randomized controlled clinical trial* [RCT]): A clinical study that uses a randomization process to assign subjects to either an experimental group(s) or a control (or comparison) group. Subjects in the experimental group receive the intervention or preventive measure of interest and then are compared to the subjects in the control (or comparison) group who did not receive the experimental manipulation.[5]

Research validity: "The degree to which a study appropriately answers the question being asked."[8(p.225)]

Systematic review: A method by which a collection of individual research studies is gathered and critically appraised in an effort to reach an unbiased conclusion about the cumulative weight of the evidence on a particular topic[9]; also referred to as a "synthesis."[3]

CLINICAL SCENARIO

Will This Clinical Practice Guideline Help You Manage My Elbow Pain?

© Photographee.eu/Shutterstock

Anne's internet search for information about how to manage her elbow pain revealed a clinical practice guideline about a variety of problems with this joint complex.* Given the breadth of its review, she is uncertain if it is even relevant to her situation. You confirm for her that the guideline includes the type of elbow pain she is experiencing and that a significant body of evidence was reviewed. However, you also note minimal involvement of patient or caregiver perspective in the consensus-building process for the recommendations.

How will you explain the strengths and limitations of this guideline and your potential use of it to aid your management decisions?

* Hegmann KT, Hoffman HE, Belcourt RM, et al. ACOEM practice guidelines: elbow disorders. *J Occup Environ Med*. 2013;55(11): 1365-1374.

Introduction

This chapter focuses on evidence that has been pre-appraised and summarized to create clinical practice guidelines (CPGs). CPGs are designed to improve the efficiency and effectiveness of health care through the use of summary recommendations about patient/client management. As a result, these synthesized collections of evidence may be an efficient place to look for answers to clinical questions. However, just like individual studies, CPGs may be flawed in terms of their design, execution, and timeliness. Results from these lower quality products may be less trustworthy as a result.

This chapter discusses the nature and potential benefits of CPGs and provides methods by which they may be appraised for their quality, meaningfulness, and usefulness.

Clinical Practice Guidelines

CPGs are defined as ". . . statements that include recommendations intended to optimize patient care. They are informed by a systematic review of evidence and an assessment of the benefits and harms of alternative care options."[2] They may focus on the management of conditions or on specific aspects of care (**Table 18-1**).[10-16] If developed appropriately, CPGs reflect findings from current best evidence, as well as expert clinical judgment and health care consumer opinion or perspective. Often they are issued in two formats: one for health care professionals and one for the general public. **Figure 18-1** depicts the recommendations included in a CPG about physical therapist management of nonarthritic hip pain.[17]

CPGs are a phenomenon of contemporary health care. They tend to be issued by government agencies or by professional societies; however, they may be developed by anyone with the motivation to organize the necessary resources to produce them. In the 1990s, the primary source of CPGs in the United States was the Agency for Health Care Policy and Research (AHCPR), now known as the Agency for Healthcare Research and Quality (AHRQ).[18]

Physical therapists and their patients or clients can locate CPGs by using electronic evidence databases or by using online resources, such as government agency or professional society websites. As of this publication, the U.S. National Library of Medicine's electronic search engine, PubMed, indexes 335 English-language CPGs about human subjects published in the last 5 years.[19] The Physiotherapy Evidence Database, PEDro, lists 614 English and non–English-language CPGs relevant to physical therapist practice.[20] An important resource is the National Guideline Clearinghouse (www.guideline. gov), maintained by AHRQ, which offers a weekly email notification of changes in their catalog, as well as new CPGs under development.[21] The American Physical Therapy Association's PTNow platform

TABLE 18-1	Examples of Clinical Practice Guidelines Relevant to Physical Therapist Practice

Conditions

- Evidence-based guidelines for the secondary prevention of falls in older adults [with systematic review].[10]
- Heel pain-plantar fasciitis: CPGs linked to the international classification of function, disability, and health from the Orthopaedic Section of the American Physical Therapy Association.[11]
- Guidelines for stroke rehabilitation and recovery.[12]
- Ottawa Panel evidence-based CPGs for the management of osteoarthritis in adults who are obese or overweight.[13]

Aspects of Patient/Client Management

- Increasing physical activity: a report on recommendations of the Task Force on Community Preventive Services [quick reference guide for clinicians].[14]
- ATS statement: guidelines for the 6-minute walk test.[15]
- Ottawa Panel evidence-based CPGs for electrotherapy and thermotherapy interventions in the management of rheumatoid arthritis in adults [with systematic review].[16]

FIGURE 18-1 Summary of recommendations regarding physical therapist management of nonarthritic hip pain.

NONARTHRITIC HIP JOINT PAIN: CLINICAL PRACTICE GUIDELINES

CLINICAL GUIDELINES

Summary of Recommendations

F **RISK FACTORS**

Clinicians should consider the presence of osseous abnormalities, local or global ligamentous laxity, connective tissue disorders, and nature of the patient's activity and participation as risk factors for hip joint pathology.

C **DIAGNOSIS/CLASSIFICATION - NONARTHRITIC HIP JOINT PAIN**

Clinicians should use the clinical findings of anterior groin or lateral hip pain or generalized hip joint pain that is reproduced with the hip flexion, adduction, internal rotation (FADIR) test or the hip flexion, abduction, external rotation (FABER) test, along with consistent imaging findings, to classify a patient with hip pain into the International Statistical Classification of Diseases and Related Health Problems (ICD) categories of **M25.5 Pain in joint, M24.7 Protrusio acetabula, M24.0 Loose body in joint,** and **M24.2 Disorder of ligament,** and the associated International Classification of Functioning, Disability and Health (ICF) impairment-based categories of hip pain **(b28016 Pain in joints)** and mobility impairments **(b7100 Mobility of a single joint; b7150 Stability of a single joint).**

F **DIFFERENTIAL DIAGNOSIS**

Clinicians should consider diagnostic categories other than non-arthritic joint pain when the patient's history, reported activity limitations, or impairments of body function and structure are not consistent with those presented in the Diagnosis/Classification section of this guideline or when the patient's symptoms are not diminishing with interventions aimed at normalization of the impairments of body function.

A **EXAMINATION – OUTCOME MEASURES**

Clinicians should use a validated outcome measure, such as the Hip Outcome Score (HOS), the Copenhagen Hip and Groin Outcome Score (HAGOS), or the International Hip Outcome Tool (iHOT-33), before and after interventions intended to alleviate the impairments of body function and structure, activity limitations, and participation restrictions in individuals with nonarthritic hip joint pain.

B **EXAMINATION – PHYSICAL IMPAIRMENT MEASURES**

When evaluating patients with suspected or confirmed hip pathology over an episode of care, clinicians should assess impairments of body function, including objective and reproducible measures of hip pain, mobility, muscle power, and movement coordination.

F **INTERVENTION – PATIENT EDUCATION AND COUNSELING**

Clinicians may utilize patient education and counseling for modifying aggravating factors and managing pain associated with nonarthritic hip joint pain.

F **INTERVENTION – MANUAL THERAPY**

In the absence of contraindications, joint mobilization procedures may be indicated when capsular restrictions are suspected to impair hip mobility, and soft tissue mobilization procedures may be indicated when muscles and their related fascia are suspected to impair hip mobility.

F **INTERVENTION – THERAPEUTIC EXERCISES AND ACTIVITIES**

Clinicians may utilize therapeutic exercises and activities to address joint mobility, muscle flexibility, muscle strength, muscle power deficits, deconditioning, and metabolic disorders identified during the physical examination of patients with nonarthritic hip joint pain.

F **INTERVENTION – NEUROMUSCULAR RE-EDUCATION**

Clinicians may utilize neuromuscular re-education procedures to diminish movement coordination impairments identified in patients with nonarthritic hip joint pain.

Reprinted with permission from Cibulka MT, White DM, Woehrle J, et al. Hip pain and mobility deficits – hip osteoarthritis: clinical practice guidelines linked to the International Classification of Functioning, Disability, and Health from the Orthopaedic Section of the American Physical Therapy Association. *J Orthop Sports Phys Ther*. 2009;39:A1-A25. https://doi.org/10.2519/jospt.2009.0301.

also offers association members access to full text versions of over 270 CPGs relevant to physical therapist practice.[22] The variability in number and focus of CPGs indexed on these different websites means evidence-based physical therapists may have to access several to ensure they have completed a comprehensive search to address their clinical questions.

The proliferation of CPGs has prompted some concrete recommendations regarding their development. Evidence-based CPGs are preferred over expert-based products because the latter are likely to reflect practitioners' habits and preferences, as well as biases inherent in their professions.[23] Shekelle et al. have outlined the following steps specific to creating evidence-based CPGs:

- Identify and refine the topic and scope of the CPGs;
- Identify and convene the appropriate stakeholders—such as clinicians, patients, caregivers, researchers, and technical support staff—to participate;
- Conduct or locate a systematic review of the evidence;
- Develop recommendations based on the systematic review, as interpreted by clinical expertise and patient experience, as well as on feasibility issues such as cost; and
- Submit the CPG for external review.[24]

Central to this process is the quantity and quality of the evidence relating to the CPG topic. The number of studies addressing an aspect of patient/client management may be insufficient to create a true *systematic review*. In addition, the studies located may have varying degrees of *bias* associated with different research designs. As a result, authors of CPGs tend to rely on a "levels of evidence" approach to characterize the strength of their recommendations.

There is considerable variability in evidence hierarchy definitions, a situation that may create inconsistencies among CPGs addressing the same topics. **Table 18-2** provides two contrasting examples of "levels of evidence" classification schemes. In an effort to simplify matters, the GRADE (Grading of Recommendations Assessment, Development and Evaluation) working group published the classification system in **Tables 18-3**[25] and **18-4**.[26] The apparent simplicity of this approach is somewhat deceptive because there are additional steps required to arrive at these grades. To develop a recommendation, CPG developers must integrate what is known about the quality and results of available evidence with the realities of the current practice environment, as well as patient and/or caregiver preferences and values. This process is characterized in **Figure 18-2**.[27]

All CPGs are not created equal. Physical therapists using CPGs should assess them in the same way that they assess individual research studies. The following questions and methods are provided to help organize one's thoughts as the CPG is considered.

Is the Guideline Valid?

Although CPGs are not research studies, they may still suffer from credibility issues. One of the first concerns is whether the CPG remains current. CPGs may become outdated as a result of the following:

1. The introduction of new patient/client management techniques;
2. New evidence clarifying beneficial or harmful consequences of current patient/client management techniques;
3. Changes in which outcomes of care are considered important clinically and socially;
4. Full compliance with current CPGs, thus no longer necessitating their use; or
5. Changes in health care resources.[28]

The range of publication dates for the sample of CPGs in Table 18-1 lends face validity to the concern about currency. Shekelle et al. conducted a review of ACHPR CPGs and discovered that 75% were

TABLE 18-2 Examples of Levels of Evidence in Clinical Practice Guidelines

Classification Scheme #1	Classification Scheme #2
Recommendation is supported by:	**Category of Evidence**
A. Scientific evidence provided by well-designed, well-conducted, controlled trials (randomized and nonrandomized) with statistically significant results that consistently support the guideline recommendation.	**1a.** Evidence for *meta-analysis* of randomized controlled trials
	1b. Evidence from at least one *randomized controlled trial*
	2a. Evidence from at least one controlled study without randomization
	2b. Evidence from at least one other type of *quasi-experimental* study
B. Scientific evidence provided by observational studies or by controlled trials with less consistent results to support the guideline recommendation.	**3.** Evidence from *nonexperimental* descriptive studies, such as comparative studies, correlation studies, and case-control studies
	4. Evidence from expert committee reports or opinions or clinical experience of respected authorities or both
C. Expert opinion that supports the guideline recommendation because the available scientific evidence did not present consistent results, or controlled trials were lacking.	**Strength of Recommendation**
	A. Directly based on category 1 evidence
	B. Directly based on category 2 evidence or extrapolated recommendation from category 1 evidence
	C. Directly based on category 3 evidence or extrapolated recommendation from category 1 or 2 evidence
	D. Directly based on category 4 evidence or extrapolated recommendation from category 1, 2, or 3 evidence

TABLE 18-3 Evidence Grading System from the GRADE Working Group

Quality of Evidence	
High	Further research is very unlikely to change our confidence in the estimate of effect.
Moderate	Further research is likely to have an important impact on our confidence in the estimate of effect and may change the estimate.
Low	Further research is very likely to have an important impact on our confidence in the estimate of effect and is likely to change the estimate.
Very Low	Any estimate of effect is very uncertain.

TABLE 18-4	Guideline Recommendation System from the GRADE Working Group
Guideline Recommendation	
Strong For	Highly confident that the desirable consequences outweigh the undesirable consequences (of implementing the patient/client management element)
Weak For	Less confident that the desirable consequences outweigh the undesirable consequences (of implementing the patient/client management element)
Weak Against	Less confident that undesirable consequences outweigh the desirable consequences (of implementing the patient/client management element)
Strong Against	Highly confident that undesirable consequences outweigh the desirable consequences (of implementing the patient/client management element)

Reprinted from *Journal of Clinical Epidemiology*, 66(7), Andrews J, Guyatt G, Oxman AD, et al., GRADE guidelines: 14. Going from evidence to recommendations: the significance and presentation of recommendations, 719–725, Copyright 2013, with permission from Elsevier.

FIGURE 18-2	Overview of the process for developing and grading guidelines.

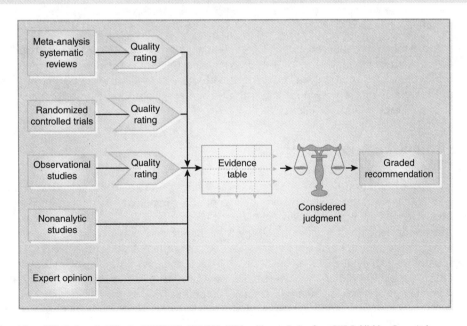

Reproduced from *BMJ*, Harbour R, Miller J., 323(7308), 334–336, 2001, with permission from BMJ Publishing Group Ltd.

outdated at the time of their study. Survival analysis indicated that 10% of the CPGs reviewed were outdated at 3.6 years and 50% were lost at 5 years. These authors conservatively recommended that CPGs be reviewed every 3 years and updated as necessary.[29] Physical therapists using evidence-based CPGs should consider whether the age of the product makes its application unreasonable or inappropriate in the current practice environment. If not, then age alone should not be a reason to reject the CPG.

A second issue is the overall quality of the CPG. Hasenfeld and Shekelle compared AHCPR CPGs with subsequently developed products.[30] Using a 30-item checklist to determine the relative quality of the CPGs they located, these authors found that newer CPGs did not meet most of the quality criteria. A more recent systematic review by Alonso-Coello et al. indicated that the quality of CPGs remains "moderate to low."[31] These results suggest that therapists must analyze CPGs carefully and use clinical judgment to determine their appropriateness for use with an individual patient or client.

In 2003, an international working group—the Appraisal of Guidelines Research and Evaluation Collaboration (AGREE)—published a 23-item CPG assessment instrument whose reliability and validity was established prior to its release.[32,33] The updated instrument (AGREE II) is composed of the following six domains:

1. Scope and purpose: "the overall aim of the guideline, the specific health questions, and the target population."
2. Stakeholder involvement: "the extent to which the guideline was developed by the appropriate stakeholders and represents the views of its intended users."
3. Rigor of development: "the process used to gather and synthesize the evidence, the methods to formulate the recommendations, and to update them."
4. Clarity and presentation: "the language, structure, and format of the guideline."
5. Applicability: "the likely barriers and facilitators to implementation, strategies to improve uptake, and resource implications of applying the guideline."
6. Editorial independence: "the formulation of recommendations not being unduly biased with competing interests."[33(p.10)]

The AGREE II tool has become the international standard for reporting the development and evaluation of CPGs. Authors creating more recent CPGs typically reference use of the instrument in their publication as verification that they have complied with this standard. The tool is publicly available so physical therapists may download it and use it as an appraisal form when reviewing CPGs for possible use with their patients or clients.

Is the Guideline Applicable?

Once the credibility of a CPG has been determined, the question of its applicability should be explored. Whether implementation of the CPG is appropriate depends on factors related to the condition of interest, the specificity of the recommendations it contains, the patient or client in question, other options available, and the practice environment in which the physical therapist is operating.

First, the condition of interest covered by the CPG should have enough impact to make implementation worth the investment in time, resources, and energy. Impact may be determined by a high prevalence rate, as is the case with arthritis, or by the seriousness of the consequences it creates, such as falls in the elderly, or both. Evidence-based physical therapists determine the potential level of impact when they consider a patient or client's risk for the condition and its potential outcomes.

Second, the decision to implement the guideline depends on the specificity of its recommendations. CPGs that address the use of particular patient/client management techniques are more likely to provide actionable details than those that address the overall management of a condition. For example, Brousseau et al. developed a CPG addressing the use of thermal and electrotherapeutic modalities to manage symptoms of rheumatoid arthritis. This CPG detailed evidence for, or against, the use of specific techniques such as lower level laser therapy, therapeutic ultrasound, and transcutaneous electrical nerve stimulation.[16] On the other hand, Moreland et al. recommended general categories of interventions (e.g., balance exercises, walking programs) in their CPG addressing fall risk in individuals 65 years and older who sustained a previous fall.[10] These authors did not specify the types of balance exercises or parameters for walking programs as a standard of care. In addition, neither CPG provided detailed recommendations regarding the frequency or dose of the interventions included. As a result, physical therapists often must return to the scientific literature for evidence of effectiveness of the techniques they want to employ in a plan of care. Fortunately, the CPG itself can expedite the search for individual studies because authors usually itemize this information in tables in the body and/or appendices of the published guideline.

Third, physical therapists must consider the congruence between a CPG's recommendations and the individual patient or client's preferences and values. Unlike research studies, CPGs may be produced in user-friendly formats that members of the general public will find easier to read and understand. For example, the American Academy of Otolaryngology—Head and Neck Surgery Foundation—provides a "plain language summary" about benign paroxysmal positional vertigo (BPPV) based on its CPG addressing this disorder of the inner ear.[34] As a result, it may be easier for physical therapists to provide information about CPG recommendations for patients or clients to consider during the decision-making process. Ideally, the CPGs will be explicit about what (and whose) preferences and values informed the development process. Assessment of preferences and values is a process that may take many forms. An evaluation of the trade-offs between the risks and benefits of various options for patient/client management is a common approach to this task. In effect, judgment in favor of, or opposed to, a particular option is determined based on its relative usefulness and ability to achieved stated wants or needs.[6] The challenge is to reconcile the utilities assumed in the CPG with those expressed by the individual patient or client.

Fourth, adoption of a CPG should be considered in terms of the outcomes achieved relative to the investment made. Comprehensive CPGs may require significant reorganization and reengineering in terms of the numbers and qualifications of health care staff, the type and amount of equipment and supplies, the methods and frequency with which care is delivered, and so forth. These changes may require considerable amounts of time, money, education, and training. If the anticipated outcomes are only incrementally better than current practice, then adoption of the CPG may not be worthwhile. Alternatively, even if the CPG is deemed beneficial, its adoption may be delayed or refused based on the nature and extent of local resource constraints.

Finally, successful CPG implementation depends on the willingness of those involved to change their current behaviors and practice. The mere presence of a CPG will not ensure its use, no matter how well it is supported by high-quality evidence. Potential barriers to change include provider preferences, habits, and concerns regarding loss of autonomy.[4,35] CPGs also appear to contradict the mandate to individualize patient/client management. This last obstacle to implementation is perhaps the most legitimate—a health care consumer's autonomy to make an informed decision to refuse a guideline recommendation should be respected. Strategies to overcome provider attitudes and behaviors are as complex as those used to encourage patients or clients to change their lifestyles. Whether to implement a guideline may depend on the extent of the effort required to facilitate this cultural shift, as well as the availability of resources to make it happen.

Summary

CPGs are statements developed to facilitate patient and provider decision making and to enhance quality of care. In their best form, these products combine a systematic review of the evidence with expert clinical judgment and health care consumer preferences and values. Some evidence suggests that guideline quality is moderate at best. In addition, recommendations included in CPGs typically do not provide detailed descriptions of specific patient/client management techniques or parameters. An instrument has been published by an international collaboration to facilitate the evaluation of guideline quality. Physical therapists should access this publicly available tool to assess a guideline's validity and relevance to their patients or clients and practice.

Exercises

1. Discuss the potential benefits of using CPGs to inform clinical decision making. Provide a clinical example relevant to physical therapist practice to illustrate your points.
2. Discuss the role of evidence in CPG development and the challenges associated with linking evidence to recommendations.
3. Discuss potential barriers to clinical guideline implementation among physical therapists. Identify one strategy for each barrier you might implement in an effort to facilitate change.
4. Consider your own practice preferences and habits or those observed in your practice colleagues. What internal barriers can you identify regarding your (their) willingness to adopt a CPG? Will any of the strategies you identified in question 3 help you (them) to change?
5. Use one of the electronic search engines to locate a CPG of interest. Then download the AGREE II tool and evaluate the CPG's quality. Assuming adoption of the guideline in practice was "easy," would you use it with individuals who have the condition addressed by the CPG? Justify your answer.

References

1. Helewa A, Walker JM. *Critical Evaluation of Research in Physical Rehabilitation: Towards Evidence-Based Practice.* Philadelphia, PA: W.B. Saunders; 2000.
2. Graham R, Mancher M, Wolman DM, Greenfield S, Steinberg E, eds. *Clinical Practice Guidelines We Can Trust.* Available at: http://www.nap.edu/catalog/13058/clinical-practice-guidelines-we-can-trust. Accessed July 31, 2016.
3. DiCenso A, Bayley L, Haynes RB. Accessing pre-appraised evidence: fine-tuning the 5S model into a 6S model. *Evid Based Nurs.* 2009;12(4):99-101.
4. Herbert R, Jamtvedt G, Hagen KB, Mead J. *Practical Evidence-Based Physiotherapy.* 2nd ed. Edinburgh, Scotland: Elsevier Butterworth-Heinemann; 2011.
5. Carter RE., Lubinsky J, Domholdt E. *Rehabilitation Research: Principles and Applications.* 4th ed. St. Louis, MO: Elsevier Saunders; 2011.

6. Straus SE, Richardson WS, Glaziou P, Haynes RB. *Evidence-Based Medicine: How to Practice and Teach EBM.* 3rd ed. Edinburgh, Scotland: Elsevier Churchill Livingstone; 2005.

7. Cook TD, Campbell DT. *Quasi-Experimentation: Design and Analysis Issues for Field Settings.* Boston, MA: Houghton Mifflin; 1979.

8. Guyatt G, Rennie D. *Users' Guides to the Medical Literature: A Manual for Evidence-Based Clinical Practice.* Chicago, IL: AMA Press; 2002.

9. Higgins JPT, Green S, eds. Cochrane Handbook for Systematic Reviews of Interventions, version 5.1.0 [updated March 2011]. The Cochrane Collaboration, 2011. Available at: http://training.cochrane.org/handbook. Accessed March 1, 2017.

10. Moreland J, Richardson J, Chan DH, et al. Evidence-based guidelines for the secondary prevention of falls in older adults [with systematic review]. *Gerontology.* 2003;49(2):93-116.

11. McPoil TG, Martin RL, Cornwall MW, et al. Heel pain-plantar fasciitis: clinical practice guidelines linked to the international classification of function, disability, and health from the orthopaedic section of the American Physical Therapy Association. *J Orthop Sports Phys Ther.* 2008;38(4):A1-A18.

12. Guidelines for Adult Stroke Rehabilitation and Recovery. American Academy of Neurology Website. Available at: https://www.aan.com/Guidelines/Home/GetGuidelineContent/744. Accessed March 1, 2017.

13. Brousseau L, Wells GA, Tugwell P, et al. Ottawa Panel evidence-based clinical practice guidelines for the management of osteoarthritis in adults who are obese or overweight. *Phys Ther.* 2011;91(6):843-861.

14. Kahn EB, Ramsey LT, Heath GW, Howze EH [Task Force on Community Preventive Services and the Centers for Disease Control and Prevention (CDC)]. Increasing physical activity: a report on recommendations of the Task Force on Community Preventive Services [quick reference guide for clinicians]. *MMWR.* 2001;50(RR-18):i-18.

15. Crapo RO, Casaburi R, Coates AL, et al. ATS statement: guidelines for the six-minute walk test. *Am J Respir Crit Care Med.* 2002;166(1):111-117.

16. Ottawa Panel. Ottawa Panel evidence-based clinical practice guidelines for electrotherapy and thermotherapy interventions in the management of rheumatoid arthritis in adults [with systematic review]. *Phys Ther.* 2004;84(11):1016-1043.

17. Enseki E, Harris-Hayes M, White DM, et al. Nonarthritic hip joint pain. *J Orthop Sports Phys Ther.* 2014;44(6):A1-32.

18. Agency for Healthcare Research and Quality website. United States Department of Health and Human Services. Available at: www.ahrq.gov. Accessed March 1, 2017.

19. PubMed. National Library of Medicine website. Available at: www.ncbi.nlm.nih.gov/pubmed. Accessed March 1, 2017.

20. Physiotherapy Evidence Database. Centre for Evidence-Based Physiotherapy. Available at: www.pedro.org.au. Accessed March 1, 2017.

21. National Guideline Clearing House website. Agency for Healthcare Research and Quality. Available at: www.guideline.gov. Accessed March 1, 2017.

22. PTNow. Available at: http://www.ptnow.org/Default.aspx. Accessed September 1, 2016.

23. Scalzitti DA. Evidence-based guidelines: application to clinical practice. *Phys Ther.* 2001;81(10):1622-1628.

24. Shekelle PG, Woolf SH, Eccles M, Grimshaw J. Developing guidelines. *BMJ.* 1999;318(7183):593-596.

25. GRADE Working Group. Grading quality of evidence and strength of recommendations. *BMJ.* 2004;328(7454):1490-1498.

26. Andrews J, Guyatt G, Oxman AD, et al. GRADE guidelines: 14. Going from evidence to recommendations: the significance and presentation of recommendations. *J Clin Epidemiol.* 2013;66(7):719-725.

27. Harbour R, Miller J. A new system for grading recommendations in evidence-based guidelines. *BMJ.* 2001;323(7308):334-336.

28. Shekelle P, Eccles MP, Grimshaw JM, Woolf SH. When should guidelines be updated? *BMJ.* 2001;323(7305):155-157.

29. Shekelle PG, Ortiz E, Rhodes S, et al. Validity of the Agency for Healthcare Research and Quality clinical practice guidelines. *JAMA.* 2001;286(12):1461-1467.

30. Hasenfeld R, Shekelle PG. Is the methodological quality of guidelines declining in the US? Comparison of the quality of US Agency for Health Care Policy and Research (AHCPR) guidelines with those published subsequently. *Qual Saf Health Care.* 2003;12(6):428-434.

31. Alonso-Coello P, Irfan A, Sola I, et al. The quality of clinical practice guidelines over the last two decades: a systematic review of guideline appraisal studies. *Qual Saf Health Care*. 2010;19(6):1-7.

32. AGREE Collaboration. Development and validation of an international appraisal instrument for assessing the quality of clinical practice guidelines: the AGREE project. *Qual Saf Health Care*. 2003;12(1):18-23.

33. The AGREE Collaboration website. Appraisal of Guidelines for Research & Evaluation. AGREE II Instrument. Available at: http://www.agreetrust.org/wp-content/uploads/2013/10/AGREE-II-Users-Manual-and-23-item-Instrument_2009_UPDATE_2013.pdf. Accessed March 1, 2017.

34. Bhattacharyya N, Hollingsworth DB, Mahoney K, O'Connor S. Plain language summary: benign paroxysmal positional vertigo. *OtolaryngolHead Neck Surg*. 2017;156(3):417-425.

35. Flodgren G, Hall AM, Goulding L, et al. Tools developed and disseminated by guideline producers to promote the uptake of their guidelines. *Cochrane Database of Systematic Reviews*. 2016;8:CD010669.

CHAPTER 19

APPRAISING QUALITATIVE RESEARCH STUDIES

OBJECTIVES

Upon completion of this chapter, the student/practitioner will be able to do the following:

1. Discuss the contribution of qualitative research studies to physical therapist clinical decision making for patients and clients.

2. Critically evaluate qualitative research studies, including the

   a. Important questions to ask related to study credibility;

   b. Meaning of study results in the context of the methodologic approach used.

3. Discuss considerations related to the application of qualitative research studies to individual patients or clients.

TERMS IN THIS CHAPTER

Bias: Results or inferences that systematically deviate from the truth "or the processes leading to such deviation."[1 (p.251)]

Data saturation: The point at which no new information can be obtained, no new data codes can be applied, and no new themes can be identified. Replicating the original study may be possible at this point.[2]

Discourse analysis: A qualitative research design that uses analysis of the form, content, and rules of conversations.[3,4]

Ethnography: A qualitative research design that uses a holistic analysis of a culture to understand shared systems of meaning.[3,4]

Ethology: A qualitative research design that uses observation of behaviors in a natural context.[4]

Grounded theory: A qualitative research design that uses analysis of social, psychological, and structural processes within a social setting to generate a theoretical understanding of subjects' perspectives and experiences.[3,4]

Historical analysis: A qualitative research design that uses analysis and interpretation of historical events.[4]

Patient-centered care: Health care that "customizes treatment recommendations and decision making in response to patients' preferences and beliefs. . . This partnership also is characterized by informed, shared decision making, development of patient knowledge, skills needed for self-management of illness, and preventive behaviors."[5(p.3)]

Phenomenology: A qualitative research design that uses analysis of experiences, interpretations, and meanings to understand the "lived experience" of the individuals studied.[3,4]

Purposive sampling: A nonprobabilistic sampling method in which investigators handpick specific individuals to participate based on characteristics important to the researchers.

Qualitative research paradigm: A research model that seeks to understand the nature of a phenomenon from the perspective and social context of the subjects who are studied, with the assumption that multiple realities may be possible and may evolve as the subjects interact with the researchers.[1,4]

Quantitative research paradigm: A research model that assumes an objective reality exists that is observable and can be measured through systematic, bias-free methods.[1,4]

Reflexivity: A principle of qualitative research methods that suggests researchers should reflect on and continually test their assumptions in each phase of the study.[4]

Triangulation: A method to confirm a concept or perspective generated through the qualitative research process.[4,6]

CLINICAL SCENARIO

My Body is Breaking Down: I Guess I Am Getting Older.

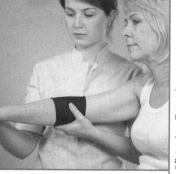

© Photographee.eu/Shutterstock

Over the course of your work with Anne, she has intermittently expressed anxiety about the impact aging will have on her body. She views this episode of elbow pain as an omen of future problems and wonders how that will impact her physical capacity over time. She prides herself on her fitness level and overall health and views this problem as a bit of a betrayal.

You have recently read a qualitative study that speaks to concerns people have about recovery from musculoskeletal injuries.*

How will you use this information as part of your plan of care for Anne?

*Carroll LJ, Lis A, Weiser S, Torti J. How well do you expect to recover, and what does recovery mean, anyway? Qualitative study of expectations after a musculoskeletal injury. *Phys Ther*. 2016;96(6):797-807.

Introduction

Qualitative research studies investigate subjects' thoughts, perceptions, opinions, beliefs, attitudes, and/or experiences.[3,4] They often focus on the perspectives and interactions of patients or clients, family members, caregivers, providers, and others engaged in the health care enterprise. The investigations are intended to capture in the subjects' own words and/or through the researchers' direct observations the experiences that unfold in their natural context.

Evidence-based physical therapists can use qualitative research studies to answer questions they have about the following:

- How individuals experience and manage health, disease, and/or disability;
- Lived cultural influences that shape perceptions and use of the health care system;
- The meaning that individuals ascribe to their roles in a health care encounter;
- Individuals' preferences and values with respect to options available for identifying and managing or remediating the conditions that impact their health;
- Individuals' beliefs and attitudes regarding their potential for recovery or adaptation through physical therapist patient/client management;
- Individuals' motivations to participate in physical therapists' plans of care.

Incorporation of this type of evidence in clinical decision making represents a holistic approach to patient/client management that is consistent with *patient-centered care.*[5] **Table 19-1** provides some examples of qualitative studies relevant to physical therapist practice.

The intent and design of qualitative research studies challenge physical therapists to find a suitable method for critically appraising them. Application of a *qualitative research paradigm* assumes that knowledge and understanding are contextual and relative to each individual studied.[1,4] Investigators

TABLE 19-1	**Examples of Qualitative Research Studies Relevant to Physical Therapist Practice**

- Timothy EK, et al. Transitions in the embodied experience after stroke: grounded theory study. *Phys Ther.* 2016;96(10):1565-1575.
- Bunzli S, et al. Patient perspectives on participation in cognitive functional therapy for chronic low back pain. *Phys Ther.* 2016;96(9):1397-1407.
- Fieril KP, et al. Experiences of exercise during pregnancy among women who perform regular resistance training: a qualitative study. *Phys Ther.* 2014;94(8):1135-1143.
- Merlo AR, et al. Participants' perspectives on the feasibility of a novel, intensive, task-specific intervention for individuals with chronic stroke: a qualitative analysis. *Phys Ther.* 2013;93(2):147-157.
- Gudfinna Bjornsdottir G, et al. Facilitators of and barriers to physical activity in retirement communities: experiences of older women in urban areas. *Phys Ther.* 2012;92(4):551-562.
- Blaney J, et al. The cancer rehabilitation journey: barriers to and facilitators of exercise among patients with cancer-related fatigue. *Phys Ther.* 2010;90(8):1135-1147.
- Levins SM, et al. Individual and societal influences on participation in physical activity following spinal cord injury: a qualitative study. *Phys Ther.* 2004;84(6):496-509.

and subjects are thought to influence each other while the researchers gather information about subjects' "lived experiences" and worldviews. Methods of control relative to extraneous environmental influences are irrelevant in this approach because it assumes that cause and effect relationships, if present, should be identified as they naturally occur. Similarly, minimization of potential subject *bias* is not required for studies in which an objective "truth" cannot be identified in the first place. As a result, researchers do not introduce experimental interventions or controls that limit knowledge or behavior in an artificial context (i.e., a laboratory). Rather, they attempt to capture how subjects construct meaning about naturally occurring phenomena and interactions within their environment. Finally, the analyses aim to identify patterns or themes in the data (i.e., words or descriptive observations) rather than determine the statistical significance of objective measurements.

This fundamentally different approach to research design requires physical therapists to consider alternative criteria by which to judge the quality of the evidence they uncover. The following approach is based on a combination of recommendations from several authors and evidence-based practice groups who have pondered this challenge.[3,7-10]

Study Credibility

Quantitative research designs assume that there is one objective truth that can be captured through properly designed and implemented methods. An investigator's ability to avoid or mitigate threats to research credibility in his or her study determines the degree to which the findings are considered "believable." However, the concept of "believability" appears inconsistent with the paradigm upon which qualitative research designs are based. Reality and meaning depend on the unique perspective of everyone engaged in the investigation, and therefore can take on multiple forms. Avoiding or minimizing threats to a study's credibility in these designs seems unnecessary, if not counterproductive. However, the need to answer critics who discount the value of qualitative research findings as subjective and anecdotal has prompted qualitative researchers to develop strategies to affirm the trustworthiness of their designs.[4] The questions itemized in **Table 19-2** inform appraisal of the credibility of a qualitative study related to physical therapist patient/client management.

1. Did the investigators use a qualitative research methodology that was consistent with their research question?

Qualitative studies—like their quantitative counterparts—start with a research question the investigators want to answer. The phrasing of that question signals the methodologic approach required to answer it. For example, a study about how individuals make sense of their disability after a job-related injury lends itself to one form of qualitative research known as *phenomenology*. Alternatively, a *grounded theory* approach would be an appropriate methodology when investigators want to explore theoretical underpinnings of differences in resilience among cancer survivors. **Table 19-3** outlines a variety of methodologies qualitative researchers may use to address their questions. Given the subjective nature of qualitative research, the credibility of these types of studies hinges on the investigators' application of the correct approach.

2. Did the investigators include individuals whose background and attributes were consistent with their research question?

Selection of subjects for prospective study in a qualitative research project is accomplished through *purposive sampling*. The research question identifies the population(s) of interest. Investigators must then identify more specifically the characteristics that would qualify an individual to participate. For example, if researchers want to conduct an ethnographic study to understand cultural influences on low-income parents of children with cerebral palsy, they would need a way to identify the financial

TABLE 19-2   Questions to Assess Qualitative Research Studies

1. Did the investigators use a qualitative research methodology that was consistent with their research question?
2. Did the investigators include individuals whose background and attributes were consistent with their research question?
3. Did the investigators use data collection methods that were consistent with their research methodology?
4. Did the investigators collect data in a context sufficient to thoroughly address their research question?
5. Did the investigators implement methods to confirm initial findings generated through their data collection processes?
6. Did the investigators interpret the data in a manner consistent with their research methodology?
7. Did the investigators explicitly examine their own beliefs, values, and assumptions in relation to their findings?
8. Did the investigators explicitly examine their influence on the research process and outcomes?

TABLE 19-3   Commonly Used Qualitative Research Methodologies

Qualitative Research Methodology	Type of Question Addressed
Discourse analysis	How do individuals in this setting communicate with one another under these circumstances or conditions?
Ethnography	How are individuals' behaviors shaped by the culture of this setting under these circumstances or conditions?
Ethology	How do individuals behave in this setting under these circumstances or conditions?
Grounded theory	How do individuals make sense of their experiences in this setting under these circumstances or conditions?
Historical analysis	How did individuals behave or interpret their experiences in this setting under these previous circumstances or conditions?
Phenomenology	How do individuals make sense of interactions with others and/or with their setting under these circumstances or conditions?

status of individuals who had children with this developmental disability. Once that profile is completed, a direct invitation to a small number of these study candidates can be made. The volume of data generated by the subjects' own words and/or the investigators' observations precludes the need for a large sample size. However, a study's credibility will be threatened if the subjects included are not representative of the population described in the research question.

Retrospective qualitative research (i.e., *historical analysis*) commonly relies on information obtained from previously created documents, data files, and/or artifacts. Interviews with purposefully selected participants in, or witnesses to, historical events may also be included. The same concerns apply with respect to congruence with the research question and representativeness of the population of interest.

3. Did the investigators use data collection methods that were consistent with their research methodology?

Qualitative research is an exercise in divining patterns and themes from words. How those words are captured depends on the research methodology applied (**Table 19-4**). For example, *ethnography* is an approach in which the investigators record their observations of subjects in their natural context to understand cultural dynamics. Phenomenology, on the other hand, requires researchers to capture the subjects' perceptions, beliefs, attitudes, and/or values in their own words. Interview formats include semi-structured, in-depth, and narrative approaches that may be applied with each individual subject or during focus group sessions. Questions are posed in an open-ended manner rather than selecting from a preestablished set of options or being confined to "yes" or "no" so that the subjects' "lived experience" is reflected. Blending researcher observation and subject interview is a common strategy in studies using a grounded theory methodology. As with the prior questions, a qualitative study's credibility will be threatened if the data collection methods used do not fit within the framework driven by the research question.

TABLE 19-4   Commonly Used Qualitative Data Collection Approaches

Qualitative Research Methodology	Data Collection Approach
Discourse analysis	Analysis of the form, content, and rules of conversations via capture of subjects' written and spoken words
Ethnography	Holistic analysis of a culture via observation
Ethology	Observation of behaviors in a natural context
Grounded theory	Analysis of social, psychological, and structural processes within a social setting via observation and/or interview
Historical analysis	Analysis and interpretation of historical events via review of previously created records (e.g., archival documents/correspondence/audiovisual recordings) and/or past or recently recorded interviews/oral histories
Phenomenology	Analysis of experiences, interpretations, meanings via interview

4. Did the investigators collect data in a context sufficient to thoroughly address their research question?

This question alludes to the holistic nature of qualitative studies. All research methodologies in the qualitative research paradigm are focused on revealing the meaning that people generate from experiences that occur in a social context. The research question determines how narrow or broad that context is. Using the example of low-income parents of children with cerebral palsy, the context may be limited to the home environment if the research question is about family dynamics in response to the impact of disability on self-care and daily routines. The social context will be wider if the question includes community-level influences. Qualitative researchers should specify where data were collected so that study readers can verify the congruence of settings with the research question.

5. Did the investigators interpret the data in a manner consistent with their research methodology?

This question speaks of the methods by which investigators transformed their data into codes, categories, and/or themes. Review of field notes, transcribed interviews, and/or historical records may be accomplished manually or with sophisticated software programs. An essential feature is a description of the decision rules used and clear evidence of an inductive process. Inductive reasoning honors the qualitative research paradigm's philosophy regarding "truth" as a subjective phenomenon that is generated by individuals through their observations, experiences, and interactions. Theory may emerge from the data that informs understanding of a phenomenon or worldview.

Interpretations that are consistent with the research question and associated qualitative research methodology also are essential to study credibility. For example, a study examining the meaning to which individuals attribute their experiences with stroke should result in interpretations that reflect the subjects' words and perspectives. Alternatively, a study that captured patterns of behavior in individuals with stroke should result in themes that are reflective of the investigators' perceptions and observations.

6. Did the investigators implement methods to confirm initial findings generated through their data collection processes?

Triangulation is a method to confirm a concept or perspective generated through the qualitative research process.[4,6] Investigators have several options available to achieve this validation. First, they may use multiple sources of data, such as patients and caregivers, to describe a phenomenon. Second, they may use data collection methods such as interviews and direct observations that focus on the same issues or phenomena. Third, they may involve multiple researchers who, through discussion of the data they have collected, provide confirmatory or contradictory information. Inherent to these approaches is an iterative process in which conceptual categories, or themes, are generated and refined through successive cycles of data gathering and analysis until a "saturation point" is reached. *Data saturation* may be indicated by the inability to obtain new data, apply new codes, and identify new themes.[2] The consistency of concepts, themes, and perspectives gleaned using these different approaches lends credibility to the findings that are reported.

7. Did the investigators explicitly examine their own beliefs, values, and assumptions in relation to their findings?

Reflexivity is a principle of qualitative designs that suggests researchers should reflect on and continually test their assumptions in each phase of the study.[4] Investigators who formally implement this principle in their work may document their preconceived notions about a phenomenon and the study participants, subject their analyses to repeated testing as new data are obtained, and challenge their interpretations from known theoretical perspectives. The intention is not to eliminate bias as would be attempted in quantitative research designs. Rather, reflexive scrutiny helps investigators place their biases in purposeful relationship to the context of their study and its participants. Engaging in this discipline is essential to addressing concerns about the inherent subjectivity in qualitative research and is often used to support a study's credibility.

8. Did the investigators explicitly examine their influence on the research process and outcomes?

An issue related to the context of the study (question #4) is the placement and role of investigators in the subjects' environment. The qualitative research paradigm assumes that meaning is generated when individuals interact with one another, even in scenarios where one person is standing in the background observing another person in action. Subjects often are predisposed to change their behavior in response to the perceived or actual expectations of the investigators (referred to by Carter et al. as "experimenter expectancies").[11(p.86)] In this situation, subjects respond to what they anticipate the investigator wants (also known as the Hawthorne effect),[6] or to subtle cues the investigator provides during data collection. In some qualitative methodologies, researchers are active participants in the social context of their study and have a more direct influence on their subjects as a result. Regardless of proximity or distance, qualitative study credibility is undermined if investigators do not explicitly consider their contribution to the meaning of the outcomes of their research.

Additional Considerations

The previous questions serve as an initial screening of the evidence to determine its potential usefulness—that is, its trustworthiness. From an evaluative standpoint, a "no" answer to any of them may so undermine the research design as to cause it to be set aside.

In addition to the eight questions itemized above, concerns pertaining to qualitative research studies include the presence or absence of a detailed description of the following:

1. Characteristics of the sample obtained;
2. Setting(s) in which the research was conducted;
3. Interactions between the researcher(s) and subjects, and the subjects with each other if relevant; and,
4. Specific data collection methods and context.

This information allows evidence-based physical therapists to determine (a) if the subjects and their settings resemble the patient or client (and his or her situation) about whom there is a question (1–2); (b) whether the themes identified are likely to be reproducible in the therapist's and/or individual's context; and, (c) whether elements of the data collection process can be incorporated into the therapist's interactions with a patient or client. Well-designed studies may have limited usefulness when these details are lacking.

Study Results

Results in qualitative research studies typically are a combination of investigator-identified themes supported by excerpts from field notes and/or interview transcriptions. Depending on the research questions, themes may be organized into proposed theoretical frameworks that may be the basis for further exploration of a phenomenon or for adaptations of clinical practice in new ways. In all cases, the results should clearly demonstrate a logical flow from the raw data to the patterns identified (rather than the other way around). In addition, the "voice" of the population of interest identified in the research question (e.g., parents of low-income children with cerebral palsy, individuals who have suffered a stroke, cancer survivors) should be clearly represented in the excerpts of data provided.

By definition, statistical analysis is not relevant in qualitative research. However, studies using a mix of quantitative and qualitative approaches will include data analysis consistent with the *quantitative research paradigm*.

Evidence and the Patient or Client

As with all evidence, a qualitative research study must be examined to determine if the subjects and their experiences resemble closely enough the patient or client, as well as the clinical context, to whom the results may be applied. Unlike evidence about other elements of the patient/client management model, qualitative studies suggest possible explanations for a patient's or client's preferences, values, motivations, perspectives, and concerns. Qualitative researchers would be the first to say that any "truth" derived from their work is inherent to the subjects studied and cannot be relied on as an objective fact against which an individual should be compared. This is where clinical judgment comes into play, because therapists must decide whether their patient's or client's interpretation of their situation is unique to him or her or resembles themes uncovered through subjects in the study. That conclusion, as well as the patient's or client's values, will provide guidance to therapists about how to use results from qualitative research studies in the patient/client management process.

Evidence Appraisal Tools

Table 19-5 provides a checklist to guide the evaluation of qualitative research studies. Alternatively, readers might consider accessing appraisal resources available online. A strategy worth considering is the creation of reference notebooks that contain completed checklists or worksheets along with their associated research articles. These compendia could facilitate the use of evidence that informs patient or client preferences, values, motivations, perspectives, and concerns by all physical therapists in a particular setting (as long as there is a commitment to keeping them up to date).

TABLE 19-5	Qualitative Research Studies—Quality Appraisal Checklist
Credibility of the Study	
Did the investigators use a qualitative research methodology that was consistent with their research question?	___ Yes ___ No ___ Insufficient detail
Did the investigators include individuals whose background and attributes were consistent with their research question?	___ Yes ___ No ___ Insufficient detail
Did the investigators use data collection methods that were consistent with their research methodology?	___ Yes ___ No ___ Insufficient detail
Did the investigators collect data in a context sufficient to thoroughly address their research question?	___ Yes ___ No ___ Insufficient detail

(*continues*)

TABLE 19-5	Qualitative Research Studies—Quality Appraisal Checklist (*Continued*)

Did the investigators interpret the data in a manner consistent with their research methodology?	___ Yes ___ No ___ Insufficient detail
Did the investigators implement methods to confirm initial findings generated through their data collection processes?	___ Yes ___ No ___ Insufficient detail
Did the investigators explicitly examine their own beliefs, values, and assumptions in relation to their findings?	___ Yes ___ No ___ Insufficient detail
Did the investigators explicitly examine their influence on the research process and outcomes?	___ Yes ___ No ___ Insufficient detail
Do you have enough confidence in the credibility of this study to consider using this evidence with your patient or client?	___ Yes ___ Undecided ___ No

Relevant Study Findings

Results reported that are specific to your clinical question: _____

Application of the Evidence to Your Patient or Client

Are there clinically meaningful differences between the subjects in the study and your patient or client?	___ Yes ___ No ___ Mixed results ___ Insufficient detail
Can you apply the results of this study in an ethical, culturally appropriate way given your current knowledge, skills, experience, and clinical context?	___ Yes ___ No
Will application of the results of this study fit within the patient's or client's expressed values and preferences?	___ Yes ___ No ___ Mixed results
Will you incorporate the results of this study in your clinical decision making with this patient or client?	___ Yes ___ No

Summary

Qualitative research studies investigate subjects' thoughts, perceptions, opinions, beliefs, attitudes, and/or experiences. The investigations are intended to capture in the subjects' own words and/or through the researchers' direct observations the experiences that unfold in their natural context. Findings from this type of evidence can inform physical therapists' understanding of the meaning their patients or clients attribute to experiences with health, disease, injury, and disability, as well as with the health care system. Verification of the credibility of these studies, as well as their relevance to the individual patient or client, is essential to determining whether the information can be applied during the patient/client management process while also respecting the individual's own preferences and values.

Exercises

1. Describe the purpose and general features of the qualitative research paradigm. Provide an example of a research question relevant to physical therapist practice that might be answered by this approach.
2. Use the research question from the previous answer and identify
   a. the qualitative research methodology you might use;
   b. potential data collection methods you might use.
   Explain why you are proposing these approaches.
3. Explain why inductive reasoning is an essential component of data analysis in qualitative research studies. Provide an example relevant to physical therapist practice to illustrate your points.
4. Describe the process of triangulation. Why is it important to a qualitative research study's credibility? Provide an example relevant to physical therapist practice to illustrate your points.
5. Describe the process of reflexivity. Why is it important to a qualitative research study's credibility? Provide an example relevant to physical therapist practice to illustrate your points.
6. Review one of the qualitative research articles cited in Table 19-1. Briefly describe how you might use the findings from that article with a patient or client resembling the subjects in the study. What challenges might you face applying this evidence in your clinical decision making?

References

1. Helewa A, Walker JM. *Critical Evaluation of Research in Physical Rehabilitation: Towards Evidence-Based Practice.* Philadelphia, PA: W.B. Saunders; 2000.
2. Fusch PI, Ness LR. Are we there yet? Data saturation in qualitative research. *The Qualitative Report.* 2015;20(9):1408-1416.
3. Hoffman T, Bennet S, Del Mar C. *Evidence-Based Practice Across the Health Professions.* Chatswood NSW, Australia: Churchill Livingstone; 2010.
4. Green J, Thorogood N. *Qualitative Methods for Health Research.* 2nd ed. London, England: Sage; 2009.
5. Greiner AC, Knebel E, eds. Health Professions Education: A Bridge to Quality. Institute of Medicine website. Available at: https://www.nap.edu/read/10681/chapter/1. Accessed July 16, 2016.
6. Portney LG, Watkins MP. *Foundations of Clinical Research: Applications to Practice.* 3rd ed. Upper Saddle River, NJ: Prentice Hall Health; 2009.
7. Law M, MacDermid D, eds. *Evidence-Based Rehabilitation: A Guide to Practice.* 2nd ed. Thorofare, NJ: Slack, Incorporated; 2008.
8. Kuper A, Lingard L, Levinson W. Critically appraising qualitative research. *BMJ.* 2008;337:A1035.
9. Giacomini MK, Cook DJ. Qualitative research in health care. Are the results of the study valid? *JAMA.* 2000;284(3):357-362.
10. Giacomini MK, Cook DJ. Qualitative research in health care. What are the results and how do they help me care for my patients? *JAMA.* 2000;284(4):478-482.
11. Carter RE, Lubinsky J, Domholdt E. *Rehabilitation Research: Principles and Applications.* 4th ed. St. Louis, MO: Elsevier Saunders; 2011.

EVIDENCE IN PRACTICE

CHAPTER 20

PATIENT OR CLIENT PREFERENCES AND VALUES

OBJECTIVES

Upon completion of this chapter, the student/practitioner will be able to do the following:

1. Discuss the relationship among evidence, clinical judgment and expertise, and patient or client preferences and values.

2. Describe patient-centered care and its relationship to evidence-based physical therapist (EBPT) practice.

3. Discuss the ethical principles of autonomy, beneficence, and nonmaleficence and their relationship to EBPT practice.

4. Differentiate between shared decision making and the traditional biomedical model for determining a plan of care.

5. Discuss the incorporation of evidence into the shared decision-making process.

6. Differentiate among patient or client preferences, expectancies, and values.

7. Describe strategies for eliciting information about patient or client preferences, expectancies, and values.

8. Explain how subject preferences, expectancies, and values may undermine the research validity of a study.

9. Describe potential strategies investigators may implement to deal with subject preferences, expectancies, and values.

TERMS IN THIS CHAPTER

Autonomy: An ethical principle that affirms an individual's right to make decisions about his or her health care.

Beneficence: An ethical principle that affirms the physical therapist's obligation to act in the best interests of the patient or client.

Biologic plausibility: The reasonable expectation that the human body could behave in the manner predicted.

Clinical expertise: Proficiency of clinical skills and abilities, informed by continually expanding knowledge, that individual clinicians develop through experience, learning, and reflection about their practice.[1,2]

Clinical practice guideline: ". . . statements that include recommendations intended to optimize patient care. They are informed by a systematic review of evidence and an assessment of the benefits and harms of alternative care options."[3] Also referred to as summaries.[4]

Cultural competence: The knowledge, skills, and abilities needed to interact with individuals from different cultures in an appropriate, relevant, and sensitive manner.[5]

Expectancy: The belief that a process or outcome possesses certain attributes.[6]

Informed consent: An individual's authorization of a procedure or technique following a conversation between the health care provider and patient or client about a proposed course of action, alternative courses of action, no action, and the risks and benefits of each of these options.[7]

Nonmaleficence: An ethical principle that affirms the physical therapist's obligation to avoid actions that cause harm to the patient or client.

Patient-centered care: Health care that "customizes treatment recommendations and decision making in response to patients' preferences and beliefs. . . . This partnership also is characterized by informed, shared decision making, development of patient knowledge, skills needed for self-management of illness, and preventive behaviors."[8(p.3)]

Placebo effect: A change in an outcome measure (usually an improvement) that is demonstrated by subjects in a control group who are receiving a placebo (or sham) intervention in a study.

Preference: The difference in the perceived desirability of two (or more) options related to health care.[6]

Research validity: "The degree to which a study appropriately answers the question being asked."[9(p.225)]

Resentful demoralization: A threat to research validity (internal validity) characterized by subjects in the control (comparison) group who, in response to knowledge about group assignment, limit their efforts in the study.

Shared decision making: An exchange of ideas between a health care provider and patient or client and collaboration in the decision itself.[7]

Values: Concepts or beliefs about desirable behaviors or states of being that are prioritized relative to one another.[10]

Introduction

Clinicians must integrate evidence with their *clinical expertise* and judgment, as well as with individual patient or client preferences and values. EBPT practice is achieved only when these three information sources contribute to the final decision about how to address a patient's or client's needs.[1] On one level, this integration process may sound counterintuitive given the emphasis on high-quality evidence that has minimized bias. After all, both clinicians and patients or clients bring a level of subjectivity to their decision making that may result in choices that contradict valid and important findings from well-designed research. Nevertheless, health care is a human

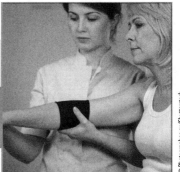

© Photographee.eu/Shutterstock

CLINICAL SCENARIO

I Am Tired of This Pain; I Think I Just Need to Push Through It!

Your initial interview with Anne indicates she is impatient with her elbow pain. She cannot exercise, do her job, or manage her household to her satisfaction. She understands that refusing oral or intramuscular medication potentially results in a longer recovery period, but she is clear about her preference to use nonpharmaceutical treatment methods. Her comment about "pushing through it" also suggests she will be susceptible to relapses that will slow her progress if she tries to accelerate your plan of care according to her own timeline.

How will you weave your assessment of her preferences and potential behaviors into your clinical decision making?

endeavor that, for many people, cannot and should not be reduced to complete dependence on science in the absence of clinician or patient or client perspective and experience. In addition, the highest quality evidence usually provides information about groups rather than individuals, a fact that reinforces reluctance to accept the relevance of even the best evidence.[11]

The challenge for physical therapists, therefore, is to gather information from all three sources in the EBPT practice triad and to discuss all of it explicitly with the patient or client so that the relative merits of available options may be considered in a holistic fashion prior to establishing a plan of care. For physical therapists to be explicit about the nature and contribution of their expertise and judgment, they must routinely engage in self-reflection and appraisal. This process includes an acknowledgment of practice preferences and habits that have developed over the years, gaps in knowledge that would benefit from additional education or training, and enablers and barriers to change in their approach to patient/client management.[12] Patients and clients, in contrast, require the opportunity to express their preferences and values in a decision-making process that traditionally has deemphasized their involvement. Physical therapists must provide this invitation early and often with each individual, as well as with family and/or caregivers, to facilitate this collaborative process. Meanwhile, evidence must be located and evaluated and its findings translated into meaningful information that all partners in the decision-making process can understand.

Needless to say, this integrated approach to patient/client management is probably easier to describe than to execute. Dierckx and colleagues found that the physical therapists they studied did not recognize the patients' desire to participate in decision making in 64% of the consultations that occurred.[13] Even when a collaborative relationship is established, there is no guarantee that patients or clients will respond to the available information in the same manner as their physical therapists. The stakes may be especially high when disagreement results between the provider and the individual over desired management approaches that are contrary to those supported by high-level evidence. Potential conflict is not a reason to avoid the process, however. This chapter discusses the involvement of patients and clients in health care decision making and the contribution of their preferences and values to EBPT practice.

Patient-Centered Care

Patient contribution to EBPT practice is an essential ingredient of patient-centered care. According to the Institute of Medicine, *patient-centered care* "is characterized by informed, shared decision making, development of patient knowledge, skills needed for self-management of illness, and preventive behaviors."[8(p.3)] This concept rejects the traditional biomedical model in which providers (e.g., physicians, physical therapists) make choices for patients based on superior knowledge and understanding of health-related issues and the options with which to address them.[14] Many patients and their families (caregivers) no longer accept their role as passive recipients of biomedical expertise and skill; rather, they increasingly view themselves as partners in a health care system that should acknowledge and accept their unique culture and perspectives.[8,15]

Several factors are responsible for this shift of focus away from providers and onto patients and their families (caregivers). First, advances in biomedical technology and pharmaceuticals have transformed uniformly fatal diseases into chronic conditions with which individuals may live for decades.[7] Examples include heart failure, chronic obstructive pulmonary disease, diabetes, many forms of cancer, and acquired immune deficiency syndrome (AIDS), to name a few. The increased costs associated with the care of these long-term problems have resulted in disease management models focused on secondary prevention through patient and family education, self-management, and adherence to preventive treatment routines.[15] By definition, these approaches depend on an informed partnership between the health care team and the patient and family (caregivers) rather than a unilateral decision-making structure.

Second, the Internet has increased the access of the general public to information about diseases and their management options. Numerous professional, patient advocacy, and government entities provide medical information in layperson's terms through free websites. The National Library of Medicine,[15] the American Heart Association,[16] the American Diabetes Association,[19] the American Medical Association,[20] and the American Physical Therapy Association[21] are just a few of the many groups offering this service. Many more sites from a variety of sources are available, the quality and accuracy of which vary considerably. Nevertheless, patients and their families (caregivers) are arriving at health care appointments armed with information, including research findings that may reduce their reliance on medical professionals for understanding about their situation.

Finally, the evidence itself indicates that increased availability of information and participation in health care decision making may enhance patient satisfaction, adherence to prescribed regimens, confidence in health care providers, adjustment to changes in health, and, in some cases, psychological and physiologic outcomes.[14] These findings are not conclusive because additional investigation is needed to determine patients' preferred level of participation in decision making, clinician characteristics and behaviors that influence participation, and the impact of that involvement across a wider range of diseases and disorders.[22-24] In addition, the role of cultural and societal context in patient management and outcomes requires further study.

Despite these knowledge gaps, patient-centered care is a concept that appears firmly embedded in contemporary health care. Patient participation during the development of *clinical practice guidelines* and self-report outcomes measures reflects this emphasis on the incorporation of the patient's point of view at all stages of the health care encounter. A similar focus may be applied to health promotion and primary prevention arenas if the phrase is changed to "client-centered care." Both terms reinforce the notion that EBPT practice is a collaborative and integrative process between the clinician and the patient or client.

Ethical Considerations

Beyond the epidemiologic and societal changes promoting patient-centered care is a more fundamental obligation for physical therapists—patient/client management that is informed by a professional code of ethics (**Figure 20-1**).[25] These statements are consistent with the concept of *autonomy*, which recognizes an individual's right to make decisions about his or her health care. By definition, the patient or client is at the center of this ethical principle, and physical therapists are duty bound to honor this position. Describing and interpreting findings from the best available evidence can be argued to support autonomy by providing patients or clients with essential information to consider before making a final choice.[15] Similarly, therapists may view the use of evidence as consistent with two additional ethical principles: beneficence and nonmaleficence. *Beneficence* instructs physical therapists to make decisions with the patient or client's best interests in mind, whereas *nonmaleficence* states that harm should be avoided. Both of these dictates may be supported by well-designed research with compelling findings demonstrating a beneficial or harmful effect, respectively. However, therapists may find that these principles conflict with autonomy when high-quality evidence recommends (or discounts) a management option that the patient or client is refusing (or requesting). Also at play in these situations are the therapist's clinical judgment and expertise and the patient or client's preferences and values, all of which influence perceptions about the meaning and relevance of the evidence beyond its stated results. Resolution of this potential dilemma is contingent on a successful negotiation of a mutually agreeable plan of care.

Informed Consent and Shared Decision Making

Patient or client self-determination depends on access to information. The opportunity to learn about the details relevant to a health care decision is the first step in the process referred to as informed consent. *Informed consent* requires formal conversations between physical therapists and patients or clients that result in unambiguous instructions regarding what services (e.g., procedures, techniques) will be accepted or refused.[7] During these conversations, evidence-based physical therapists should supply details about the patient or client's diagnosis, prognosis, treatment options, and associated risks and benefits. In addition, therapists are responsible for translating available research findings into meaningful information that is applicable to the individual. In return, patients or clients hopefully will share their perceptions regarding their condition; understanding of, and preferences for different management options and their potential impact on daily life, as well as goals to be achieved at the conclusion of physical therapy. Respect for patient or client autonomy requires that this information exchange occur in an explicit manner.

The ability to exercise one's autonomy in health care implies an understanding of the potential consequences of the different choices outlined during the consent process. From a legal perspective, informed consent is particularly focused on the potential risk associated with elements of the plan of care. Risk in this sense reflects both the likelihood that harm will occur, as well as the severity of the adverse outcome itself, both of which may be defined by the provider's clinical experience and/or the available evidence.[7] Patients or clients may evaluate this risk within their sociocultural context and in reference to available evidence or perceived knowledge about the situation.

This potentially high-stakes evaluation process is most evident for surgical procedures. For example, the statement "arteriovenous (AV) malformation surgery is associated with an 8% risk of death"[26] suggests a low probability of a serious event occurring as a result of a proposed intervention. Whether 8% is low enough, however, is an individual decision that may be influenced by a patient's definition of acceptable risk,[14] as well as by cultural and social reactions to uncertainty about the future. Similarly, willingness to risk death to repair the AV defect may also depend on a patient's perspective

FIGURE 20-1	Code of ethics for the physical therapist.

Code of Ethics for the Physical Therapist

✚APTA
American Physical Therapy Association™

HOD S06-09-07-12 [Amended HOD S06-00-12-23; HOD 06-91-05-05;HOD 06-87-11-17;
HOD 06-81-06-18; HOD 06-78-06-08; HOD 06-78-06-07; HOD 06-77-18-30; HOD 06-77-17-27;
Initial HOD 06-73-13-24] [Standard]

Preamble

The Code of Ethics for the Physical Therapist (Code of Ethics) delineates the ethical obligations of all physical therapists as determined by the House of Delegates of the American Physical Therapy Association (APTA). The purposes of this Code of Ethics are to:

1. Define the ethical principles that form the foundation of physical therapist practice in patient/client management, consultation, education, research, and administration.

2. Provide standards of behavior and performance that form the basis of professional accountability to the public.

3. Provide guidance for physical therapists facing ethical challenges, regardless of their professional roles and responsibilities.

4. Educate physical therapists, students, other health care professionals, regulators, and the public regarding the core values, ethical principles, and standards that guide the professional conduct of the physical therapist.

5. Establish the standards by which the American Physical Therapy Association can determine if a physical therapist has engaged in unethical conduct.

No code of ethics is exhaustive nor can it address every situation. Physical therapists are encouraged to seek additional advice or consultation in instances where the guidance of the Code of Ethics may not be definitive.

This Code of Ethics is built upon the five roles of the physical therapist (management of patients/clients, consultation, education, research, and administration), the core values of the profession, and the multiple realms of ethical action (individual, organizational, and societal). Physical therapist practice is guided by a set of seven core values: accountability, altruism, compassion/caring, excellence, integrity, professional duty, and social responsibility. Throughout the document the primary core values that support specific principles are indicated in parentheses. Unless a specific role is indicated in the principle, the duties and obligations being delineated pertain to the five roles of the physical therapist. Fundamental to the Code of Ethics is the special obligation of physical therapists to empower, educate, and enable those with impairments, activity limitations, participation restrictions, and disabilities to facilitate greater independence, health, wellness, and enhanced quality of life.

Principles

Principle #1: Physical therapists shall respect the inherent dignity and rights of all individuals.
(Core Values: Compassion, Integrity)

1A. Physical therapists shall act in a respectful manner toward each person regardless of age, gender, race, nationality, religion, ethnicity, social or economic status, sexual orientation, health condition, or disability.

1B. Physical therapists shall recognize their personal biases and shall not discriminate against others in physical therapist practice, consultation, education, research, and administration.

Principle #2: Physical therapists shall be trustworthy and compassionate in addressing the rights and needs of patients/clients.
(Core Values: Altruism, Compassion, Professional Duty)

2A. Physical therapists shall adhere to the core values of the profession and shall act in the best interests of patients/clients over the interests of the physical therapist.

2B. Physical therapists shall provide physical therapy services with compassionate and caring behaviors that incorporate the individual and cultural differences of patients/clients.

2C. Physical therapists shall provide the information necessary to allow patients or their surrogates to make informed decisions about physical therapy care or participation in clinical research.

2D. Physical therapists shall collaborate with patients/clients to empower them in decisions about their health care.

2E. Physical therapists shall protect confidential patient/client information and may disclose confidential information to appropriate authorities only when allowed or as required by law.

Principle #3: Physical therapists shall be accountable for making sound professional judgments.
(Core Values: Excellence, Integrity)

3A. Physical therapists shall demonstrate independent and objective professional judgment in the patient's/client's best interest in all practice settings.

3B. Physical therapists shall demonstrate professional judgment informed by professional standards, evidence (including current literature and established best practice), practitioner experience, and patient/client values.

3C. Physical therapists shall make judgments within their scope of practice and level of expertise and shall communicate with, collaborate with, or refer to peers or other health care professionals when necessary.

3D. Physical therapists shall not engage in conflicts of interest that interfere with professional judgment.

3E. Physical therapists shall provide appropriate direction of and communication with physical therapist assistants and support personnel.

FIGURE 20-1   Code of ethics for the physical therapist. (*Continued*)

Principle #4: Physical therapists shall demonstrate integrity in their relationships with patients/clients, families, colleagues, students, research participants, other health care providers, employers, payers, and the public.

(Core Value: Integrity)

4A. Physical therapists shall provide truthful, accurate, and relevant information and shall not make misleading representations.

4B. Physical therapists shall not exploit persons over whom they have supervisory, evaluative or other authority (eg, patients/clients, students, supervisees, research participants, or employees).

4C. Physical therapists shall discourage misconduct by health care professionals and report illegal or unethical acts to the relevant authority, when appropriate.

4D. Physical therapists shall report suspected cases of abuse involving children or vulnerable adults to the appropriate authority, subject to law.

4E. Physical therapists shall not engage in any sexual relationship with any of their patients/clients, supervisees, or students.

4F. Physical therapists shall not harass anyone verbally, physically, emotionally, or sexually.

Principle #5: Physical therapists shall fulfill their legal and professional obligations.

(Core Values: Professional Duty, Accountability)

5A. Physical therapists shall comply with applicable local, state, and federal laws and regulations.

5B. Physical therapists shall have primary responsibility for supervision of physical therapist assistants and support personnel.

5C. Physical therapists involved in research shall abide by accepted standards governing protection of research participants.

5D. Physical therapists shall encourage colleagues with physical, psychological, or substance-related impairments that may adversely impact their professional responsibilities to seek assistance or counsel.

5E. Physical therapists who have knowledge that a colleague is unable to perform their professional responsibilities with reasonable skill and safety shall report this information to the appropriate authority.

5F. Physical therapists shall provide notice and information about alternatives for obtaining care in the event the physical therapist terminates the provider relationship while the patient/client continues to need physical therapy services.

Principle #6: Physical therapists shall enhance their expertise through the lifelong acquisition and refinement of knowledge, skills, abilities, and professional behaviors.

(Core Value: Excellence)

6A. Physical therapists shall achieve and maintain professional competence.

6B. Physical therapists shall take responsibility for their professional development based on critical self-assessment and reflection on changes in physical therapist practice, education, health care delivery, and technology.

6C. Physical therapists shall evaluate the strength of evidence and applicability of content presented during professional development activities before integrating the content or techniques into practice.

6D. Physical therapists shall cultivate practice environments that support professional development, lifelong learning, and excellence.

Principle #7: Physical therapists shall promote organizational behaviors and business practices that benefit patients/clients and society.

(Core Values: Integrity, Accountability)

7A. Physical therapists shall promote practice environments that support autonomous and accountable professional judgments.

7B. Physical therapists shall seek remuneration as is deserved and reasonable for physical therapist services.

7C. Physical therapists shall not accept gifts or other considerations that influence or give an appearance of influencing their professional judgment.

7D. Physical therapists shall fully disclose any financial interest they have in products or services that they recommend to patients/clients.

7E. Physical therapists shall be aware of charges and shall ensure that documentation and coding for physical therapy services accurately reflect the nature and extent of the services provided.

7F. Physical therapists shall refrain from employment arrangements, or other arrangements, that prevent physical therapists from fulfilling professional obligations to patients/clients.

Principle #8: Physical therapists shall participate in efforts to meet the health needs of people locally, nationally, or globally.

(Core Value: Social Responsibility)

8A. Physical therapists shall provide pro bono physical therapy services or support organizations that meet the health needs of people who are economically disadvantaged, uninsured, and underinsured.

8B. Physical therapists shall advocate to reduce health disparities and health care inequities, improve access to health care services, and address the health, wellness, and preventive health care needs of people.

8C. Physical therapists shall be responsible stewards of health care resources and shall avoid overutilization or underutilization of physical therapy services.

8D. Physical therapists shall educate members of the public about the benefits of physical therapy and the unique role of the physical therapist.

Proviso: The Code of Ethics as substituted will take effect July 1, 2010, to allow for education of APTA members and nonmembers.

about alternative outcomes without surgery—namely a 2–4% risk of stroke and associated loss of function.[26] Each of these factors may be influenced further by results from studies about prognostic factors associated with AV malformation rupture, or survival after repair, as well as by varying clinical judgments about the appropriateness of surgery, given a patient's clinical history and examination findings. The surgeon's job is to help the patient understand and consider all of this information thoroughly before making a decision. Physical therapists may find themselves in similar situations when proposed procedures are invasive (e.g., vaginally applied treatments for urinary incontinence) or potentially risky (e.g., cervical manipulation).

Once the information exchange has occurred, a clear voluntary decision about the elements of patient/client management must be determined. How that decision is reached depends on how the physical therapist and patient or client view the nature of their relationship. In the traditional biomedical model, physical therapists are the experts who evaluate the risks and benefits of each management option on behalf of the patient and recommend (or make) the decision within their frame of reference about what is in the best interests of the patient. Their evaluation may be derived from their clinical experience and judgment, and/or available evidence, depending on the therapists' practice habits. The patient's or client's sociocultural context and contribution to the decision is marginalized in this scenario. As stated earlier, this approach is the antithesis of patient-centered care.

Shared decision making, in contrast, is a process that supports an active partnership between therapists and patients or clients. *Shared decision making* is defined as "an exchange of ideas between a health care provider and patient and collaboration in the decision itself."[7(p.55)] In other words, the therapist and the patient or client explore together their understanding of the clinical situation and the management options available as well as any preferences they have. They then mutually accept responsibility for the decision and its consequences.[13] In this model, all information relevant to the decision is incorporated, including culturally based patient or client preferences and values.[11] Moreover, in situations in which relatively equal management options exist, preferences and values may be the deciding factor in the selection process. When preferences and values are in conflict with the best available evidence, it is the physical therapist's responsibility to negotiate a suitable management option with the individual in a manner that is consistent with ethical codes and standards of conduct. To do that, therapists need to understand where preferences and values come from and how they may affect participation in, and outcomes of, care.

Preferences, Expectancies, and Values

For the purposes of this text, *preferences* are defined as the differences in the perceived desirability of two (or more) options related to health care.[6] These perceptions may be derived objectively from evidence, education, and observation, or they may be based on subjective interpretations and imprecise information about the potential benefits and risks of each choice. Unfortunately, the lack of quality control for the plethora of medical information on the Internet may contribute to patient or client misunderstandings of available evidence. Physical therapists often try to address detected inaccuracies in patient or client understanding through education, as well as through discussions about the best available evidence. Nevertheless, an individual's inner conviction about what is "right for me" may prevail, particularly when there is a high level of uncertainty about the outcomes of care. Bower et al. also point out that the strength of patient or client preferences may be more important than whether they are based on valid information.[6]

The desirability of one option over another may be stimulated in part by what patients or clients anticipate will happen when they participate in, or receive, health care.[27] This anticipation is reflected in the term *expectancy*, which is defined as the belief that a process or outcome possesses certain attributes.[6] Patients and clients reveal their expectancies in an explicit fashion when they define their goals for treatment. Physical therapists also may detect implicit expressions of expectancies when a patient guards an injured extremity during efforts to examine it or when clients perform more repetitions of an exercise than prescribed. In the first scenario, the patient likely anticipates (expects) pain when the extremity is moved; in the second scenario, the client likely believes that a higher volume of exercise will produce either a quicker result or a higher level of performance. In both situations, expectancies have helped to define the desirability (or lack thereof) of the examination technique or intervention.

Preferences about health care also may be shaped by the values patients or clients and their families (caregivers) use to guide their decisions and actions.[27] *Values* are defined as concepts or beliefs about desirable behaviors or states of being that are prioritized relative to one another.[10] Values may be global in perspective, as exemplified by beliefs in the importance of honesty, integrity, fairness, and so on. Values also may be defined more narrowly with reference to health care. Examples of patient or client values relevant to physical therapy may include, but are not limited to, the following

- Meaning of symptoms such as pain, shortness of breath, or fatigue;
- Importance of healthy lifestyles;
- Ability to minimize or avoid suffering;
- Preservation or restoration of self-image;
- Importance of work, school, and/or household responsibilities;
- Ability to care for and be involved with family and/or friends;
- Quality and consistency of the therapist-patient (or client) relationship; and
- Importance and usefulness of research in health care decision making.

By definition, all values are not equally important, although there is no uniformly accepted order for these beliefs. Individuals will prioritize them based on their own experiences and understanding of the world, as well as in response to sociocultural norms and expectations. The order also may shift depending on the patient's or client's health and/or psychological and emotional status at a given point in time.[10] Understandably, physical therapist management options are more likely to be desirable if they are consistent with a patient's or client's values.

Assessment of Preferences and Values

The challenge for physical therapists, therefore, is to ascertain a patient's or client's preferences, expectancies, and values, so that this information may be integrated with clinical judgment and the best available evidence. Accessing research about patient or client perspectives and experiences is an evidence-based approach to this task. Well-designed qualitative studies may provide insight into specific issues or concerns about which the physical therapist was not previously aware. **Table 20-1** provides some examples of qualitative research about patient preferences and values related to physical therapist management.

From a therapeutic relationship perspective, the process starts during the initial contact with the patient or client during which specific interview questions and/or spontaneous revelations might provide the necessary details. Family members and caregivers also may lend some insight into these issues; however, the inaccuracy of those speaking on behalf of the patient or client (e.g., the proxy) has been noted in several studies.[10] This disconnect may be attributable to a lack of knowledge about the individual's wishes or to the influence of the proxy's own preferences, expectancies, and values. This substitution of one set of preferences, expectancies, and values for another may be purposeful, as is the case in cultures in which family members are expected to make health care decisions for loved ones, or they may be subliminal. In either case, physical therapists must determine whose preferences, expectancies, and values are to be respected when finally deciding how to proceed with a plan of care.

TABLE 20-1	Examples of Qualitative Studies About Patient Preferences in Physical Therapy
<ul><li>Sander AP, et al. Factors that affect decisions about physical activity and exercise in survivors of breast cancer: a qualitative study. *Phys Ther.* 2012;92(4):525–536.</li><li>Gibson BE, et al. Children's and parents' beliefs regarding the value of walking: rehabilitation implications for children with cerebral palsy. *Child Care Health Dev.* 2012;38(1):61–69.</li><li>Bulley C, et al. User experiences, preferences and choices relating to functional electrical stimulation and ankle foot orthoses for foot drop after stroke. *Physiotherapy.* 2011;97(3): 226–233.</li><li>Slade SC, et al. People with non-specific chronic low back pain who have participated in exercise programs have preferences about exercise: a qualitative study. *Aust J Physiother.* 2009;55(2):115–121.</li></ul>

Assessment tools such as rating scales, questionnaires, and decision aids also are available to facilitate the specification of preferences, expectancies, and values. For example, Straus et al. include a 0 to 1 numerical rating scale in which 0 represents death and 1 represents complete health. Patients are asked to rate the relative value of the intended outcome of treatment on this scale in a fashion similar to that used with a visual analog scale for pain (**Figure 20-2**).[28] Inferences about preferences, expectancies, and values also may be drawn from quality of life self-report instruments, depending on the phrasing of the survey items. However, when the information is gathered it must be discussed and interpreted with respect to the patient's or client's sociocultural context, as is consistent with culturally competent health care.

Use of decision aids is another method that may assist patients and clients during their consideration of potential management options for a given condition or disorder. These tools are available in a variety of forms including pamphlets, videos, and computer-based instruments. Their goal is the same: to provide individuals with information about the risk–benefit trade-offs of their different choices and to help them understand and express their preferences regarding these options. Greater knowledge and understanding theoretically should facilitate the shared decision-making process. A systematic review by O'Connor et al. reported that use of decision aids

- Increased patients' knowledge about their options;
- Reduced patients' feelings about being uninformed or unclear about their personal values;
- Reduced patients' tendency to adopt passive decision-making roles;
- Increased the accuracy of patients' risk assessment when probabilities were included in the decision aids; and
- Reduced the rates of selection of certain elective procedures and medications.[29]

However, these authors also found that use of decision aids was no better than alternative methods for affecting change in patients' satisfaction with decision making, expressed anxiety levels, or realized health outcomes. These findings reinforce the notion that participation in decision making and the act of making a decision itself may be distinct phenomena that require further study.[22,23]

At the same time, physical therapists also must be aware of their own preferences, expectancies, and values and evaluate how they influence clinical decision making. For example, therapists may indicate a preference for treatment techniques based on theory or *biologic plausibility*, regardless of

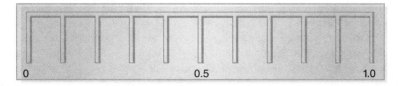

FIGURE 20-2   Rating scale for assessing values.

Reproduced from Straus SE, Richardson WS, Glaziou P, Haynes RB. *Evidence-Based Medicine: How to Practice and Teach EBM*. Copyright © Elsevier 2005. Reprinted with Permission from Elsevier.

what the evidence indicates. Other clinicians may willingly use evidence about interventions but only if it comes from randomized clinical trials. Experience also gives therapists an anecdotal perception about "what works," which can develop into an expectancy that is conveyed when describing a potential management option. Finally, physical therapists may value the achievement of a patient's or client's full potential more than the individual with whom they are working. The issue is not the existence of these tendencies per se, but rather the potential lack of purposeful deliberation about their appropriateness for a specific patient or client. In the absence of such self-awareness and analysis, physical therapists may impose their own preferences and values relevant to the plan of care on the individual rather than negotiate the outcome in an explicit fashion.

Incorporating evidence into this discussion requires physical therapists to clarify how the research findings are relevant to this specific individual. Of course, this task will be easier if the evidence includes subjects and circumstances that resemble the individual patient or client and his or her clinical situation. The manner in which the information is presented also matters. For therapists this means that explanations should be free from jargon and should be delivered in a way that accommodates individual patient or client learning needs and styles. Therapists must also be prepared to offer their objective opinion about the role the evidence plays in their decision making in general and in the specific situation. When evidence is inconclusive, or nonexistent, then decisions will be reached based on some combination of clinical judgment and patient or client preferences and values. Ultimately, the goal is to engage the individual in shared decision making in a *culturally competent* manner in an effort to minimize conflict between competing value systems and priorities and to reach a mutually agreeable approach to the plan of care.

Quantitative Evidence About Preferences, Expectancies, and Values

As it turns out, preferences, expectancies, and values are both the focus of, and a potential concern for, health care research. Understanding preferences, expectancies, and values from a scientific point of view is consistent with evidence-based practice and has revealed some interesting findings. For example, Erkan et al. surveyed physicians to determine their preferences for rheumatoid arthritis medications and to evaluate whether cost influenced their choices.[30] The authors used three different patient scenarios to examine whether physicians were adopting more aggressive treatment strategies by using newly established drugs. The results indicated that 65% of the time physicians chose long-established medications for the mild case scenario but preferred the newest medications, in combination with established regimens, for cases of increasing severity. However, this proportion dropped to 14% when cost was factored into the decision.

A subsequent study by Fraenkel et al. evaluated patient preferences for rheumatoid arthritis treatment.[31] These authors used an interactive computer program to elicit subject preferences for four drugs based on trade-offs between treatment side effects, effectiveness, and cost within different risk-benefit scenarios. Their results indicated that, on average, patients preferred drugs that reduced both rare and common side effects more than drugs with known benefits. Interestingly, the drug that was selected most often because of this characteristic was the same drug that physicians in the previous study reserved primarily for severe cases, and only when cost was not a factor.

These projects were conducted independently and did not include the same trade-off questions for each sample. More recently, Gu et al. simultaneously surveyed orthopedic surgeons and patients regarding time trade-offs related to infected total hip arthroplasty outcomes. These authors reported statistically different preference ratings between the surgeons and patients for trade-offs related to 5 of the 10 health states described in the survey.[32] Similarly, Bederman et al. surveyed orthopedic and neurosurgeons, family practitioners, and patients in Ontario, Canada, regarding preferences for lumbar surgery. These authors found differences in preferences among all three groups, with family practitioners having a higher preference for surgery than the surgeons! Each group also used a different constellation of factors in support of their decision for surgery.[33] This study reflects an important dynamic in contemporary health care: multiple providers with different points of view engaging with the same patient. When considered together, all of these studies point to a potential disconnect between providers and patients that may interfere with informed consent and shared decision-making processes.

An additional concern about preferences, expectancies, and values is their potential influence on research outcomes. Specifically, these characteristics are assumed to be potential threats to *research validity* of intervention studies when subjects are aware of their group assignment.[6,27,34,35] Two mechanisms are proposed to explain the potential impact of preferences, expectancies, and values. First, subjects who receive their desired intervention may exhibit a response in excess of the actual treatment effect. This response is thought to share the same mechanism as the *placebo effect* and may be enhanced by higher-than-average compliance with the treatment protocol. Second, allocation to an undesired intervention may produce *resentful demoralization*, thereby resulting in decreased adherence to the group protocol. This point is particularly salient when an experimental intervention is being compared to another treatment approach. King et al. outlined the proposed causal mechanisms that may produce exaggerated treatment effects (**Figure 20-3**).[27] Direct influences are attributed to purposeful changes in behavior (e.g., increased compliance), whereas indirect influences are attributed to the biopsychological effects of expectancies about preferred treatments.

Evidence about the extent of preference effects actually occurring in research is equivocal.[35] Several authors have described research designs that take subject preference into account. One approach is to identify which subjects have strong preferences for the treatment options in the study and assign them to those groups while randomizing everyone else who is preference free. This method requires larger sample sizes because of the increased number of groups and is likely to be logistically and financially prohibitive. An alternative approach is to identify subject preferences before randomization and then use this data as an adjustment factor in subsequent analyses. Two studies pertinent to physical therapist practice used the latter approach. Klaber Moffett et al. found that preference did not influence clinical outcomes following interventions for lower back pain,[36] but they subsequently reported a potential (although nonsignificant) influence on outcomes following treatment of neck pain.[37]

The reality is that most studies that inform patient/client management do not address the potential influence of subject preferences on outcomes. Therefore, physical therapists should consider whether preferences may have played a role in individual studies. Designs in which subjects are randomly

FIGURE 20-3   The proposed effects of subject preferences on research
studies.

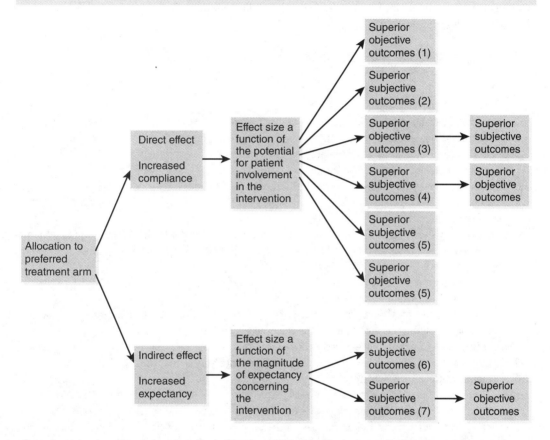

Causal mechanisms for preference effects. Numbers (1) to (7) refer to examples in text.

Reprinted from King M, Nazareth I, Lampe F, Bower P, et al. Conceptual framework and systematic review of the effects of participants' and professionals' preferences in randomised controlled trials. *Health Technol Assess*. 2005;9(35):1-191. http://www.journalslibrary.nihr .ac.uk/hta/volume-9/issue-35. With permission from the NIHR Evaluation, Trials, and Studies Coordinating Center.

allocated and remain blind to group assignment are least vulnerable to this potential problem. Studies with unmasked assignment are at greater risk; however, until there is a better understanding of the extent of this effect, studies should not be rejected based on this issue alone.

Summary

EBPT practice integrates the best available evidence with clinical judgment and expertise, as well as with patient or client preferences and values. This definition is consistent with patient (or client)-centered care and supports the ethical principle of autonomy. Informed consent and shared decision making are the processes by which this integration occurs in practice. Determination of an evidence-based plan of care requires physical therapists to elicit and understand patient or client preferences and values within each individual's sociocultural context. Therapists also must be aware of their own preferences and values and how they shape clinical decision making. Finally, the nature of preferences in clinical practice and their influence on research validity requires further study to better understand their contribution to outcomes.

Exercises

1. Define patient-centered care in your own words. Explain how EBPT practice is consistent with this definition. Provide an example relevant to physical therapist practice to illustrate your points.
2. Discuss the ethical considerations related to EBPT practice. Provide an example relevant to physical therapist practice to illustrate your points.
3. Describe the elements of informed consent. Discuss the implications for presenting evidence to patients or clients during the consent process. Provide an example relevant to physical therapist practice to illustrate your points.
4. Differentiate shared decision making from the traditional biomedical model of determining a plan of care. Explain how this process relates to EBPT practice. Provide an example relevant to physical therapist practice to illustrate your points.
5. Define the concept of patient or client preferences and provide two examples relevant to physical therapist practice to support your answer.
6. For each preference described in question 5, identify two potential expectancies and two potential values that may influence the nature of the preference.
7. Identify one of your preferences, along with associated expectancies and values, related to patient/client management. Discuss how these issues may influence your approach to EBPT practice.
8. An elderly patient with a history of falls tells you she will not remove the area rugs in her home or change the shoes she wears despite numerous studies that indicate an increased fall risk due to these factors. During this exchange you learn that she values appearance and views these changes as concessions to old age and frailty. Discuss strategies you will use to help the patient understand the evidence under these circumstances. Discuss what you will do if she continues to disagree with your recommendations.
9. Explain why individual preferences may be a threat to the research validity of a study. Describe one strategy with which investigators might address the challenge of subject preferences. Provide an example relevant to physical therapist practice to illustrate your points.

References

1. Sackett DL, Rosenberg WMC, Gray JAM, et al. Evidence-based medicine: what it is and what it isn't. *BMJ.* 1996;312(7023):71–72.
2. Higgs J, Jones M, Loftus S, Christensen N, eds. *Clinical Reasoning in the Health Professions.* 3rd ed. Oxford, England: Butterworth-Heinemann; 2008.

3. Graham R, Mancher M, Wolman DM, Greenfield S, Steinberg E, eds. *Clinical Practice Guidelines We Can Trust.* Available at: http://www.nap.edu/catalog/13058/clinical-practice-guidelines-we-can-trust. Accessed July 31, 2016.

4. DiCenso A, Bayley L, Haynes RB. Accessing pre-appraised evidence: fine-tuning the 5S model into a 6S model. *Evid Based Nurs.* 2009;12(4):99–101.

5. Purtilo RB, Jensen GM, Royeen CB. *Educating for Moral Action: A Sourcebook in Health and Rehabilitation Ethics.* Philadelphia, PA: F.A. Davis; 2005.

6. Bower P, King M, Nazareth I, et al. Patient preferences in randomised controlled trials: conceptual framework and implications for research. *Soc Sci Med.* 2005;61(3):685–695.

7. Whitney SN, McGuire AL, McCullough LB. A typology of shared decision making, informed consent, and simple consent. *Ann Intern Med.* 2003;140(1):54–59.

8. Greiner AC, Knebel E, eds. Health Professions Education: A Bridge to Quality. Institute of Medicine website. Available at: https://www.nap.edu/read/10681/chapter/1. Accessed July 16, 2016.

9. Guyatt G, Rennie D. *Users' Guides to the Medical Literature: A Manual for Evidence-Based Clinical Practice.* 3rd ed. Chicago, IL: AMA Press; 2014.

10. Karel MJ. The assessment of values in medical decision making. *J Aging Studies.* 2000;14(4):403–422.

11. Hasnain-Wynia R. Is evidence-based medicine patient-centered and is patient-centered care evidence-based? *Health Serv Res.* 2006;41(1):1–8.

12. American Physical Therapy Association. Guide to Physical Therapist Practice 3.0. Available at: http://guide toptpractice.apta.org. Accessed July 16, 2016.

13. Dierckx K, Deveugele M, Roosen P, Devisch I. Implementation of shared decision making in physical therapy: observed level of involvement and patient preference. *Phys Ther.* 2013;93(10):1321–1330.

14. Ford S, Schofield T, Hope T. What are the ingredients for a successful evidence-based patient choice consultation? A qualitative study. *Soc Sci Med.* 2003;56(3):589–602.

15. Slowther A, Ford S, Schofield T. Ethics of evidence-based medicine in the primary care setting. *J Med Ethics.* 2004;30(2):151–155.

16. Definition of Disease Management. Wikepedia website. Available at: https://en.wikipedia.org/wiki /Disease_management_(health). Accessed March 1, 2017.

17. MedlinePlus. The National Library of Medicine website. Available at: https://medlineplus.gov/. Accessed March 1, 2017.

18. Diseases and Conditions. The American Heart Association website. Available at: www.heart.org/HEARTORG /Conditions/Conditions_UCM_001087_SubHomePage.jsp. Accessed March 1, 2017.

19. The American Diabetes Association website. Available at: http://www.diabetes.org/. Accessed March 1, 2017.

20. Resources for Patients. The American Medical Association website. Available at: www.ama-assn.org/ama /pub/patients/patients.page. Accessed August 18, 2013.

21. Information for Consumers. American Physical Therapy Association website. Available at: www.moveforward pt.com/Default.aspx. Accessed March 1, 2017.

22. Edwards A, Elwyn G. Inside the black box of shared decision making: distinguishing between the process of involvement and who makes the decision. *Health Expect.* 2006;9(4):307–320.

23. Swenson SL, Buell S, Zettler P, et al. Patient-centered communication: do patients really prefer it? *J Gen Intern Med.* 2004;19(11):1069–1079.

24. Street RL Jr, Gordon HS, Ward MM, et al. Patient participation in medical consultations: why some patients are more involved than others. *Med Care.* 2005;43(10):960–969.

25. Code of Ethics for Physical Therapists. American Physical Therapy Association website. Available at: www .apta.org/uploadedFiles/APTAorg/About_Us/Policies/Ethics/CodeofEthics.pdf#search=%22code of ethics%22. Accessed March 1, 2017.

26. Arteriovenous Malformations and Other Vascular Lesions of the Central Nervous System Fact Sheet. National Institute of Neurological Disorders and Stroke. National Institutes of Health website. Available at: https://www .ninds.nih.gov/Disorders/All-Disorders/Arteriovenous-Malformation-Information-Page Accessed March 1, 2017.

27. King M, Nazareth I, Lampe F, et al. Conceptual framework and systematic review of the effects of participants' and professionals' preferences in randomised controlled trials. *Health Technol Assess.* 2005;9(35):1–191.

28. Straus SE, Richardson WS, Glaziou P, Haynes RB. *Evidence-Based Medicine: How to Practice and Teach EBM.* 3rd ed. Edinburgh, Scotland: Elsevier Churchill Livingstone; 2005.

29. O'Connor AM, Bennett CL, Stacey D, et al. Decision aids for people facing health treatment or screening decisions. *Cochrane Database Syst Rev.* 2009;(3):CD001431.

30. Erkan D, Yazici Y, Harrison MJ, Paget SA. Physician treatment preferences in rheumatoid arthritis of differing disease severity and activity: the impact of cost on first-line therapy. *Arthritis Rheum.* 2002;47(3):285–290.

31. Fraenkel L, Bogardus ST, Concato J, Felson DT, Wittink DR. Patient preferences for treatment of rheumatoid arthritis. *Ann Rheum Dis.* 2004;63(11):1372–1378.

32. Gu NY, Wolff C, Leopold S, et al. A comparison of physician and patient time trade-offs for post-operative hip outcomes. *Value Health.* 2009;12(4):618–620.

33. Bederman SS, Mahomed NN, Kreder HJ, et al. In the eye of the beholder: preferences of patients, family physicians, and surgeons for lumbar spinal surgery. *Spine.* 2010;35(1):108–115.

34. Torgerson D, Sibbald B. Understanding controlled trials: what is a patient preference trial? *BMJ.* 1998;316(7128):360.

35. McPherson K, Britton A. Preferences and understanding their effects on health. *Qual Health Care.* 2001;10(suppl I):i61–i66.

36. Klaber Moffett J, Torgerson D, Bell-Syer S, et al. Randomised controlled trial of exercise for low back pain: clinical outcomes, costs and preferences. *BMJ.* 1999;319(7205):279–283.

37. Klaber Moffett JA, Jackson DA, Richmond S, et al. Randomised trial of a brief physiotherapy intervention compared with usual physiotherapy for neck pain patients: outcomes and patients' preference. *BMJ.* 2005;330(7482)1–6.

CHAPTER 21

PUTTING IT ALL TOGETHER

OBJECTIVES

Upon completion of this chapter, the student/practitioner will be able to do the following:
1. Use a hypothetical patient example to model the formulation of a clinical question, as well as the search for and evaluation of evidence pertaining to the following:

   a. A diagnostic test;

   b. A clinical measure;

   c. A prognostic (risk) factor;

   d. An intervention;

   e. A self-report outcomes instrument; and

   f. An individual's perspective about his or her health.

Use a hypothetical patient example to model the use of physiologic studies to answer a clinical question pertaining to interventions.

Introduction

This chapter uses hypothetical patient cases to illustrate the process of evidence-based physical therapist practice. The first section contains brief scenarios focusing on a diagnostic test, a clinical measure, a prognostic (risk) factor, an intervention, a self-report outcomes instrument or an individual's perspective about his or her health. Cases reflect patients across the life span in a variety of clinical settings. At the conclusion of each scenario, a clinical question is presented followed by a figure that illustrates the search strategies used. For the sake of chapter length, only one article from each search is appraised using the relevant quality appraisal checklist. Worksheets adapted from the Oxford Centre for Evidence Based Medicine also are presented.[1]

The second section illustrates the use of several physiologic studies as evidence during patient/client management. Physiologic studies rank lower on the various evidence hierarchies because these works focus on anatomy, physiology, and pathophysiology rather than on the "whole patient." The subjects of these studies are cells, tissues, or organ systems and their properties and functions under healthy and diseased states. Observations and experimental manipulation usually are conducted in well-controlled laboratory conditions. As a result, it is often difficult to generalize findings from these studies directly to patients or clients in clinical settings. Despite these potential drawbacks, physiologic studies may be the only form of evidence that is available to answer particular questions. Therefore, it is important for evidence-based physical therapists to understand how physiologic studies may inform their clinical decisions.

This chapter comes with an important caveat. These examples are illustrations only. They are not intended to serve as practice guidelines or standards of care for the conditions described. Remember also that there are multiple ways to search for evidence, a fraction of which can be included here.

Section One: Clinical Case Examples Using Evidence

Case #1   Evidence About a Diagnostic Test

This patient is a 67-year-old African American man who had elective double coronary artery bypass surgery using an internal mammary artery graft 1 day ago. His mediastinal chest tubes were removed early this morning. He is awake and anxious to get out of bed. He indicates that his previous limitations to activity over the last 6 months were pressure in his chest, as well as occasional fatigue and cramping in his legs. His goal is to return to his previous occupational and leisure activities as soon as possible. The physical therapist's initial clinical examination in the intensive care unit reveals the following:

- *Initial Observation:* Moderately overweight man supine in bed with head elevated to 45 degrees. He is receiving 3 liters of oxygen via nasal cannula. His sternal incision is dressed and dry. There is an arterial line placed in the left radial artery. Bedside telemetry monitoring is in place. He has a Foley catheter that is draining clear yellow urine.
- *Social History:* He is a widower and lives in a two-story home. He operates the family farm raising soybeans and corn. He also maintains goats and chickens. His son, daughter-in-law, and two grandchildren live with him and help him with the farm duties. He enjoys bird hunting.
- *Significant Medical History:* Left anterior descending coronary artery disease treated with percutaneous transluminal angioplasty twice in the last 5 years. He has a 25 pack year smoking habit that was discontinued 8 years ago and hyperlipidemia. He has been overweight for at least 15 years. He denies history of arthritis, previous trauma, or other documented neuromusculoskeletal disorders related to his lower extremities.
- *Medications:* Oxycodone (pain), metoprolol (blood pressure and heart rate), and lovastatin (hyperlipidemia).
- *Mental Status:* He is alert and oriented to person, place, and time. He follows multiple-step commands and answers questions appropriately.
- *Pain at Rest (Numeric Pain Rating Scale):* 4/10 for his chest incision.
- *Vital Signs at Rest:* Heart rate = 84 beats/min with regular rhythm; Blood pressure = 122/74 mmHg;
- *Respiratory rate* = 16 breaths/min; Oxygen saturation = 97%.
- *Body Mass Index (BMI)* = 28.4 kg/m^2.
- *Auscultation:* Heart sounds = normal S1 and S2; Lung sounds = clear in the upper and midzones, but crackles are present in both bases.
- *Breathing Pattern:* He demonstrates shallow inspirations with guarding due to incisional discomfort.
- *Active Range of Motion:* All joints in both upper and lower extremities are within normal limits except for shoulder elevation, which is voluntarily restricted to 90 degrees of flexion due to incisional discomfort.
- *Mobility:* He performs 75% of the effort to come to sitting at the edge of the bed and to execute a stand pivot transfer to a chair with assistance of one person.
- *Vital Signs with Activity:* Heart rate = 96 beats/min; Blood pressure = 138/82 mmHg; Respiratory rate = 24 breaths/min; Oxygen saturation = 94%. Rating of perceived exertion = 5 on a 10 point scale.
- *Pain with Activity (Numeric Pain Rating Scale):* 7/10.

- *Palpation:* No edema is noted in his lower extremities while in the dependent position. His dorsal pedal pulse is absent on the right. Both posterior tibial pulses and his left dorsal pedal pulse are barely detectable.

The diminished lower extremity pulses and this patient's complaint of prior leg fatigue and cramping suggest that he is developing peripheral arterial disease; however, the physical therapist wonders how well palpation of peripheral pulses correctly identifies an individual with this problem. He decides to search the literature to answer the following clinical question:

Is manual palpation of lower extremity pulses during a physical exam as accurate as the ankle-brachial index (ABI) for detecting potential peripheral arterial disease in a 67-year-old man with coronary artery disease?

Figure 21-1 illustrates a literature search using the National Library of Medicine's PubMed Clinical Queries function and the search phrase "pedal pulse palpation" (limits = English, Humans). Four articles are identified, all of which appear to address the clinical question based on their titles and abstracts. One article includes only patients with diabetes, a condition that is not present in this patient. A second article compares pulse palpation with tests (including the ABI) conducted in a vascular laboratory rather than during a standard physical exam. The most recent article (2016) compares the utility of pedal pulse palpation with the ABI as part of a vascular screening study of over 18,000 Danish men. The large sample size suggests the potential for greater accuracy of statistical findings. However, the Collins et al. article[2] is selected for review because the authors performed a similar comparison of the two examination techniques in a sample of American men who more closely resemble this patient.

FIGURE 21-1 Search results for evidence related to a diagnostic test for a patient with diminished lower extremity pulses (using the PubMed Clinical Queries function).

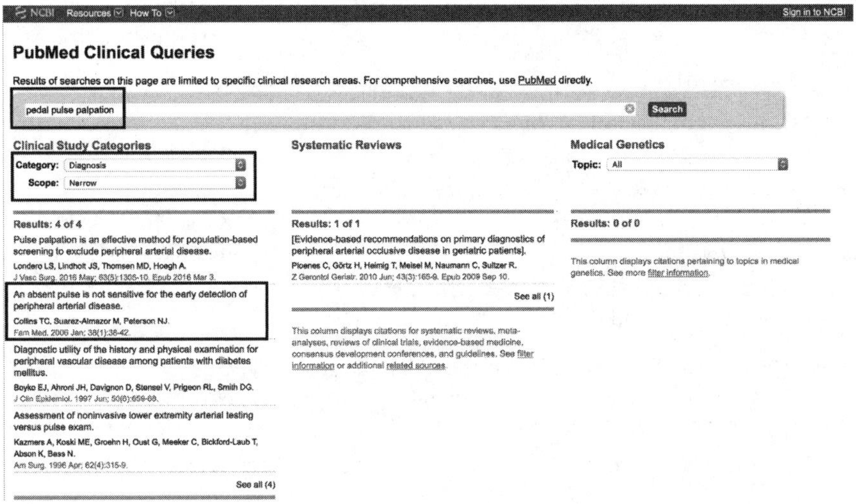

Table 21-1 provides a critique of the Collins et al. article[2] using the quality appraisal checklist for evidence about diagnostic tests. Based on his analysis of the study, the physical therapist decides that the absence of a pulse on manual palpation is sufficient to rule in peripheral arterial disease (high specificity), but that the presence of a pulse is not useful for ruling out this condition (low sensitivity).

TABLE 21-1	**Quality Appraisal Checklist for an Article About a Diagnostic Test for a Man with Diminished Lower Extremity Pulses**

Research Validity of the Study

Did the investigators evaluate (or provide a citation for) the reliability of the index diagnostic test? Study personnel measuring pulses were trained and practiced until they consistently obtained the same results as the investigator; correlation coefficients were not provided.	X Yes ___ No ___ Insufficient detail
Did the investigators include subjects with all levels or stages of the condition being evaluated by the index diagnostic? N = 403 (37.3% = no symptoms; 55.2% = "atypical symptoms"; 7.5% = "classic intermittent claudication").	X Yes ___ No ___ Insufficient detail
Did the investigators compare results from the index diagnostic test to results from a gold standard diagnostic test? Pedal pulses were compared to a bedside ankle-brachial index (ABI), but not to a vascular laboratory assessment.	___ Comparison to a "gold standard" test was performed X Comparison to another test was performed ___ Comparison to another test was performed ___ Comparison was performed but the description is inadequate ___ No comparison was made
Were all subjects evaluated with the comparison diagnostic test? All subjects underwent the ABI.	X Yes ___ No ___ Insufficient detail
Were the individuals performing and interpreting each test's results unaware of the other test's results (i.e., were they masked, or blinded)? The same trained research assistants performed both the pedal pulse assessments and the ABIs.	___ Yes X No ___ Insufficient detail
Was the time between application of the index test and the gold standard comparison diagnostic test short enough to minimize the opportunity for change in the subjects' condition?	X Yes ___ No ___ Insufficient detail
Did the investigators confirm their findings with a new set of subjects?	___ Yes X No ___ Insufficient detail

TABLE 21-1	Quality Appraisal Checklist for an Article About a Diagnostic Test for a Man with Diminished Lower Extremity Pulses (*Continued*)

Do you have enough confidence in the research validity of this paper to consider using this evidence with your patient or client?

___ Yes
_X_ Undecided
___ No

Limitations include lack of a true "gold standard" comparison test, the potential for tester bias, and lack of validation in a second set of subjects.

Relevant Study Findings

Results reported that are specific to your clinical question:

- True positive = absent pulse in a subject with PAD
- True negative = present pulse in a subject without PAD

Sensitivity of pulse palpation = 18% (left leg) and 32% (right leg)

Specificity of pulse palpation = 99% (left leg) and 98% (right leg)

Positive predictive value(s) of pulse palpation = 67% (left leg) and 63% (right leg)

Negative predictive value(s) of pulse palpation = 89% (left leg) and 93% (right leg)

+ Likelihood ratio(s) of nonpalpable pulse in patient with PAD (vs. without PAD) = 18 (left leg) and 16 (right leg)

_ Likelihood ratio(s) of palpable pulse in patient with PAD (vs. without PAD) = 0.83 (left leg) and 0.69 (right leg)

Statistical significance and/or precision of the relevant study results:

Obtained p values for each relevant statistic reported by the authors: Not reported for the measures listed above.

Obtained confidence intervals for each relevant statistic reported by the authors: Not reported for the measures listed above.

Is the index diagnostic test reliable?

The authors state that the research assistants performed the pedal pulse assessments reliably, but statistical confirmation was not provided.

___ Yes
___ No
_X_ Mixed results
___ Insufficient detail

Is the index diagnostic test valid? If yes, continue below.

The results indicate that pedal pulse palpation is valid for ruling in PAD but not for ruling out the condition.

___ Yes
___ No
_X_ Mixed results
___ Insufficient detail

What is the pretest probability that your patient or client has the condition of interest?

~10-13% (based on the sample in the article)

What is the posttest probability that your patient or client has the condition of interest if you apply this test?

~64-73% if pulse is absent;
~7-11% if pulse is present

(continues)

TABLE 21-1   **Quality Appraisal Checklist for an Article About a Diagnostic Test for a Man with Diminished Lower Extremity Pulses (*Continued*)**

Application of the Evidence to Your Patient or Client

Are there clinically meaningful differences between the subjects in the study and your patient or client?

___ Yes
_X_ No
___ Mixed results
___ Insufficient detail

Mean age = 63.8 (SD = 0.36) years; sample included African American males and individuals with a history of smoking and hyperlipidemia.

Can you perform the index diagnostic test safely and appropriately in your clinical setting given your current knowledge and skill level and your current resources?

_X_ Yes
___ No
___ Insufficient description of the techniques used

Both manual palpation of pulses and the ABI are performed easily at the bedside by physical therapists.

Application of the Evidence to Your Patient or Client

Does the index diagnostic test fit within the patient's or client's expressed values and preferences?

___ Yes
_X_ No
___ Mixed results

The patient wants to resume an active lifestyle so he would benefit from the more accurate test (ABI) to help determine the underlying cause of his leg cramping.

Will you use the index diagnostic test for this patient or client?

___ Yes
_X_ No

The physical therapist will use the ABI instead of relying on manual pulses.

Your Calculations

Left LE		PAD Present (ABI < 0.90)	PAD Absent (ABI ≥ 0.90)	Totals
Palpation of Pedal Pulses	Positive (Absent pulse)	a 8	b 4	a + b 12
	Negative (Present pulse)	c 37	d 304	c + d 341
	Totals	a + c 45	b + d 308	a + b + c + d 353

Left Lower Extremity

Sensitivity = a/(a + c) = 8/45 = 18%

Specificity = d/(b + d) = 304/308 = 99%

Positive predictive value = a/(a + b) = 8/12 = 67%

Negative predictive value = d/(c + d) = 304/341 = 89%

TABLE 21-1	Quality Appraisal Checklist for an Article About a Diagnostic Test for a Man with Diminished Lower Extremity Pulses (*Continued*)

Likelihood ratio for a positive test result = LR+ = sens/(1 − spec) = 0.18/1 − 0.99 = 18

Likelihood ratio for a negative test result = LR− = (1 − sens)/spec = 1 − 0.18/0.99 = 0.83

Change in Probabilities if Test Is Performed:

Pretest probability (prevalence) = (a + c)/(a + b + c + d) = 45/353 = 13%

Pretest odds = prevalence/(1 _ prevalence) = 0.13/0.87 = 0.15

Posttest odds (LR+) = pretest odds × LR+ = 0.15 = 18 = 2.7

Posttest probability = posttest odds/(posttest odds + 1) = 2.7/3.7 = 73%

Posttest odds (LR−) = pretest odds × LR− = 0.15 = 0.83 = 0.12

Posttest probability = posttest odds/(posttest odds + 1) = 0.12/1.12 = 11%

Left LE		PAD		Totals
		Present (ABI < 0.90)	**Absent (ABI ≥ 0.90)**	
Palpation of Pedal Pulses	Positive (Absent pulse)	**a** 12	**b** 7	**a + b** 19
	Negative (Present pulse)	**c** 25	**d** 314	**c + d** 339
	Totals	**a + c** 37	**b + d** 321	**a + b + c + d** 358

Right Lower Extremity

Sensitivity = a/(a + c) = 12/37 = 32%

Specificity = d/(b + d) = 314/321 = 98%

Positive predictive value = a/(a + b) = 12/19 = 63%

Negative predictive value = d/(c + d) = 314/339 = 93%

Likelihood ratio for a positive test result = LR+ = sens/(1 _ spec) = 0.32/1 _ 0.98 = 16

Likelihood ratio for a negative test result = LR− = (1 _ sens)/spec = 1 _ 0.32/0.98 = 0.69

Change in Probabilities if Test Is Performed:

Pretest probability (prevalence) = (a + c)/(a + b + c + d) = 37/358 = 10%

Pretest odds = prevalence/(1 _ prevalence) = 0.10/0.90 = 0.11

Posttest odds (LR+) = pretest odds × LR+ = 0.11 = 16 = 1.8

Posttest probability = posttest odds/(posttest odds + 1) = 1.8/2.8 = 64%

Posttest odds (LR−) = pretest odds × LR− = 0.11 = 0.69 = 0.08

Posttest probability = posttest odds/(posttest odds + 1) = 0.08/1.08 = 7.4%

Data from Collins TC, Suarez-Almazor M, Petersen NJ. An absent pulse is not sensitive for the early detection of peripheral arterial disease. *Fam Med.* 2006;38(1):38_42.

Given that three out of four pulses are detectable, the physical therapist plans to measure this patient's ABI in both lower extremities. In light of the patient's desire to return to an active lifestyle, as well as his favorable rehabilitation potential, the physical therapist will report his findings to the attending physician with a recommendation for additional lower extremity vascular competency tests should the ABI results suggest the presence of peripheral arterial disease.

Case #2 Evidence About a Clinical Measure

This patient is a 23-year-old Native American man who suffered a high-caliber gunshot wound to his left lower extremity during combat operations 2 weeks ago. He underwent a transtibial amputation that was complicated by infection requiring intravenous antibiotics and revision of the incision site. He is eager to begin acute inpatient rehabilitation because he wants to return to his unit as soon as possible. The physical therapist's initial clinical examination reveals the following:

- *Initial Observation:* Athletic young man sitting on an elevated mat in the rehabilitation gym. His lower extremity incision is approximated, open to room air and dry. Residual ecchymosis is present without observable erythema.
- *Social History:* He is single and serves as a staff sergeant in the U.S. Army. He was on his second tour in theater when he was wounded.
- *Significant Medical History:* None.
- *Medications:* Oxycodone as needed (pain).
- *Mental Status:* Alert and oriented to person, place, and time. He follows multiple-step commands and answers questions appropriately.
- *Pain (Numeric Pain Rating Scale):* 7/10 without pain medication; 3/10 with pain medication (taken 1 hour prior to his physical therapy appointment).
- *Vital Signs at Rest:* Heart rate = 66 beats/min with regular rhythm; Blood pressure = 114/64 mmHg; Respiratory rate = 14 breaths/min; Oxygen saturation = 99% on room air.
- *Body Mass Index (BMI)* = 21.8 kg/m2.
- *Palpation:* He complains of tenderness around the incision site. The peri-incisional skin feels slightly warmer to the touch than the skin on the superior aspect of the tibia, and 2+ edema is noted distally.
- *Active Range of Motion:* Normal for all joints of both lower extremities with complaint of incisional discomfort during left knee flexion and extension.
- *Passive Range of Motion:* Normal for all joints in both lower extremities.
- *Mobility:* He maneuvers around the mat independently. He performs 75% of the effort to come from sitting to standing on his right lower extremity with assistance of one person. He stands using a walker or parallel bar with close supervision of one person for 2 minutes before complaint of fatigue. He ambulates approximately 50 feet hopping on his right leg using a standard walker and contact guard of one person.
- *Vital Signs with Activity:* Heart rate = 84 beats/min with regular rhythm; Blood pressure = 130/60 mmHg; Respiratory rate = 22 breaths/min; Oxygen saturation = 99%.
- *Pain with Activity (Numeric Pain Rating Scale):* 5/10.

The physical therapist wants to collect quantitative data regarding residual limb volume so she can track this patient's progress with limb-shaping intervention strategies. She is aware of a variety of methods for measuring lower extremity volume in patients with venous insufficiency, lymphedema, or swelling after a noninvasive injury but wonders whether these techniques are appropriate for patients with lower extremity amputations. She decides to search the literature to answer the following clinical question:

Is circumferential measurement of limb girth a reliable and valid method for quantifying the amount of edema in the residual limb of a 23-year-old man with a transtibial amputation?

Figure 21-2 illustrates a literature search using the National Library of Medicine's PubMed basic search box function. The initial search string, "residual limb" and measurement (limits = English, Humans), returns 86 articles, among which are those related to quantification of pain rather than edema. Limiting the search by adding "NOT pain" to the search string identifies 45 articles, 6 of which appear to address the clinical question based on their titles and abstracts. Several of the remaining articles investigated computerized measurement devices commonly used by prosthetists rather than physical therapists in acute rehabilitation settings. One citation is a systematic review that includes articles pertaining to residual limb measurement. However, there are only three articles relevant to the clinical question and analysis of their quality is limited. The physical therapist decides to review one of these articles[3] in more detail because it examined the reliability and validity of circumferential measurements as compared to another accepted measure of edema, water volume displacement, in patients with lower extremity amputations.

Table 21-2 provides a critique of the Boonhong et al. article[3] using the quality appraisal checklist for evidence about clinical measures. Based on her analysis of the study, the physical therapist decides that circumferential measurement using either the cylinder or cone estimation formula will

FIGURE 21-2   Search results for evidence related to a clinical measure for a patient with a transtibial amputation (using the PubMed Basic Search function).

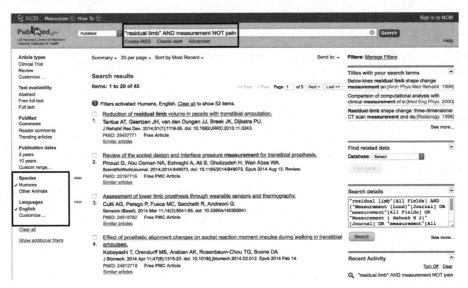

TABLE 21-2	Quality Appraisal Checklist for an Article About a Clinical Measure for a Man with a Transtibial Amputation

Research Validity of the Study

Did the investigators include subjects with all levels or stages of the condition being evaluated by the index clinical measure?

   ___ Yes
   _X_ No
   ___ Insufficient detail

Exclusion criteria did not specify individuals with acute amputations; however, the convenience sample resulted in subjects with lower extremity amputations of at least 4 months' duration.

Did the investigators evaluate (or provide a citation for) the reliability of the index clinical measure?

   _X_ Yes
   ___ No
   ___ Insufficient detail

Initial circumferential and water volume displacement measures were collected and then repeated 5 minutes later to assess reliability. The authors did not indicate whether intra- or interrater reliability was assessed.

Did the investigators compare results from the index clinical measure to results from a gold standard measure?

   ___ Comparison to a gold standard measure was performed
   _X_ Comparison to another measure was performed
   ___ Comparison to another measure was performed
   ___ Comparison was performed but the description is inadequate
   ___ No comparison was made

Circumferential girth measures using two geometric estimation methods (cylinder and cone) were compared to water volume displacement measures.

Were all subjects evaluated with the comparison measure?

   _X_ Yes
   ___ No
   ___ Insufficient detail

All subjects were measured using the water volume displacement technique.

Were the individuals performing and interpreting each measure's results unaware of the other measure's results (i.e., were they masked, or blinded)?

   ___ Yes
   ___ No
   _X_ Insufficient detail

The authors did not describe who collected or documented the results for any of the measures performed.

Was the time between application of the index clinical measure and the gold standard measure short enough to minimize the opportunity for change in the subjects' condition?

   _X_ Yes
   ___ No
   ___ Insufficient detail

Subjects were measured within the same session with 5-minute intervals between each measure.

Did the investigators confirm their findings with a new set of subjects?

   ___ Yes
   _X_ No
   ___ Insufficient detail

TABLE 21-2	Quality Appraisal Checklist for an Article About a Clinical Measure for a Man with a Transtibial Amputation (*Continued*)

Do you have enough confidence in the research validity of this paper to consider using this evidence with your patient or client?

___ Yes
_X_ Undecided
___ No

The authors' description of the measurement techniques used indicate reasonable efforts to minimize error; however, it is unclear what type of reliability was assessed and what role tester bias may have played.

Relevant Study Findings

Results reported that are specific to your clinical question:

Correlation coefficient(s): Pearson's r for circumferential and water volume displacement measures: final residual volume = 0.987; change in residual volume = 0.921

Other: Repeated measures for circumferential measures: (cylinder) = 700.23 ($\pm$289) cm^3 and 704.48 ($\pm$290) cm^3; (cone) = 700.74 ($\pm$289) cm^3 and 704.97 ($\pm$290) cm^3

Other: Change in volume over 30-day follow-up period: (cylinder) = 36.18 ($\pm$80.02) cm^3; (cone) = 36.25 ($\pm$80.07) cm^3; mean difference in change between water volume displacement method and circumferential measures: (cylinder) = 3.88 ($\pm$32.34) cm^3; (cone) = 3.81 ($\pm$32.25) cm^3

Statistical significance and/or precision of the relevant study results:

Obtained p values for each relevant statistic reported by the authors:

p = 0.01 for Pearson correlations between circumferential and water volume displacement measures (both final residual volume and change in residual volume)

Obtained confidence intervals (CIs) for each relevant statistic reported by the authors:

95% CI for mean difference in change between water volume displacement method and circumferential measure (cylinder) = -7.99, 15.74

95% CI for mean difference in change between water volume displacement method and circumferential measure (cone) = -8.02, 15.64

Is the index clinical measure reliable?

_X_ Yes
___ No
___ Mixed results
___ Insufficient detail

Is the index clinical measure valid?

Circumferential measures (cylinder or cone) produced results comparable to the water volume displacement technique within the same time frame (criterion and concurrent validity).

___ Yes
___ No
_X_ Mixed results
___ Insufficient detail

Is the index clinical measure responsive?

The ability to detect change in volume over time was not evaluated using the circumferential techniques.

___ Yes
_X_ No
___ Mixed results
___ Insufficient detail

(continues)

TABLE 21-2   Quality Appraisal Checklist for an Article About a Clinical Measure for a Man with a Transtibial Amputation (*Continued*)

Application of the Evidence to Your Patient or Client

Are there clinically meaningful differences between the subjects in the study and your patient or client?	_X_ Yes ___ No ___ Mixed results ___ Insufficient detail
All of the subjects (n = 51; 69% male) had transtibial amputations. However, the mean age was 55 (SD = 18) years and the mean duration since amputation was 5.5 months.	
Can you perform the index clinical measure safely and appropriately in your clinical setting given your current knowledge and skill level and your current resources?	_X_ Yes ___ No ___ Insufficient description of the techniques used
The authors provide explicit descriptions of all of the measurement techniques used.	
Does the index clinical measure fit within the patient's or client's expressed values and preferences?	_X_ Yes ___ No ___ Mixed results
The patient understands that residual limb volume control is essential to appropriate prosthetic fit. He wants accurate measurement so that his progress is evident both to him and to the prosthetist who will be manufacturing his new limb.	
Will you use the index clinical measure for this patient or client?	_X_ Yes ___ No
Despite the study's limitations, the physical therapist decides to use the circumferential measurement technique because it is sufficiently reliable and valid to provide absolute quantifiable data and minimizes the risk of incisional contamination due to immersion in water.	

Data from Boonhong J, Osiri M, Werawatganon T. Validity and reliability of girth measurement (circumference measurement) for calculating residual limb volume in below-knee amputees. *Chula Med J.* 2007;51(2):77_88.

provide objective data that are more helpful than the pitting edema grades she has used so far. She notes the possibility that change in residual limb volume may not be detected with this technique, but decides to compare the data she collects with changes in the stump shrinker fit for this patient to draw her own conclusions.

Case #3   Evidence About Prognostic (Risk) Factors

This patient is a 78-year-old Caucasian woman diagnosed with Parkinson's disease 7 years ago. Her modified Hoehn and Yahr stage score reported at her last neurologist's visit was 3.0. Her Unified

Parkinson's Disease Rating Scale total score was 48. She fell for the first time turning from the counter to the kitchen table 1 week ago, resulting in a contusion and an extensive hematoma on her left hip. She denies any dizziness or other precipitating symptoms. Her primary complaint is increased difficulty coming to standing and walking because of pain with movement of her left lower extremity. Her family has expressed concern about her safety because of increasing loss of balance and near falls leading up to this recent event. However, they are committed to keeping her at home for as long as possible. The patient is worried that her declining function is a burden to her husband and wants to know what options are available to help them at home. The home health physical therapist's initial clinical examination reveals the following:

- *Initial Observation:* Frail elderly woman accompanied by her 80-year-old husband.
- *Social History:* Her home is a split-level ranch style with five steps to the bedroom and bathroom. Handrails are located on both sides of the stairs. Tight pile wall-to-wall carpets are in all rooms except the kitchen and bathroom. The entrance to the home is at ground level.
- *Significant Medical History:* Hypertension and depression.
- *Medications:* Levodopa-carbidopa (Parkinson's), hydrochlorothiazide (hypertension), and citalopram (depression).
- *Mental Status:* She is alert and oriented to person, place, and time. She follows two-step commands with delayed motor response.
- *Pain at Rest (Numeric Pain Rating Scale):* 2/10.
- *Vital Signs at Rest:* Heart rate = 76 beats/min with regular rhythm; Blood pressure = 124/66 mmHg; Respiratory rate = 16 breaths/min; Oxygen saturation = 98% on room air.
- *Mobility:* She performs 50% of the effort to come to standing with assistance of one person. She stands using a rolling walker with a forward flexed posture and contact guard of one person. She ambulates with a festinating gait pattern, with decreased stance time on the left lower extremity due to pain, for a total distance of 50 feet. She performs 75% of this task with assistance of one person to change directions and recover balance when turning.
- *Vital Signs with Activity:* Heart rate = 92 beats/min with regular rhythm; Blood pressure = 140/60 mmHg; Respiratory rate = 28 breaths/min; Oxygen saturation = 97%.
- *Pain with Activity (Numeric Pain Rating Scale):* 8/10.

As the physical therapist considers this case, he recognizes that the patient has several characteristics that have been identified as risk factors for falls in the elderly. However, the physical therapist is not sure which of these factors is specifically relevant to individuals with Parkinson's disease. He decides to search for evidence to address the following clinical question:

> *Which risk factors predict future fall risk for a 78-year-old woman with Parkinson's disease who has suffered a recent fall at home?*

Figure 21-3 illustrates a literature search using the National Library of Medicine's PubMed Medical Subject Headings (MeSH) search function (limits = English, Humans, Title/Abstract). The original search terms crosswalk to terms in the MeSH library as follows: falls = accidental falls; risk = risk factors; Parkinson's = Parkinson's disease. Of the 77 citations returned, the therapist selects 10 to review (**Figure 21-4**) and identifies a potential article related to his clinical question.[4]

FIGURE 21-3 Search results for evidence related to prognostic (risk) factors for a patient with Parkinson's disease who has suffered a recent fall (using the PubMed MeSH Search function).

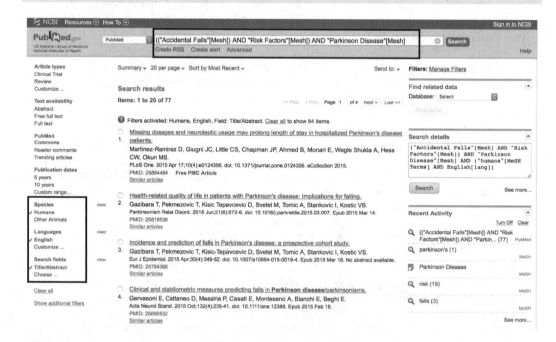

Screenshot from PubMed (www.pubmed.gov), the U.S. National Library of Medicine, Bethesda, MD, USA, and the National Institutes of Health. Accessed May 23, 2016.

Table 21-3 provides a critique of the Matinolli et al. article[4] using the quality appraisal checklist appropriate for evidence about prognostic (risk) factors. Based on his analysis of the study, the physical therapist decides to inquire about the patient's activities of daily living subscale score on the Unified Parkinson's Disease Rating Scale. He will inform the patient and her family about her increased risk for future falls like the one suffered the previous week. The physical therapist also decides to instruct the family on movement and guarding techniques designed to reduce that risk. Finally, he will explore the possibility of a personal care attendant in view of the husband's age and everyone's desire for the patient to remain at home for as long as possible.

FIGURE 21-4 Narrowed selection of articles for evidence related to prognostic (risk) factors for a patient with Parkinson's disease who has suffered a recent fall (using the PubMed MeSH Search function).

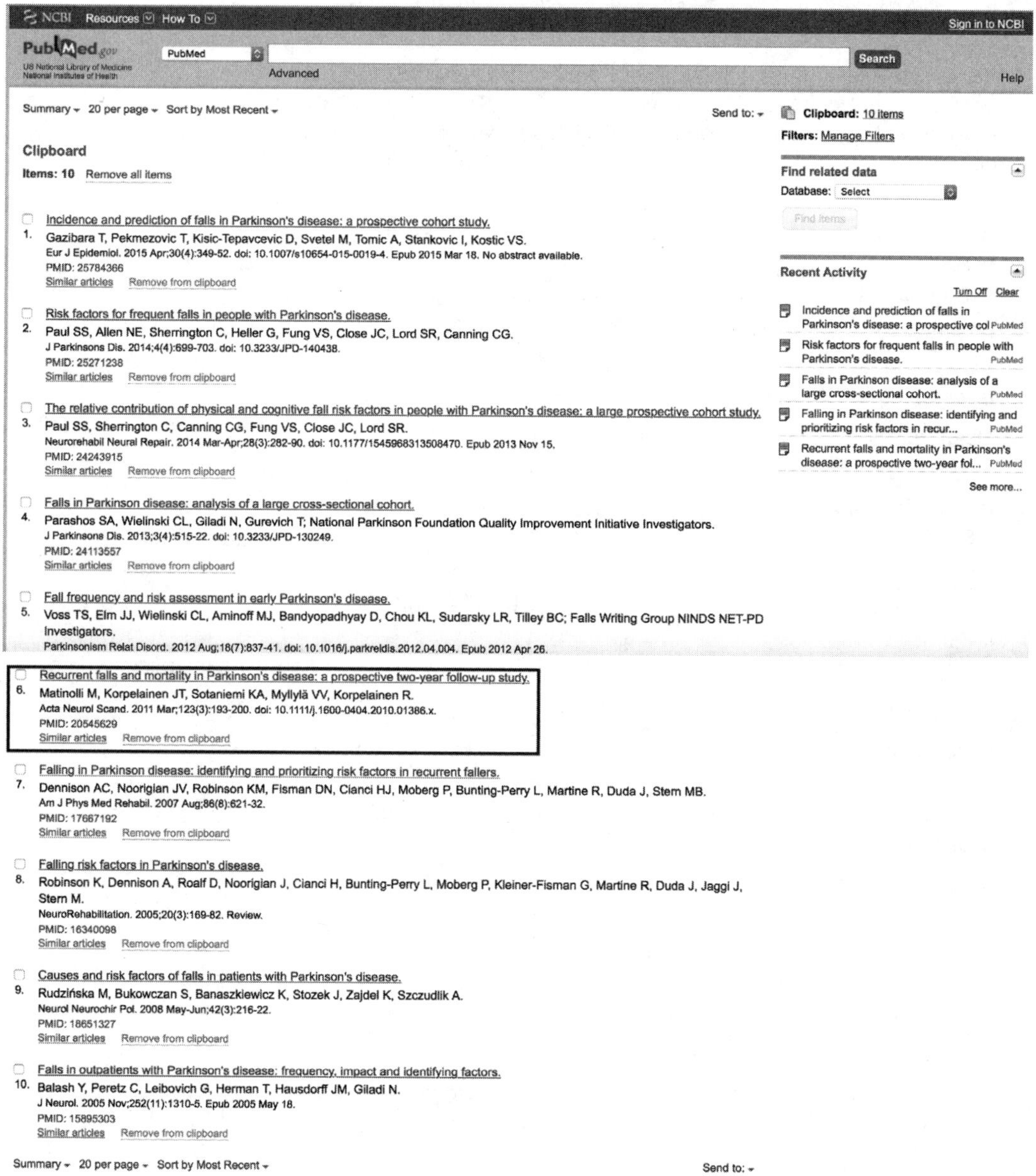

Screenshot from PubMed (www.pubmed.gov), the U.S. National Library of Medicine, Bethesda, MD, USA, and the National Institutes of Health. Accessed May 23, 2016.

TABLE 21-3	Quality Appraisal Checklist for an Article About Prognostic (Risk) Factors for a Woman with Parkinson's Disease

Research Validity of the Study

Did the investigators operationally define the sample in their study?

Total n = 125

Recurrent Fallers (n = 59) (mean age = 68.9 ± 10.4 years; 36% female; mean Hoehn and Yahr stage score = 2.4 ± 0.7 [2 = bilateral involvement without impairment of balance; 5 = wheelchair bound or bedridden]; mean Unified Parkinson's Disease Rating Scale score = 51.6 ± 21 (0 = no disability).

X Yes
___ No
___ Insufficient detail

Were the subjects representative of the population from which they were drawn?

The subjects included were younger and had shorter duration disease than those who were excluded.

___ Yes
X No
___ Insufficient detail

Did all subjects enter the study at the same (preferably early) stage of their condition?

Mean duration of Parkinson's disease in the recurrent fallers = 7.5 ± 5.7 years

___ Yes
X No
___ Insufficient detail

Was the study time frame long enough to capture the outcome(s) of interest?

2 years

X Yes
___ No
___ Insufficient detail

Did the investigators collect outcome data from all of the subjects enrolled in the study?

X Yes
___ No
___ Insufficient detail

Were outcome criteria operationally defined?

Specific definitions of a "fall" were provided to subjects.

X Yes
___ No
___ Insufficient detail

Did the sample include subgroups of patients for whom prognostic estimates will differ?

Subjects who fell once were analyzed separately from subjects who fell multiple times.

X Yes
___ No
___ Insufficient detail

Were the individuals collecting the outcome measures masked (or blinded) to the status of prognostic factors in each subject?

Falls were measured by self-report of the subjects and/or caregivers.

___ Yes
X No
___ Insufficient detail

Research Validity of the Study

Did the sample include subgroups of patients for whom prognostic estimates will differ? If so, did the investigators conduct separate subgroup analyses or statistically adjust for these different prognostic factors?

Predictive factors for recurrent fallers were analyzed separately.

X Yes
___ No
___ Insufficient detail

TABLE 21-3   **Quality Appraisal Checklist for an Article About Prognostic (Risk) Factors for a Woman with Parkinson's Disease (*Continued*)**

Did investigators confirm their findings with a new set of subjects?	___ Yes _X_ No ___ Insufficient detail
Do you have enough confidence in the research validity of this paper to consider using this evidence with your patient or client?	_X_ Yes ___ Undecided ___ No

Relevant Study Findings

Results reported that are specific to your clinical question:

Correlation coefficient(s):_____

Coefficient(s) of determination:_____

Odds ratio(s): _____

Odds ratio (OR) for recurrent falls:

History of falling: OR = 3.2

Unified Parkinson's Disease Rating Scale _ Activities of Daily Living Subscale: OR = 1.13

Other important findings for recurrent fallers with Parkinson's disease:

Compared to nonrecurrent fallers, recurrent fallers had a higher prevalence of:

   Freezing of gait

   Falls unrelated to freezing of gait

   Walking aid use

   Slow performance on the Timed Up and Go test

Statistical significance and/or precision of the relevant study results:

   Obtained p values for each relevant statistic reported by the authors:

   Freezing of gait: $p = 0.027$

   Falls unrelated to freezing of gait: $p < 0.001$

   Walking aid use: $p = 0.011$

   Slow performance on the Timed Up and Go test: $p = 0.020$

Obtained confidence intervals for each relevant statistic reported by the authors:

   History of falling: 95% CI: 1.23, 7.44

   Unified Parkinson's Disease Rating Scale _ Activities of Daily Living Subscale: 95% CI: 1.04, 1.22

   Both 95% CIs indicate reasonably precise estimates of risk.

Application of the Evidence to Your Patient or Client

How likely are the outcomes over time (based on your experience or on the proportion of subjects in the study who achieved the outcome)?	47.2% of subjects reported recurrent falls

(continues)

TABLE 21-3   Quality Appraisal Checklist for an Article About Prognostic (Risk) Factors for a Woman with Parkinson's Disease (*Continued*)

Are there clinically meaningful differences between the subjects in the study and your patient or client?	___ Yes ___ No
Compared to recurrent fallers in the study, she is on the high end of the age range but has a similar duration of disease and a similar Unified Parkinson's Disease Rating Scale stage score.	_X_ Mixed results ___ Insufficient detail
Will sharing information from this study about prognostic indicators or risk factors help your patient or client given his or her expressed values and preferences?	_X_ Yes ___ No ___ Mixed results

How will you use this information with your patient or client?

The patient and her family would benefit from understanding the nature of fall risk in Parkinson's disease. Specifically, the patient can be instructed regarding movement techniques to avoid center of mass falls while the family can be instructed in guarding techniques during at risk movements. The possibility of a personal care attendant also should be explored, given her husband's age.

Data from Matinolli M, Korpelainen JT, Sotaniemi KA, et al. Recurrent falls and mortality in Parkinson's disease: a prospective two-year follow-up study. *Acta Neurol Scand*. 2011;123(3):193_200.

Case #4   Evidence About an Intervention (Randomized Clinical Trial)

This patient is a 43-year-old right-handed woman of Asian descent who presents to an outpatient physical therapy clinic with progressive pain and stiffness that prevents her from lifting her right arm above her head to wash and dry her hair and to reach up into cabinets for dishes. She also complains of sudden sharp pain when she reaches to her right side at her desk or tries to reach into the backseat of her car. She denies previous trauma or similar problems but does recall an incident 3 months earlier in which her Labrador retriever nearly "pulled my arm out of its socket" trying to chase a cat during a morning walk. The physical therapist's initial clinical examination reveals the following:

- *Initial Observation:* Fit-looking woman who maneuvers independently from the waiting room to the exam room guarding her right upper extremity.
- *Social History:* She is married with two children ages 11 and 14 years. She works as a grant reviewer for a charitable foundation where she spends an average of 5 hours a day on her computer. She attends the gym 4 to 5 days a week for strength and aerobic training but has discontinued upper extremity activities.
- *Significant Medical History:* Type I diabetes diagnosed at age 12 years and hyperlipidemia.
- *Medications:* Insulin (diabetes) and simvastatin (hyperlipidemia). Prescription-strength ibuprofen "just takes the edge off" her shoulder pain.
- *Mental Status:* Alert and oriented to person, place, and time.
- *Pain (Numeric Pain Rating Scale):* worst: 9/10; average: 5/10; today: 5/10.
- *Vital Signs at Rest:* Heart rate = 60 beats/min with regular rhythm; Blood pressure = 110/58 mmHg; Respiratory rate = 10 breaths/min; Oxygen saturation = 99% on room air.
- *Palpation:* She complains of general tenderness over the right rotator cuff tendons with point tenderness at the subacromial space.

- *Cervical Spine:* No restrictions are noted in active or passive motion or in segmental vertebral mobility. The therapist is unable to reproduce the patient's upper extremity symptoms during this portion of the examination.
- *Active Range of Motion:* Her left glenohumeral joint is normal in all planes. Her right glenohumeral joint demonstrates 90 degrees of flexion, 70 degrees of abduction, 30 degrees of external rotation with her arm at her side, and 35 degrees of extension. When she tries to reach behind her back, she can only get to her pants pocket. All limitations are in response to increased pain provoked at the end of the achieved ranges.
- *Passive Range of Motion:* Her left glenohumeral joint is normal in all planes. Her right glenohumeral joint demonstrates 100 degrees of flexion, 82 degrees of abduction, 35 degrees of external rotation with her arm at her side, 40 degrees of extension with all limitations due to pain, producing an empty end feel.
- *Motor Control:* She initiates right shoulder elevation through activation of her upper trapezius in a hiking maneuver.
- *Accessory Joint Motion:* The left glenohumeral joint has normal accessory motion. Restriction to movement is noted with posterior and inferior glides of the right humeral head. Pain is reproduced when the humeral head is mobilized into the restriction.
- *Disability of Arm, Shoulder and Hand Scale (DASH) Score:* 79 of 100 possible points (higher score represents greater disability).

The physical therapist concludes that her examination findings are consistent with adhesive capsulitis of the right shoulder. The patient tells her that her physician recommended a corticosteroid injection for her shoulder, but she declined that option as she already has to inject herself with insulin daily. She also found information on the Internet that indicates that corticosteroids are "not good" for people with diabetes. She wants to know what the physical therapist can do to speed up her recovery. After considering the list of interventions that have potential to address this patient's problem, the physical therapist decides to review the evidence to answer the following clinical question:

Which combination of interventions will produce the quickest improvement in pain and function for a 43-year-old woman with diabetes and adhesive capsulitis of the shoulder: (1) joint mobilization and exercise or (2) joint mobilization, exercise, and physical agents?

Figure 21-5 illustrates a literature search using the Cochrane Library online database and the search string "adhesive capsulitis" AND (physical therapy OR physiotherapy). The search is limited to Cochrane reviews. Of the seven citations returned, three appear relevant to her clinical question. The Page et al. article is a systematic review and meta-analysis of evidence regarding the use of electrotherapeutic modalities, alone and in combination with other interventions, for shoulder pain. Several of the articles reviewed focus on patients with adhesive capsulitis, but they were analyzed individually because they addressed different interventions and outcome measures. The remaining evidence includes patients with other disorders of the shoulder, such as rotator cuff tendonitis and subacromial bursitis. As a result, the physical therapist decides to retrieve an original article by van der Windt et al.[5] and review it to answer her question. The article compares physical therapy (exercise and joint mobilization, as well as electrical stimulation, hot or cold packs as needed for pain) to corticosteroid injections.

Table 21-4 provides a critique of the van der Windt et al. article[5] using the quality appraisal checklist appropriate for evidence about interventions. Based on her analysis of the study, the physical therapist decides to inform the patient that the available evidence is limited and does not include patients with diabetes. Diabetes is known to delay healing time in general and may adversely influence this patient's prognosis in ways that cannot be estimated because subjects like her were not studied. However, she will discuss the findings from van der Windt et al., including (1) the use of exercise and joint mobilization techniques as the primary physical therapy intervention methods; (2) the potential for a longer recovery time during the first 2 to 3 months, as compared to corticosteroid injections; and (3) the potential that her eventual improvement may be comparable over the long term to that achieved with injections. Based on the evidence and her prior experience with patients similar to this one, the physical therapist also will offer electrical stimulation combined with ice for pain management as needed during treatment.

FIGURE 21-5   Search results for evidence related to interventions for a patient with adhesive capsulitis of the shoulder (using the Cochrane Library).

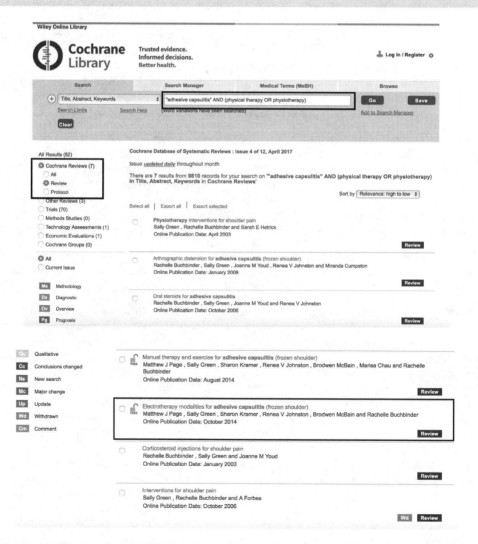

TABLE 21-4 Quality Appraisal Checklist for an Article About Interventions for a Woman with Adhesive Capsulitis of the Shoulder

Research Validity of the Study

Did the investigators randomly assign (or allocate) subjects to groups?
The authors used a random number generator.

_X_ Yes
___ No
___ Insufficient detail

Was each subject's group assignment concealed from the people enrolling individuals in the study?

_X_ Yes
___ No
___ Insufficient detail

Did the groups have similar sociodemographic, clinical, and prognostic characteristics at the start of the study?
More subjects in the physical therapy group were female and had:

• concomitant neck pain;

• an acute onset of shoulder pain and stiffness; and

• involvement of their dominant upper extremity.

In comparison, more subjects in the corticosteroid group had:

• previous episodes of shoulder pain and stiffness;

• a higher rating of severity of pain associated with their main complaint; and

• a higher rating of severity of pain at night.

___ Yes
_X_ No
___ Insufficient detail

Were subjects masked (or blinded) to their group assignment?

___ Yes
_X_ No
___ Insufficient detail

Were clinicians and/or outcome assessors masked (or blinded) to the subjects' group assignment?

_X_ Yes
___ No
___ Insufficient detail

Were the instruments used to measure outcomes reliable and valid?

_X_ Yes
___ No
___ Insufficient detail

Did the clinicians and/or outcomes assessors have demonstrated competence applying the outcomes measures?
A citation was provided regarding the reliability of the digital goniometer used to measure glenohumeral range of motion, but the reliability of the examiner was not addressed.

___ Yes
___ No
_X_ Insufficient detail

Did the investigators manage all of the groups in the same way except for the experimental intervention(s)?
Medication use and additional treatments outside of the study were not controlled.

___ Yes
_X_ No
___ Insufficient detail

(continues)

TABLE 21-4	Quality Appraisal Checklist for an Article About Interventions for a Woman with Adhesive Capsulitis of the Shoulder (*Continued*)

Did the investigators apply the study protocol and collect follow-up data on all subjects over a time frame long enough for the outcomes of interest to occur?	X Yes ___ No ___ Insufficient detail
Measures were collected at 3, 7, 13, 26, and 52 weeks, respectively.	
Did subject attrition (e.g., withdrawal, loss to follow-up) occur over the course of the study?	X Yes ___ No ___ Insufficient detail
Two patients withdrew from the physical therapy group; four patients withdrew from the injection group. The investigators did not perform an analysis of the characteristics of those who withdrew to determine whether sampling bias had resulted.	
If attrition occurred, did the investigators perform an intention-to-treat analysis?	X Yes ___ No ___ Insufficient detail ___ Not applicable
They also analyzed their data excluding 12 patients who were not treated according to protocol for the purposes of comparison.	
Did the investigators confirm their findings with a new set of subjects?	___ Yes X No ___ Insufficient detail
Do you have enough confidence in the research validity of this paper to consider using this evidence with your patient or client?	___ Yes ___ Undecided X No
Limitations include unequal distribution of subject characteristics at baseline and the lack of control for interventions provided outside of the study.	

Relevant Study Findings

Results reported that are specific to your clinical question:

Test(s) of differences: _____

Effect size(s): Subjects in the corticosteroid group achieved a statistically significant greater improvement as compared to subjects in the PT group, for the following measures:

- Pain during the day = mean difference between groups = 12 mm on a visual analog scale
- Pain at night = mean difference between groups = 14 mm on a visual analog scale
- Shoulder disability = mean difference between groups = 25 points on a 100-point scale
- External rotation of affected shoulder = mean difference between groups = 15 degrees
- Therapist rating of success = mean difference between groups = 15 mm on visual analog scale

Subjects in the physical therapy group did not improve their range of motion during the 7 weeks of treatment:

- Mean change in external rotation = −2 degrees (SD = 14)
- Mean change in abduction = −1 degree (SD = 14)

TABLE 21-4	Quality Appraisal Checklist for an Article About Interventions for a Woman with Adhesive Capsulitis of the Shoulder (*Continued*)

- Subjects in the corticosteroid group:
- Improved their external rotation, with a mean change = 13 degrees (SD = 16)
- Did not improve their abduction, with a mean change = 4 degrees (SD = 11)

Absolute benefit increase(s): _____

Relative benefit increase(s): _____

Absolute risk reduction(s): _____

Relative risk reduction(s): _____

Number needed to treat (harm): _____

Other: _____

Statistical significance and/or precision of the relevant study results:

Obtained p values for each relevant statistic reported by the authors:

Corticosteroid group versus physical therapy group:

- Pain during the day: $p < 0.001$
- Pain at night: $p = 0.015$
- Shoulder disability: $p = 0.024$
- External rotation of affected shoulder: $p = 0.002$
- Therapist rating of success: $p < 0.001$

Obtained confidence intervals for each relevant statistic reported by the authors:

Corticosteroid group versus physical therapy group:

- Pain during the day: 95% CI: 15, 37 mm
- Pain at night: 95% CI: 3, 25 mm
- Shoulder disability: 95% CI: 14, 35 points
- External rotation of affected shoulder: 95% CI: 9, 20 degrees

Therapist rating of success: 95% CI: 7, 22 mm

Do these findings exceed a minimal clinically important difference?   X Yes

MCID = 25% improvement of treatment group over control group;   ___ No
success rate in the study = 31%.   ___ Insufficient detail

Application of the Evidence to Your Patient or Client

Are there clinically meaningful differences between the subjects in the   X Yes
study and your patient or client?   ___ No

Subjects were older and individuals with diabetes were excluded   ___ Mixed results
from the study.   ___ Insufficient detail

(*continues*)

TABLE 21-4   Quality Appraisal Checklist for an Article About Interventions for a Woman with Adhesive Capsulitis of the Shoulder (*Continued*)

Can you perform the intervention of interest safely and appropriately in your clinical setting given your current knowledge and skill level and your current resources? The investigators did not provide specific protocols for the physical therapy interventions provided in the study. However, the physical therapist already uses these types of interventions for similar patients.	___ Yes ___ No _X_ Insufficient description of the techniques used
Does the intervention of interest fit within the patient's or client's expressed values and preferences? The patient wants physical therapy rather than a corticosteroid injection.	_X_ Yes ___ No ___ Mixed results
Do the potential benefits outweigh the potential risks of using the intervention of interest with your patient or client? The primary adverse reaction noted in the study was pain lasting > 2 days in both groups.	_X_ Yes ___ No ___ Mixed results
Will you use the intervention of interest for this patient or client?	_X_ Yes ___ No

Data from Van der Windt DAWM, Koes BW, Deville W, et al. Effectiveness of corticosteroid injections versus physiotherapy for treatment of painful stiff shoulder in primary care: randomized trial. *BMJ*. 1998;317(7168):1292_1296.

Case #5   Evidence About an Intervention (Nonrandomized Trial/Outcomes Research)

This patient is a 6-year-old white male with spastic diplegia who has been referred to outpatient pediatric physical therapy to continue the progress he achieved with standing balance and gait over the school year. He was a full-term infant who was delivered vaginally without complication to a healthy 28-year-old mother following a normal pregnancy. APGAR (activity, pulse, grimace, appearance, and breathing) scores were 6 and 9 at 1 minute and 5 minutes, respectively. He was diagnosed with cerebral palsy at 16 months of age when his parents noticed that he "wasn't moving like other babies." He has not suffered any seizures and is age appropriate in his cognitive and emotional function. His primary method of locomotion is a wheelchair, but he can walk short distances in the classroom and at home using a posterior walker and bilateral solid ankle-foot orthoses (AFOs). His primary limitation to activity is fatigue and weakness. His goal is to walk without a walker back and forth to the cafeteria with his classmates when he returns to the school in the fall. The physical therapist's initial clinical examination reveals the following:

- *Initial Observation:* Slender boy seated in a custom wheelchair accompanied by his parents. He is wearing glasses and bilateral solid AFOs.
- *Social History:* He has an older sister and one younger brother. He has just completed the first grade. He is an avid baseball fan.
- *Significant Medical History:* He is being considered for botulinum toxin injections to his gastrocnemius, hamstrings, and hip adductors bilaterally. He also is nearsighted.
- *Medications:* None.

- *Mental Status:* He is alert and oriented to person, place, and time. His answers to questions are age appropriate. He follows two-step commands with motor limitations as described below.
- *Pain (Wong-Baker FACES Pain Rating Scale):* None.
- *Vital Signs at Rest:* Heart rate = 84 beats/min with regular rhythm; Blood pressure = 92/58 mmHg; Respiratory rate = 20 breaths/min; Oxygen saturation = 98% on room air.
- *Muscle Tone:* Spasticity is present in the hamstrings and hip adductors, bilaterally (Modified Ashworth Scale score = 3). Mildly increased muscle tone is noted in the quadriceps, biceps, and triceps, bilaterally (Modified Ashworth Scale score = 1).
- *Range of Motion:* He has hip flexion and plantar flexion contractures bilaterally. He is lacking 8 degrees of knee extension on the left and 5 degrees of knee extension on the right. His ankles can be dorsiflexed passively to neutral with significant resistance.
- *Mobility (Independently):* He performs the following tasks:
  - Pushing up to stand from his wheelchair
  - Standing with unilateral upper extremity support
  - Manipulating objects with his free hand while standing
  - Ambulating 65 feet with the posterior walker; he stops due to fatigue and frustration with having to use the assistive device
- *Mobility (Assisted):* He performs the following tasks with assistance of one person for 25%–50% of the effort:
  - Standing without upper extremity support
  - Walking without an assistive device
- *Gait Pattern:* His legs cross in a scissoring pattern when walking. He also has a crouched appearance, which is exaggerated further if he does not wear his AFOs. Step length is short for his age, and his upper extremities provide significant assistance for balance while advancing the swing leg.
- *Vital Signs with Activity:* Heart rate = 100 beats/min with regular rhythm; Blood pressure = 112/64 mmHg; Respiratory rate = 30 breaths/min; Oxygen saturation = 98%.
- *Gross Motor Function Classification System (GMFCS) Score:* Level III (age 4 to 6 years).

The physical therapist's clinic has just purchased a body weight suspension harness system to use for gait training over ground as well as on a treadmill. To date, the system has been used with children with incomplete spinal cord injuries and brain injuries. The physical therapist decides to review the evidence to answer the following clinical question:

Will partial body weight-supported gait training on a treadmill improve functional outcomes in a 6-year-old boy with spastic diplegia whose ambulatory ability is limited by weakness and fatigue?

Figure 21-6 illustrates the Rehabilitation Reference Center function on the American Physical Therapy Association's PTNow Web portal. The search string "cerebral palsy" AND treadmill AND harness AND (gait OR ambulation) was entered and the search was limited to children aged 6–12. Of the 12 citations returned on the "Journals" tab, one specifically addressed the effect of body weight-supported treadmill training in children with cerebral palsy. The Kurz et al. article[6] is selected for review even though its focus is on changes in gait kinematics, because it includes children with spastic diplegia within the age range and GMFCS scores of this physical therapist's patient. Most of the subjects also wore AFOs.

Table 21-5 provides an analysis of the Kurz et al. article[6] using the quality appraisal checklist appropriate for articles that are nonrandomized trials about physical therapy interventions or outcomes research. The evidence has several important design limitations, including lack of random assignment,

FIGURE 21-6 Search results for evidence related to interventions for a patient with cerebral palsy (using the PTNow Rehabilitation Reference Center).

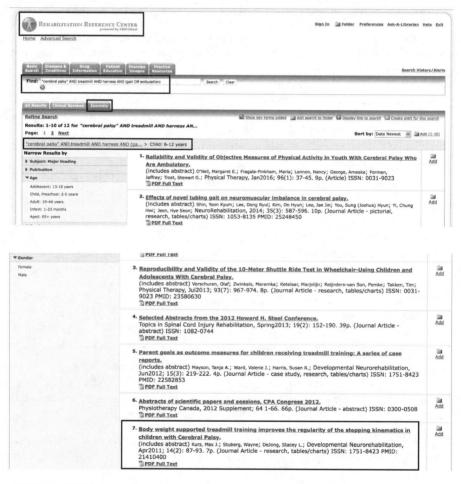

Courtesy of EBSCO host. EBSCO Industries, Inc.

lack of adjustment for confounding variables, and a small sample size. However, the physical therapist decides to recommend body weight-supported treadmill training as an element of this patient's treatment plan because (1) all subjects improved their stepping kinematics, preferred walking speed, and a dimension of the Gross Motor Function Measure (GMFM) score, and (2) the results appeared meaningful in the light of two other studies available in his clinic. Both the treadmill and the harness will allow the physical therapist to carefully titrate the patient's exertion levels to deal with his low

TABLE 21-5	Quality Appraisal Checklist for an Article That Is a Nonrandomized Trial or Outcomes Paper Related to Interventions for a Child with Spastic Diplegia

Research Validity of the Study

Was this a study with more than one group?

___ Yes
_X_ No
___ Insufficient detail

All 12 subjects participated in the body weight-supported treadmill training according to the same protocol (titration of weight support, speed, and time). However, the intensity of the training sessions was individualized to each child's heart rate.

Were the groups comparable at the start of the study?

___ Yes
___ No
___ Insufficient detail
_X_ Not applicable

If groups were not equal at the start of the study, was risk adjustment performed?

___ Yes
___ No
___ Insufficient detail
_X_ Not applicable

Were variables operationally defined and adequately measured by the data used for the study?

___ Yes
___ No
_X_ Insufficient detail

The investigators indicated the method by which treadmill speed and body weight support were adjusted; however, each regimen was specific to each child and so the comparative effectiveness of different doses could not be assessed.

Were standardized person-level outcomes instruments used?

_X_ Yes
_X_ No
___ Insufficient detail

The primary outcome measure was gait kinematics measured electronically while the children walked over ground in a laboratory. However, dimension E of the GMFM was used to assess changes in functional abilities such as walking forward/backward, kicking a ball, and walking up and down stairs.

Were standardized data collection methods implemented?

___ Yes
___ No
_X_ Insufficient detail

The gait analysis procedures were described but not details regarding administration of the GMFM.

Did the interventions of interest precede the outcomes?

_X_ Yes
___ No
___ Insufficient detail

(continues)

> **TABLE 21-5**   Quality Appraisal Checklist for an Article That Is a
> Nonrandomized Trial or Outcomes Paper Related to
> Interventions for a Child with Spastic Diplegia (*Continued*)

Research Validity of the Study

Were other potentially confounding variables accounted for in the analysis?

___ Yes
_X_ No
___ Insufficient detail

The investigators did not collect information regarding the subject's current medication regimens or current activity/fitness levels. In addition, the investigators could not evaluate differences in treatment response based on type of cerebral palsy or GMFCS level.

Were missing data dealt with in an appropriate manner?

_X_ Yes
___ No
_X_ Insufficient detail

The authors do not address if data were lost.

Did the investigators confirm their findings with a new set of subjects?

___ Yes
_X_ No
___ Insufficient detail

Do you have enough confidence in the research validity of this paper to consider using this evidence with your patient or client?

___ Yes
_X_ Undecided
___ No

The primary limitations are the lack of adjustment for confounding factors and the small sample size, both of which could have masked treatment effects.

Relevant Study Findings

Results reported that are specific to your clinical question:

Test(s) of differences: _____

Walking speed: Pre = 0.51 + 0.09 m s^{-1}; Post = 0.60 + 0.09;

Step length: Pre = 0.29 + 0.03 m s^{-1}; Post = 0.34 + 0.02 m;

GMFM score (dimension E): Pre = 17.7 + 4%; Post = 19.5 + 4%

Test(s) of relationships: _____

Effect size(s): _____

Absolute benefit increase(s): _____

Relative benefit increase(s): _____

Absolute risk reduction(s): _____

Relative risk reduction(s): _____

Number needed to treat (harm): _____

Other: _____

Statistical significance and/or precision of the relevant study results:

Obtained p values for each relevant statistic reported by the authors:

The mean change in walking speed: $p = 0.02$

The mean change in step length: $p = 0.03$

TABLE 21-5	Quality Appraisal Checklist for an Article That Is a Nonrandomized Trial or Outcomes Paper Related to Interventions for a Child with Spastic Diplegia (*Continued*)

The mean change in GMFM score (dimension E): $p = 0.01$

Obtained confidence intervals for each relevant statistic reported by the authors:

Do these findings exceed a minimal clinically important difference?

The authors do not indicate an MCID threshold for dimension E of the GMFM. However, a different article at the physical therapist's clinic reported that an MCID of 1.8 for children classified as GMFCS level III was indicative of a moderate effect.[7]

___ Yes
___ No
_X_ Insufficient detail

Application of the Evidence to Your Patient or Client

Are there clinically meaningful differences between the subjects in the study and your patient or client?

Individual subject characteristics are not provided. The general description of subjects suggests that some of them were similar to this patient (age, GMFCS level, spastic diplegia, use of AFOs).

___ Yes
___ No
___ Mixed results
_X_ Insufficient detail

Can you perform the interventions of interest safely and appropriately in your clinical setting given your current knowledge and skill level and your current resources?

_X_ Yes
___ No
___ Insufficient description of the techniques used

Do the interventions of interest fit within your patien'st or client's expressed values and preferences?

The patient is extremely enthusiastic about this option because he can "work out" like they do at his parents' fitness center and will not have to use his walker.

_X_ Yes
___ No
___ Mixed results

Do the outcomes fit within your patient's or client's expressed values and preferences?

It is unclear whether his ambulation ability in school will improve significantly, but his parents believe improved walking ability will translate into overall enhanced quality of life.

___ Yes
___ No
_X_ Mixed results

Do the potential benefits outweigh the potential risks of using the interventions of interest with your patient or client?

Adverse effects were not reported. However, the benefits appear meaningful based on their consistency with other studies accessible in the physical therapist's clinic.

___ Yes
___ No
_X_ Mixed results

Will you use the interventions of interest for this patient or client?

Despite their limitations, the findings are consistent with an earlier article addressing the same question.[8]

_X_ Yes
___ No

Data from Kurz MJ, Stuberg W, DeJong SL. Body weight supported treadmill training improves the regularity of the stepping kinematics in children with cerebral palsy. *Dev Neurorehabil.* 2011;14(2):87-93.

level of aerobic conditioning while simultaneously allowing interventions to improve his gait pattern. The physical therapist plans to search other databases for additional articles with stronger research designs to further inform his clinical decision making.

Case #6   Evidence About a Self-Report Outcomes Measure

This patient is a 31-year-old African American woman who has referred herself to an outpatient physical therapy clinic that recently advertised the addition of a women's health clinical specialist to the practice. The patient reports that she has been suffering regular episodes of urinary leaking since the birth of her twins 8 months ago. The incontinence typically occurs when she laughs, sneezes, walks briskly on her treadmill, or lifts her 2-year-old daughter. She has read about pelvic floor exercises and has tried to implement them on her own but has been unable to detect improvement. She has tried to resume her running routine but the incontinence symptoms are worse when she is more active. The physical therapist's initial clinical examination reveals the following:

- *Initial Observation:* Healthy-appearing woman with no obvious mobility limitations maneuvering from the clinic waiting area to the private examination room.
- *Social History:* She is married with three children. She enjoyed running 5 miles daily prior to her most recent pregnancy.
- *Significant Medical History:* She delivered her oldest child (8 pounds, 10 ounces) vaginally without complication. Her twins were delivered by Caesarean section. She experienced intermittent low back pain during the last trimester of her most recent pregnancy; however, these symptoms resolved as her weight has decreased and her activity levels have increased.
- *Medications:* None.
- *Mental Status:* Alert and oriented to person, place, and time. She answers questions appropriately. She is well educated about her condition through review of information on various women's health advocacy Web sites.
- *Pain (Numeric Pain Rating Scale):* 0/10.
- *Vital Signs at Rest:* Heart rate = 74 beats/min with regular rhythm; Blood pressure =126/64 mmHg; Respiratory rate = 12 breaths/min; Oxygen saturation = 99% on room air.
- *Posture:* No obvious asymmetries in standing. She has an increased anterior pelvic tilt that she can correct with verbal cues.
- *Inspection (Trunk):* Lower transverse incision scar is well healed. Rectus abdominus and oblique muscle contractions are symmetric to command.
- *Inspection (Pelvic Floor):* Perineal skin is normal in color. There is no evidence of organ prolapse but urinary leakage is noted with Valsalva maneuvers. She activates pelvic floor muscles to command.
- *Palpation:* Lower transverse incision scar is nonadherent. Vaginal soft tissue structures are normal and symmetric. The patient denies pain to palpation of any structures.
- *Pelvic Floor Manual Muscle Test Scores (Internal):* 2/5 (weak squeeze) strength with 4-second-hold endurance score.
- *Electromyography:* An internal testing protocol of 10 contractions with 4-second holds and 10-second rests resulted in resting average of 0.130 microvolts (¼), a work average score of 0.600 ¼, and a peak score of 0.685 ¼.
- *Lower Quarter Screen:* She has normal range of motion, strength, and reflexes in both lower extremities.
- *Accessory Joint Motion (Spine):* She has normal mobility for all lumbar and lumbosacral segments without pain. Sacroiliac compression and distraction maneuvers do not elicit pain.

FIGURE 21-7   Search results for a clinical question related to a self-report outcomes measure for a patient with stress urinary incontinence (using the CINAHL Advanced Search function).

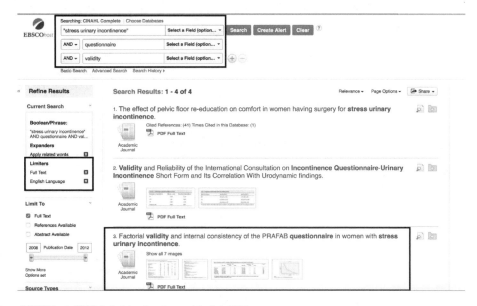

Courtesy of EBSCO host. EBSCO Industries, Inc. Accessed April 1, 2017

During the examination, the patient expresses frustration about the changes in her lifestyle that have been required to cope with her incontinence. The physical therapist recognizes that standardized measurement of the impact of urinary incontinence on this patient's quality of life would be a useful adjunct to track her responses to the interventions provided. The clinic currently only has available generic and orthopedic condition-specific health status instruments. She decides to review the literature to answer the following clinical question:

> *Which patient self-report quality of life instrument is the most valid and responsive to change following physical therapy intervention in a 31-year-old woman with stress urinary incontinence?*

Figure 21-7 illustrates a literature search using the advanced search function of the Cumulative Index of Nursing and Allied Health Literature (CINAHL) Complete database and the search string "stress urinary incontinence" AND questionnaire AND validity. Limits were set at English language and full text availability. Three citations were returned, one of which looked relevant to the question posed based on their titles and abstracts. The Hendriks et al. article[9] is selected for review because it evaluates the short-form versions of two different quality of life instruments specific to pelvic floor disorders that already have established reliability and validity.

Table 21-6 provides an analysis of the Hendriks et al. article[9] using the quality appraisal checklist appropriate for articles about self-report outcomes instruments. Based on her analysis of the study,

TABLE 21-6	Quality Appraisal Checklist for an Article About Self-Report Outcomes Measures for a Woman with Stress Urinary Incontinence

Research Validity of the Study

Instrument Development and Application

Did the investigators provide an adequate description of the index self-report instrument development process, including identification of participants and methods for item development and selection?

___ Yes
___ No
___ Insufficient detail
_X_ Separate study or studies cited

Is the index self-report instrument understandable (readable) by all patient populations?

The investigators did not report on the ease with which subjects could read and understand the questionnaires. However, 25% of the sample were classified as having a "low" educational level.

___ Yes
___ No
_X_ Insufficient detail
___ Separate study or studies cited

Does the index self-report instrument take a reasonable amount of time to administer?

The investigators did not report the actual administration times in this article.

___ Yes
___ No
___ Insufficient detail
_X_ Separate study or studies cited

Is the index self-report instrument easy to score and interpret?

_X_ Yes
___ No
___ Insufficient detail
___ Separate study or studies cited

Instrument Reliability

Did the investigators evaluate the internal consistency of the index self-report instrument?

_X_ Adequate design and method; factor analysis used; (= 0.70_0.90)
___ Inadequate description of methods used
___ Inadequate description of methods used
___ Inadequate internal consistency (< 0.70)
___ Separate study or studies cited
___ No information found on internal consistency

Did the investigators evaluate the reproducibility (test-retest reliability) of the index self-report instrument?

___ Adequate design, method, and ICC > 0.70
___ Inadequate description of methods used
___ Inadequate reliability (ICC < 0.70)
_X_ Separate study or studies cited
___ No information found on test-retest reliability

TABLE 21-6	Quality Appraisal Checklist for an Article About Self-Report Outcomes Measures for a Woman with Stress Urinary Incontinence (*Continued*)

Did the investigators evaluate the limits of agreement of the index self-report instrument?	___ Adequate design, method, and result (κ and/or SEM) ___ Inadequate description of methods used ___ Inadequate agreement X Separate study or studies cited ___ No information found on agreement

Instrument Validity

Did the investigators evaluate the content validity of the index self-report instrument?	___ Patients and investigators (or experts) involved in assessment ___ Only patients involved in assessment ___ No patients involved in assessment ___ Inadequate description of methods used ___ Separate study or studies cited X No information found on content validity
Did the investigators evaluate the construct validity of the index self-report instrument?	X Adequate design, method, and result ___ Inadequate description of methods used ___ Inadequate construct validity ___ Separate study or studies cited ___ No information found on construct validity
Did the investigators evaluate the criterion validity of the index self-report instrument?	___ Adequate design, method, and result ___ Inadequate description of methods used ___ Inadequate criterion validity ___ Separate study or studies cited X No information found on criterion validity
Did the investigators evaluate the index self-report instrument on a population other than the one for which it originally was designed?	___ Adequate design, method, and result ___ Inadequate description of methods used ___ Separate study or studies cited X Not applicable
Did the investigators evaluate the responsiveness of the index self-report instrument?	___ Adequate design, method, and result (effect size and/or standardized response mean) [for PFDI-20] ___ Adequate design, method, and result (effect size and/or standardized response mean) [for PFDI-20] ___ Inadequate description of methods used ___ Inadequate responsiveness [for PFIQ-7] X Separate study or studies cited ___ No information found on responsiveness

(*continues*)

TABLE 21-6	Quality Appraisal Checklist for an Article About Self-Report Outcomes Measures for a Woman with Stress Urinary Incontinence (*Continued*)

Did the investigators evaluate the floor and ceiling effects of the index self-report instrument?	___ No floor or ceiling effects identified ___ Floor and/or ceiling effects exceed 15% of instrument ___ Separate study or studies cited _X_ No information found on floor and/or ceiling effects
Did the investigators evaluate the interpretability of the index self-report instrument?	_X_ 2 or more types of information provided (including standard deviations) ___ Inadequate description of methods used ___ Separate study or studies cited ___ No information found on interpretation
Did the investigators evaluate the minimal clinically important difference (MCID) of the index self-report instrument?	___ MCID calculated ___ Inadequate MCID _X_ Separate study or studies cited ___ No information found on MCID
Do you have enough confidence in the research validity of this paper to consider using this evidence with your patient or client?	_X_ Yes ___ Undecided ___ No

Relevant Study Findings

Results reported that are specific to your clinical question:

Cronbach's α: 0.82

Correlation coefficient(s): 0.42-0.68 (Factor 1); 0.46 (Factor 2)

ICC: 0.96

Pearson's r: _____

Effect size(s): _____

Standardized response mean(s): _____

Other: MCID = -3.0 for low severity incontinence; -5.0 for high severity incontinence (possible score = 5 – 20).

Statistical significance and/or precision of the relevant study results:

Obtained p values for each relevant statistic reported by the authors:

$p < 0.01$–0.05 for different results

Obtained confidence intervals for each relevant statistic reported by the authors:

Not reported for the results listed

TABLE 21-6	Quality Appraisal Checklist for an Article About Self-Report Outcomes Measures for a Woman with Stress Urinary Incontinence (*Continued*)

Application of the Evidence to Your Patient or Client

Are there clinically meaningful differences be-tween the subjects in the study and your patient or client?

   _X_ Yes
   ___ No
   ___ Mixed results
   ___ Insufficient detail

She meets the exclusion criterion related to recent pregnancy or surgery (6 months). In addition, the subjects in this study speak Dutch. This patient speaks English.

Can you administer the index self-report instrument appropriately in your clinical setting given your current resources?

   _X_ Yes
   ___ No
   ___ Insufficient description of the techniques used

Does the index self-report instrument fit within the patient's or client's expressed values and preferences?

   _X_ Yes
   ___ No
   ___ Mixed results

Given the patient's frustrations about the impact of incontinence on her lifestyle, a mechanism for tracking improvement (if any) in her quality of life will provide her with valued information.

Will you use the index self-report instrument for this patient or client?

   ___ Yes
   _X_ No

Even though the authors provide an English language version, the PRAFAB has not been validated with English-speaking women with stress incontinence.

Hendriks EJ, Bernards AT, Staal JB, de Vet HC, de Bie RA. Factorial validity and internal consistency of the PRAFAB questionnaire in women with stress urinary incontinence. *BMC Urology.* 2008;8 1-1.

the physical therapist decides not to implement the PRAFAB instrument with her patient. Even though it is short, easy to administer, and has established discriminant validity and a minimally important clinical change score, it has only been validated in the Dutch language. The authors provide an English language translation but performance in English-speaking individuals has not been evaluated. Therefore, the physical therapist will use a generic self-report instrument available in her clinic until she has time to repeat her evidence search.

Case #7 Evidence Addressing a Patient's Perspective About His or Her Health

This patient is a 37-year-old male who is preparing for an allogenic stem cell transplant to address his refractory stage III non-Hodgkin's lymphoma. His younger sister is the donor. He was originally diagnosed 5 years prior and had been in remission following chemotherapy until 6 months ago. Before he is admitted to the hospital for his pretransplant conditioning process, his oncologist wants him to participate in a supervised exercise program to build his strength and endurance. The cancer rehabilitation physical therapist's initial clinical examination reveals the following:

- *Observation:* Pale, reserved Caucasian male ambulating independently but slowly into the exam room. He is wearing a surgical mask to protect him from airborne contaminants.
- *Social History:* He is married and a father of two girls, ages 7 and 5. He continues to work as a financial analyst at a local investment firm but telecommutes due to fatigue and a desire to avoid potential exposure to bacteria and viruses prior to his transplant. Before he was diagnosed, he enjoyed golfing and daily walks with his family and two Weimaraners.
- *Significant Medical History:* Non-Hodgkin's lymphoma diagnosed at age 32. Treated with cyclophosphamide, doxorubicin, vincristine (Oncovin), and prednisone. No other medical or surgical history.
- *Complete Blood Count* (sent with his referral): Hemoglobin (Hgb) = 9.8 g/dL; Hematocrit (Hct) = 38.7%; White blood cells (WBC) = 5,508 microliters.
- *Medications:* Supplemental iron to address persistent anemia.
- *Mental Status:* He is alert and oriented to person, place, and time and answers questions appropriately.
- *Pain (Numeric Pain Rating Scale):* 0/10.
- *Vital Signs at Rest:* Heart rate = 100 beats/min with regular rhythm; Blood pressure = 96/50 mmHg; Respiratory rate = 14 breaths/min; Oxygen saturation = 95% on room air.
- *Body Mass Index (BMI):* 17.6 kg/m2.
- *Auscultation:* Lungs are clear bilaterally.
- *Strength:* Lower extremities: 30-seconds chair stand test = 13 repetitions with volitional stop due to fatigue. Upper extremities: grip strength = 30.8 kg; dominant hand (right).
- *Aerobic Capacity:* Six-minute walk test = 559 meters with 1 rest due to fatigue.
- *Vital Signs with Activity:* Heart rate = 122 beats/min; Blood pressure = 110/64 mmHg; Respiratory rate = 22 breaths/min; Oxygen saturation = 93%. Rating of perceived exertion = 6 on a 10-point scale.

During the examination, the patient indicates that his main complaint is fatigue and wonders how he will manage it successfully and still prepare for his transplant. He is curious about how other individuals in his situation have felt about these issues. The physical therapist wonders whether there is evidence from other individuals with lymphoma that would assist both of them in understanding this patient's concerns. He decides to conduct a search to answer the following clinical question:

> *Does the evidence suggest a way for me to assist a 37-year-old male with non-Hodgkin's lymphoma with his experience of cancer-related fatigue?*

The physical therapist initially searches PubMed and CINAHL Complete with the search string lymphoma AND fatigue AND qualitative. He locates several relevant articles, none of which are available as free full text. **Figure 21-8** illustrates the same search using Google Scholar on recommendation from some colleagues who had success locating free full-text articles through this search engine. Over 13,000 citations are identified sorted by relevance. The first article by Spichiger et al.[10] is selected for review because it is specific to the clinical question, includes individuals with lymphoma, and is also listed in the first several citations returned by PubMed and CINAHL Complete.

FIGURE 21-8   Search results for a clinical question related to a patient's perspective about cancer-related fatigue (using Google Scholar).

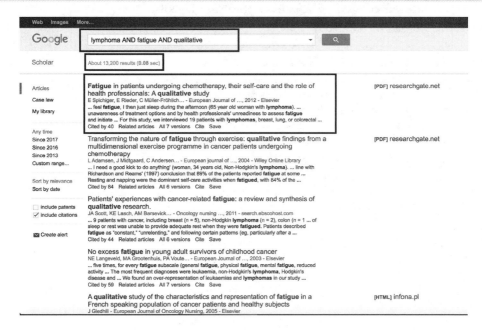

Google and the Google logo are registered trademarks of Google Inc., used with permission.

Table 21-7 provides an analysis of the Spichiger et al. article[10] using the quality appraisal checklist appropriate for qualitative research studies. The physical therapist notes several methodological strengths of the article. However, he acknowledges the authors omitted some procedural elements related to the influence of their assumptions and interactions with the subjects that are critical to high-quality evidence of this type. Despite these limitations, the physical therapist decides to share the article's findings with his patient and discuss how they both may use the information to address fatigue-related concerns. He anticipates his patient will behave like some of the subjects in the article and seek additional information on this topic via the Internet.

Section Two: Using Physiologic Studies as Evidence

Case #8   Physiologic Studies as Evidence

This patient is a 15-year-old Hispanic male soccer player who reported gradual onset of pain in the region of his right knee over the course of his participation in a weekend soccer tournament approximately 1 week ago. He denies any previous injury to his knee. His mother reports that radiographs taken at the pediatrician's office were negative. Presently, the patient complains of

TABLE 21-7	Quality Appraisal Checklist for an Article About Patient Experiences for a Man with non-Hodgkin's Lymphoma

Qualitative Research Studies—Quality Appraisal Checklist

Research Validity of the Study

Did the investigators use a qualitative research methodology that was consistent with their research question?

A grounded theory approach was implemented to "explore patients' fatigue-related interactions with professionals during chemotherapy, patients' strategies to deal with the symptoms and the perceived outcomes of their self-care activities."

X Yes
___ No
___ Insufficient detail

Did the investigators include individuals whose background and attributes were consistent with their research question?

8 men, 10 women; age range: 23–87; 5 diagnosed with lymphoma; 5 working part time; 11 with white collar positions; 2 living with partners and children;

X Yes
___ No
___ Insufficient detail

Did the investigators use data collection methods that were consistent with their research methodology?

Subject interviews ranging from 30 to 65 minutes were conducted by two trained oncology nurse research assistants, recorded and transcribed; questions were open ended and followed an initial guide.

X Yes
___ No
___ Insufficient detail

Did the investigators collect data in a context sufficient to thoroughly address their research question?

Interviews were conducted at the conclusion of the third round of chemotherapy at the treatment center.

X Yes
___ No
___ Insufficient detail

Did the investigators interpret the data in a manner consistent with their research methodology?

Themes identified related to fatigue experiences = being informed about fatigue; enduring fatigue; experiencing fatigue in relation to life and life circumstances; experiencing or lacking support; fatigue-related self-care; and handling fatigue in the absence of advice from health professionals.

X Yes
___ No
___ Insufficient detail

Did the investigators implement methods to confirm initial findings generated through their data collection processes?

An iterative data coding and analysis process is described but not clearly enough to judge if triangulation occurred. The authors acknowledge as a limitation that data saturation was not attempted or achieved.

___ Yes
___ No
X Insufficient detail

TABLE 21-7	Quality Appraisal Checklist for an Article About Patient Experiences for a Man with non-Hodgkin's Lymphoma (*Continued*)

Did the investigators explicitly examine their own beliefs, values, and assumptions in relation to their findings?	___ Yes
	X No
Reflexivity is not referenced.	___ Insufficient detail
Did the investigators explicitly examine their influence on the research process and outcomes?	___ Yes
	X No
Reflexivity is not referenced.	___ Insufficient detail
Do you have enough confidence in the credibility of this study to consider using this evidence with your patient or client?	___ Yes
	X Undecided
	___ No

Relevant Study Findings

Results reported that are specific to your clinical question:

"At the start of their chemotherapy, health professionals informed patients that common side effects included fatigue. While all participants experienced different dimensions of fatigue, all were willing to endure it for the sake of an expected improvement in their conditions. Individuals' fatigue experiences depended largely on their particular life and illness circumstances. Most engaged in fatigue-related self-care activities and managed the symptom on their own. Communication with or input from health professionals was virtually absent during chemotherapy."

Application of the Evidence to Your Patient or Client

Are there clinically meaningful differences between the subjects in the study and your patient or client?	X Yes
	___ No
Subjects were actively undergoing chemotherapy whereas this patient is in between treatment.	___ Mixed results
	___ Insufficient detail
Can you apply the results of this study in an ethical, culturally appropriate way given your current knowledge, skills, experience and clinical context?	X Yes
	___ No
Will application of the results of this study fit within the patient or client's expressed values and preferences?	X Yes
	___ No
This patient is interested in learning how others like him have managed with fatigue.	___ Mixed results
Will you incorporate the results of this study in your clinical decision making with this patient or client?	X Yes
	___ No

intermittent pain with walking and ascending and descending steps. He has not attempted a return to soccer practice or gym class. The outpatient physical therapist's initial clinical examination reveals the following:

- *Observation:* Pleasant young man who ambulates independently to the examination room with a mildly antalgic gait pattern. He is accompanied by his mother.
- *Social History:* He is in the 10th grade and works for a local grocery store several nights a week. He is a starting halfback on the high school soccer team, as well as on a town league. College scouts have been evaluating his performance to determine his recruitment potential.
- *Significant Medical History:* None.
- *Medications:* 440 mg of naproxen sodium (pain and inflammation) twice daily.
- *Mental Status:* He is alert and oriented to person, place, and time and answers questions appropriately.
- *Pain (Numeric Pain Rating Scale):* worst: 8/10; average: 5/10; today: 4/10.
- *Vital Signs at Rest:* Heart rate = 66 beats/min with regular rhythm; Blood pressure = 104/50 mmHg; Respiratory rate = 12 breaths/min; Oxygen saturation = 99% on room air.
- *Body Mass Index (BMI):* 18.9 kg/m2.
- *Palpation:* There is tenderness over the anterior aspect of the medial tibial condyle with mild, localized swelling in the same region. The tibiofemoral and patellofemoral joint lines are non-tender. No crepitus with active or passive knee flexion and extension is noted.
- *Strength:* Manual muscle testing of the hamstrings, hip adductors, and sartorius on the right reproduces pain in the region of the medial condyle. Strength is at least full range of motion against gravity, but his effort is limited by pain. His left lower extremity strength is normal.
- *Flexibility:* Indirect assessment of hamstring length in supine (passive knee extension with hip at 90 degrees) reveals a popliteal angle of approximately 30 degrees bilaterally with reproduction of pain symptoms on the right at the end of the range.
- *Gait:* He ambulates independently with decreased stance time and decreased knee flexion during the swing phase on his right.
- *Special Tests:* No laxity noted with stress tests of the medical collateral, lateral collateral, anterior cruciate, and posterior cruciate ligaments.

The physical therapist concludes that her findings are consistent with acute inflammation of the pes anserinus bursa and associated tendinous attachments secondary to overuse. Limitation in hamstring extensibility may be implicated as well. The prognosis for recovery is excellent, and the patient's goal of unrestricted return to competitive soccer without pain is realistic. As part of the overall treatment plan for this patient, low-intensity therapeutic ultrasound is considered to facilitate resolution of the acute inflammatory process. The intended treatment area, however, is in the region of the proximal tibial epiphysis, and because the patient is a 15-year-old boy the physical therapist assumes that this growth plate is open. Prior to proceeding with ultrasound treatment, she decides to review the evidence to answer the following clinical question:

> *Is therapeutic ultrasound contraindicated as an intervention for inflammation in the region of an open epiphyseal plate in a 15-year-old boy with knee pain?*

Table 21-8 details the results of an interactive literature search using the National Library of Medicine's PubMed online database. Unfortunately, none of the articles were from human studies, so the physical therapist looked for the animal studies that most closely mimicked application of

TABLE 21-8	Search Results for a Clinical Question Related to the Use of Ultrasound Over an Open Epiphyseal Plate in a Teenager with Knee Pain (Using PubMed's Basic Search Function)

Search String (Limits = English)	Results
Ultrasound AND epiphyseal plates	87 citations are returned, most of which address diagnostic ultrasound; 4 citations are noted for possible review.
Ultrasound AND epiphyseal plates NOT diagnostic	23 citations are returned; 2 of the articles identified in the first search appear again in this search.
Therapeutic ultrasound AND epiphyseal plates	5 citations are returned, 3 of which appeared in the results of the first search.
Therapeutic ultrasound AND "bone growth"	17 citations are returned, most of which address bone healing after fracture rather than the growth of immature bone; 3 new articles are identified for potential review.

Relevant Titles

El-Bialy T, et al. Growth modification of the mandible with ultrasound in baboons: a preliminary report. *Am J Orthod Dentofacial Orthop*. 2006;130(4):435.e7_e14.

Harle J, et al. Effects of ultrasound on transforming growth factor-beta genes in bone cells. *Eur Cell Mater*. 2005;10:70_76.

El-Bialy T, et al. Growth modification of the rabbit mandible using therapeutic ultrasound: is it possible to enhance functional appliance results? *Angle Orthod*. 2003;73(6):631_639.

Lyon R, et al. The effects of therapeutic vs. high-intensity ultrasound on the rabbit growth plate. *J Orthop Res*. 2003;21(5):865_871.

Zhang ZJ, et al. The influence of pulsed low-intensity ultrasound on matrix production of chondrocytes at different stages of differentiation: an explant study [published correction appears in Ultrasound Med Biol. 2003;29(8):1223]. *Ultrasound Med Biol*. 2002;28(11_12):1547_1553.

Ogurtan Z, et al. Effect of experimental therapeutic ultrasound on the distal antebrachial growth plates in one-month-old rabbits. *Vet J*. 2002;164 (3):280_287.

therapeutic ultrasound as used clinically by physical therapists on human patients. A review of the abstracts for the articles listed in the table indicated that one study did not describe the intensity of the ultrasound used, whereas another discussed the acoustic properties of ultrasound energy in bone rather than the tissue-level effects of the ultrasound energy. Four articles investigated the use of ultrasound to facilitate fracture healing. As a result, these articles were not reviewed further. Critiques of the remaining three articles are provided here.

Article 1

Lyon et al.[11] examined the effects of ultrasound treatment on the epiphyseal plates and metaphyseal regions of the knee in growing rabbits. The investigators used a contralateral control design and compared two different treatment intensities in separate groups of rabbits. The two treatment intensities (0.5 and 2.2. W/cm^2) and the frequency (1 MHz) were representative of those commonly used by physical therapists. However, the authors did not report the duty cycle used, making it impossible to calculate the total dose of ultrasound energy delivered. Following 6 weeks of treatment, the authors observed significant histologic changes in the epiphyseal plates of knees in the higher treatment intensity group relative to both the low intensity group and controls. Plate height was greater and chondrocytes were less organized. Radiographically, growth plate lines were less distinct and metaphyseal wedging deformities were noted in the high-dose group. During the course of treatment, skin burns developed in the treatment region on all the high-dose knees. No significant changes were noted relative to controls in any of the dependent variables for the lower dose group. The therapist concluded that the 1 MHz at 0.5 W/cm^2 used in the study was consistent with the dose she considered using with her patient. Nonetheless, she noted the following major differences between the study's parameters and those under consideration: (1) 20-minute daily treatments for 6 weeks versus 7- to 10-minute treatments three times a week for a few weeks at most; (2) stationary sound head versus moving sound head; and (3) pulsed mode versus continuous mode. Initially, the therapist was encouraged by the results of this study because she was considering a "low dose" for her patient, but she then realized that she really could not determine a safe dosage range from reading this paper. Because the investigators used an unspecified pulsed ultrasound duty cycle, all she could conclude was that at some finite net intensity between 50 mW/cm^2 and 0.25 W/cm^2 (assuming an available duty cycle range of 10%–50%) no deleterious changes occurred.

Article 2

Ogurtan et al.[12] also examined the effects of ultrasound treatment on the epiphyseal plates and bone growth rates in growing rabbits; however, they used the distal radius and ulna for their model. They, too, used a contralateral control design and compared two different treatment intensities in separate groups of rabbits. Groups were subdivided into those treated for 10, 15, or 20 days. The two treatment intensities (0.2 and 0.5 W/cm^2) and the frequency (1 MHz) were representative of those commonly used by physical therapists. Treatments were delivered in pulsed mode, using a 20% duty cycle for 5 minutes. The authors reported treatment dose as spatial average temporal average (SATA), meaning that the temporal peak intensity (what would have been displayed on the intensity meter of the unit) during treatment was either 1.0 W/cm^2 for the 0.2 W/cm^2 SATA group or 2.5 W/cm^2 for the 0.5 W/cm^2 SATA group. The 0.5 W/cm^2 SATA dose would be the same net energy output as a 5-minute treatment in continuous mode at 0.5 W/cm^2, a dose comparable to what the therapist was considering for her patient.

In comparison to controls, the authors found no difference in height of the growth plates, bone growth rates, or bone morphology in the radius and ulna of rabbits treated with either intensity ultrasound at any time period. However, the physical therapist realized that the treatment doses reported were not consistent with the maximum output intensity available for the ultrasound unit in the study. She concluded that the authors were reporting temporal peak intensities, which would result in SATAs that were 20% of those reported. This difference would mean that the authors examined the effects of ultrasound at either 40 mW/cm^2 or 0.1 W/cm^2, both much lower doses than the therapist was considering for use with her patient.

Article 3

Zhang et al.[13] examined the effects of very low intensity ultrasound delivered using a commercially available unit with fixed parameters designed specifically for fracture healing. The target tissue was chick embryo sternum in culture. The proximal portion of the chick embryo sternum undergoes endochondral ossification, analogous to the bone growth that occurs at epiphyseal plates in immature humans. The ultrasound frequency used in this study was 1.5 MHz provided during 20-minute daily treatments. The authors reported an anabolic effect on chondrocytes and increased matrix production relative to control specimens that were not sonicated, despite a dose/intensity that was lower than the lowest dose that can be delivered by ultrasound units typically used in physical therapy clinics (0.2 W/cm^2 at 20% duty cycle, equivalent to 40 mW/cm^2). The tissue type studied and the treatment parameters used were considerably different than the scenario with which the physical therapist was dealing. However, she was concerned about the possibility that such a low dose of ultrasound may in fact be capable of facilitating bone growth.

Physical Therapist's Decision

In her search, the physical therapist found one study in which she was unable to discern the actual ultrasound dosages used but that nonetheless demonstrated the potential for deleterious effects on the epiphyseal plate. A second study did not find any deleterious effects but appears to have examined two ultrasound dosages below that which she was considering for her patient. The final study, using an in vitro model and intensity lower than that achievable on any of the units available to her, showed a potential anabolic effect on bone growth.

In the absence of controlled studies describing human clinical trials, she would have been able to make a reasonable judgment based on animal studies had they used (or completely described the use of) similar ultrasound treatment parameters. The evidence she located suggests that very low intensity ultrasound may enhance cellular activity at the epiphyseal plate, which may, in turn, facilitate increased bone growth. At some higher, undefined threshold, ultrasound may damage the epiphyseal plate and hinder growth. There may be some point in between that is "safe," but she was not comfortable defining this dosage based on a single study in which the dosages appeared to be inconsistent with the ultrasound unit's performance. Accordingly, the physical therapist decides to exclude therapeutic ultrasound for her patient's treatment plan.

Summary

The cases in this chapter are intended to serve as models to help students and clinicians develop their own evidence-based practice skills. Note that the "best available" evidence did not always represent the highest levels of evidence indicated by various published evidence hierarchies. In spite of these challenges, conclusions were drawn based on the physical therapist's clinical judgment in conjunction with the patient's preferences and values. Remember that these examples are not intended to serve as practice guidelines or standards of care for the conditions described.

References

1. Oxford Centre for Evidence Based Medicine Web site. Available at: www.cebm.net. Accessed October 1, 2106.
2. Collins TC, Suarez-Almazor M, Petersen NJ. An absent pulse is not sensitive for the early detection of peripheral arterial disease. *Fam Med*. 2006;38(1):38-42.
3. Boonhong J, Osiri M, Werawatganon T. Validity and reliability of girth measurement (circumference measurement) for calculating residual limb volume in below-knee amputees. *Chula Med J*. 2007;51(2):77-88.
4. Matinolli M, Korpelainen JT, Sotaniemi KA, et al. Recurrent falls and mortality in Parkinson's disease: a prospective two-year follow-up study. *Acta Neurol Scand*. 2011;123(3):193-200.

5. van der Windt DAWM, Koes BW, Deville W, et al. Effectiveness of corticosteroid injections versus physiotherapy for treatment of painful stiff shoulder in primary care: randomized trial. *BMJ*. 1998;317(7168):1292-1296.

6. Kurz MJ, Stuberg W, DeJong SL. Body weight supported treadmill training improves the regularity of the stepping kinematics in children with cerebral palsy. *Dev Neurorehabil*. 2011;14(2):87-93.

7. Oeffinger D, Bagley A, Rogers S, et al. Outcome tools used for ambulatory children with cerebral palsy: responsiveness and minimal clinically important differences. *Dev Med Child Neurol*. 2008 Dec;50(12):918-25

8. Dodd KJ, Foley S. Partial body-weight-supported treadmill training can improve walking in children with cerebral palsy: a clinical controlled trial. *Dev Med Child Neurol*. 2007;49(2):101-105.

9. Hendriks EJ, Bernards AT, Staal JB, de Vet HC, de Bie RA. Factorial validity and internal consistency of the PRAFAB questionnaire in women with stress urinary incontinence. *BMC Urology*. 2008;8 1-1.

10. Spichiger E, Rieder E, Müller-Fröhlich C, Kesselring A. Fatigue in patients undergoing chemotherapy, their self-care and the role of health professionals: A qualitative study. *Eur J Oncol Nurs*. 2012;16(2):165-171.

11. Lyon R, Liu XC, Meier J. The effects of therapeutic vs. high-intensity ultrasound on the rabbit growth plate. *J Orthop Res*. 2003;21(5):865-871.

12. Ogurtan Z, Celik I, Izci C, et al. Effect of experimental therapeutic ultrasound on the distal antebrachial growth plates in one-month-old rabbits. *Vet J*. 2002;164(3):280-287.

13. Zhang ZJ, Huckle J, Francomano CA, Spencer RG. The influence of pulsed low-intensity ultrasound on matrix production of chondrocytes at different stages of differentiation: an explant study [published correction appears in *Ultrasound Med Biol*. 2003;29(8):1223]. *Ultrasound Med Biol*. 2002;28(11_12):1547-1553.

CALCULATION OF CONFIDENCE INTERVALS

TABLE A-1 Standard Errors (SEs) and Confidence Intervals (CIs) for Some Clinical Measures of Interest

Clinical Measure	Standard Error (SE)	Typical Calculation of SE and CI[a]
I. THERAPEUTIC STUDIES		
(a) Outcome is an event—one group		
In general, r events are observed among n patients, so the observed proportion is $p = r/n$. In the illustrative example, $p = 24/60 = 0.4$ (or 40%).		
Proportion (event rate in one group)[b]	$SE = \sqrt{\dfrac{p \times (1 - p)}{n}}$	If $p = 24/60 = 0.4$ (or 40%): $SE = \sqrt{\dfrac{0.4 \times 0.6}{60}} = 0.063$ (or 6.3%)
	where p is proportion and n is number of patients	95% CI is 40% ± 1.96 × 6.3% or 27.6 to 52.4%[b]
(b) Outcome is an event—comparison of two groups[c]		
In general, r_1 and r_2 events are observed among n_1 and n_2 patients in two groups, so the observed proportions are $p_1 = r_1/n_1$ and $p_2 = r_2/n_2$. In the illustrative example, $p_1 = 15/125$ (or 12%) and $p_2 = 30/120 = 0.25$ (or 25%)[d]		
Absolute risk reduction (ARR)	$SE = \sqrt{\dfrac{p_1(1 - p_1)}{n_1} + \dfrac{p_2(1 - p_2)}{n_2}}$	$ARR = p_2 - p_1 = 0.13$ (or 13%): $SE = \sqrt{\dfrac{0.12 \times 0.88}{125} + \dfrac{0.25 \times 0.75}{120}} = 0.049$ (or 4.9%)
Number needed to treat (NNT)	Not calculated	95% CI is 13% ± 1.96 × 4.9%, i.e., 3.4% to 22.6%[b] NNT = 100/ARR = 100/13 = 7.7; CI is obtained as reciprocal of CI for ARR, so 95% CI is 100/22.6 to 100/3.4 or 4.4 to 29.4[e]
Relative risk (RR)	$RR = p_2/p_2$ $SE \text{ of } \log_e RR = \sqrt{\dfrac{1}{r_1} + \dfrac{1}{r_2} - \dfrac{1}{n_1} - \dfrac{1}{n_2}}$	$RR = 0.12/0.25 = 0.48$ (48%); $\log(RR) = -0.734$; $SE \text{ of } \log_e RR = \sqrt{\dfrac{1}{15} + \dfrac{1}{30} - \dfrac{1}{125} - \dfrac{1}{120}} = 0.289$; 95% CI for $\log_e RR$ is $-0.734 \pm 1.96 \times 0.289$, i.e., -1.301 to -0.167; 95% CI for RR is 0.272 to 0.846 or 27.2% to 84.6%

Clinical Measure	Standard Error (SE)	Typical Calculation of SE and CI[a]
Relative risk reduction (RRR)	Not calculated	$RRR = 1 - RR = 1 - p_1/p_2 = 1 - 12/25 = 0.52$ (or 52%) 95% CI for RRR is obtained by subtracting CI for RR from 1 (or 100%), i.e., 0.154 to 0.728 or 15.4% to 72.8%
Odds ratio (OR)	$OR = \dfrac{r_1(n_2 - r_2)}{r_2(n_1 - r_1)}$	$OR = \dfrac{15 \times 90}{30 \times 110} = 0.409;\ \log_e OR = -0.894$
	$SE\ of\ \log_e\ OR = \sqrt{\dfrac{1}{r_1} + \dfrac{1}{r_2} + \dfrac{1}{n_1 - r_1} + \dfrac{1}{n_2 - r_2}}$	$SE\ of\ \log_e\ OR = \sqrt{\dfrac{1}{15} + \dfrac{1}{30} + \dfrac{1}{90} + \dfrac{1}{110}} = 0.347$ 95% CI for $\log_e OR$ is $-0.894 \pm 1.96 \times 0.347$, or -1.573 to -0.214; 95% CI for OR is 0.207 to 0.807

(c) Outcome is a measurement

Mean	If s is standard deviation (SD) of n observations, $SE = s/n$	95% CI is mean $\pm t \times SE^f$ If mean $= 17.2$, $s = 6.4$, $n = 38$, then $SE = 6.4/38 = 1.038$ and 95% CI is $17.2 \pm 2.026 \times 1.038$ or 15.1 to 19.3
Difference between two means	If s_1 and s_2 are SDs of n_1 and n_2 observations, $SE(\text{diff}) =$ $\sqrt{\dfrac{(n_1 - 1)s_1^2 + (n_2 - 1)s_2^2}{n_1 + n_2 - 2} \times \left(\dfrac{1}{n_1} + \dfrac{1}{n_2}\right)}$	95% CI is mean difference $\pm t \times SE(\text{difference})^f$ If mean$_1 = 17.2$, $s_1 = 6.4$, $n_1 = 38$, mean$_2 = 15.9$, $s_2 = 5.6$, $n_2 = 45$, then mean difference $= d = 17.2 - 15.9 = 1.3$, $t = 1.99^f$ $SE(\text{diff}) = \sqrt{\dfrac{37 \times 6.4^2 \times 44 \times 5.62^2}{38 + 45 - 2} \times \left(\dfrac{1}{38} + \dfrac{1}{45}\right)} = 1.317$ and 95% CI is $1.3 \pm 1.99 \times 1.317$ or -1.32 to 3.92

II. DIAGNOSTIC STUDIES

(a) A single proportion

In general, r diagnoses are observed among n patients, so the observed proportion is $p = r/n$. Using the notation of Chapter 3, the sensitivity is $a/(a + c)$, the specificity is $b/(b + d)$, the positive predictive value is $a/(a + b)$, and the negative predictive value is $d/(c + d)$. The illustrative example is from Table 3.3. The sensitivity is $731/809 = 90\%$ or 0.90, and the specificity is $1500/1770 = 85\%$ or 0.85, $p = 73/82 = 0.89$ (or 89%).

(continues)

TABLE A-1 Standard Errors (SEs) and Confidence Intervals (CIs) for Some Clinical Measures of Interest (*Continued*)

Clinical Measure	Standard Error (SE)	Typical Calculation of SE and CI[a]
Sensitivity, specificity, predictive values	$$SE = \sqrt{\frac{p \times (1-p)}{n}}$$ where p is proportion and n is number of patients	For the sensitivity, $p = 731/809 = 0.90$ (or 90%): $$SE = \sqrt{\frac{0.90 \times 0.10}{809}} = 0.0105 \ (\text{or } 1.05\%)$$ 95% CI is 90% $\pm$ 1.96 $\times$ 1.05% or 87.9% to 92.1%[b]

(b) Likelihood ratio

In general, the likelihood ratios for positive or negative test results are, respectively, obtained as either LR+ = sensitivity/(1 − specificity) and LR− = (1 − sensitivity)/specificity.

Clinical Measure	Standard Error (SE)	Typical Calculation of SE and CI[a]
Likelihood ratio (LR)	$LR+ = [a/(a+c)]/[b/(b+d)]$ $LR- = [c/(a+c)]/[d/(b+d)]$ $$SE \text{ of } \log_e LR+ = \sqrt{\frac{1}{a} + \frac{1}{b} - \frac{1}{(a+c)} - \frac{1}{(b+d)}}$$ $$SE \text{ of } \log_e LR- = \sqrt{\frac{1}{c} + \frac{1}{d} - \frac{1}{(a+c)} - \frac{1}{(b+d)}}$$	$LR+ = (731/809)/(270/1770) = 0.9/(1-0.85) = 6.0;$ $\log_e(LR+) = 1.792;$ $$SE \text{ of } \log_e LR+ = \sqrt{\frac{1}{731} + \frac{1}{270} - \frac{1}{809} - \frac{1}{1770}} = 0.05272;$$ 95% CI for $\log_e$ LR+ is 1.792 $\pm$ 1.96 $\times$ 0.0572, i.e., 1.680 to 1.904; 95% CI for LR+ is 5.37 to 6.71. A similar approach is used to derive a CI for LR−.

[a]In general a confidence interval is obtained by taking the estimate of interest and adding and subtracting a multiple of the SE. Except in the case of means or differences in means, the multiple is taken as a value from the standard normal distribution. For a 95% CI the multiplier is 1.96; for a 90% CI it is 1.645, and for a 99% CI it is 2.576. For proportions, this method is the traditional method referred to in footnote b. In some cases, such as for RR (and RRR) and OR, the CI is obtained for the logarithm of the quantity of interest and the values are antilogged (logs to base e are used in the table).

[b]The method illustrated is the traditional method. It works fine in most cases, but is not recommended when sample sizes are small and/or proportions are near either 0% or 100% (in which case it is possible for the CI to include impossible values outside the range 0% to 100%). Newer methods are recommended both for general use and especially for the circumstances described. The methods are too complex to include here; they are described in reference 8 and incorporated into the software included with it.

[c]As used in this book, p_1 corresponds to the event rate in the experimental group (EER), and p_2 to the event rate in the control group (CER).

[d]The above calculations assume that comparisons are between two independent groups. For CIs derived from paired data (e.g., from crossover trials or matched case-control studies), and also CIs for some other statistics, see reference 8.

[e]When the ARR is not significantly different from zero, one limit of the 95% CI is negative. Taking reciprocals gives a CI for the NNT with one negative value, which corresponds to a harmful effect. We can write the CI in terms of both the NNT and NNH. For example, a 95% CI for the ARR of −5% to 25% gives the 95% CI for the NNT of 10 as −20 to 4, or from NNH = 20 to NNT = 4. However, the values included in this interval are NNH from 20 to ∞ (infinity) and NNT from 4 to ∞. We can write this as NNH = 20 to ∞ to NNT = 4 (see references 8 and 9).

[f]The calculation of a CI for a mean or the difference between means the multiplier for a 95% CI is not 1.96 but a value from the t distribution with $n − 1$ or $n_1 + n_2 − 2$ degrees of freedom (df), respectively. The appropriate value of t is found from statistical tables or software. As df increases, t approaches 1.96. For df larger than 40, t is close to 2.

Reprinted from Straus SE, Richardson WS, Glaziou P, Haynes RB. *Evidence-Based Medicine: How to Practice and Teach EBM*, 3rd ed., pages 267–272. Copyright © 2005, with permission from Elsevier.

ADDITIONAL EVIDENCE APPRAISAL TOOLS AVAILABLE ON THE INTERNET

Website	Diagnostic Tests	Prognostic Factors	Interventions	Clinical Prediction Rules	Systematic Reviews	Practice Guidelines	Qualitative Studies
BestBETs: Best Evidence Topics www.bestbets.org	√	√	√	√	√	√	√
Centre for Evidence-Based Medicine—Oxford www.cebm.net	√	√	√		√		
Critical Appraisal Skills Program www.casp-uk.net	√	√	√	√	√		√
Evidence-Based Practice, Duke University http://guides.mclibrary.duke.edu/content.php?pid=274373&sid=2262222	√	√	√		√	√	√
Evidence-Based Medicine Toolkit www.ebm.med.ualberta.ca	√	√	√		√	√	
PRISMA Statement www.prisma-statement.org					√		
The Agree Collaboration www.agreetrust.org						√	
University of Bristol—QUADAS http://www.bristol.ac.uk/social-community-medicine/projects/quadas/					√		
University of South Australia www.unisa.edu.au/Research/Sansom-Institute-for-Health-Research/Research/Allied-Health-Evidence/Resources/CAT/	√	√	√		√	√	√

ADDITIONAL CALCULATIONS FOR EVIDENCE-BASED PHYSICAL THERAPIST PRACTICE

Calculations Related to Diagnostic Tests

	+ Disorder	– Disorder
+ Test Result	True Positives (a)	False Positives (b)
– Test Result	False Negatives (c)	True Negatives (d)

Sensitivity (Sn) = $\dfrac{\text{Patients with the condition who test positive (a)}}{\text{All patients with the condition (a + c)}}$

Specificity (Sp) = $\dfrac{\text{Patients without the condition who test negative (d)}}{\text{All patients without the condition (b + d)}}$

Positive predictive value (PPV) = $\dfrac{\text{Patients with the condition who test positive (a)}}{\text{All patients with positive test results (a + b)}}$

Negative predictive value (NPV) = $\dfrac{\text{Patients without the condition who test negative (d)}}{\text{All patients with negative test results (c + d)}}$

Positive likelihood ratio (LR+) = $\dfrac{\text{Sensitivity}}{1 - \text{Specificity}}$ or $\dfrac{(a/a + c)}{[1 - (d/b + d)]}$

Negative likelihood ratio (LR–) = $\dfrac{1 - \text{Sensitivity}}{\text{Specificity}}$ or $\dfrac{[1 - (a/a + c)]}{(d/b + d)}$

Pretest odds = $\dfrac{\text{Pretest probability}}{1 - \text{Pretest probability}}$

Posttest odds = Pretest odds × Likelihood ratio (LR+ or LR–)

Posttest probability = $\dfrac{\text{Posttest odds}}{\text{Posttest odds} + 1}$

Calculations Related to Prognostic Factors

	Outcome Present	Outcome Absent
Factor Present	True-Positive Relationship (a)	False-Positive Relationship (b)
Factor Absent	False-Negative Relationship (c)	True-Negative Relationship (d)

Odds ratio (OR) = [a/b]/[c/d] *or* ad/bc
Relative risk (RR) = [a/a + b]/[c/c + d]

Calculations Related to Interventions

Absolute effect size (ES) = Mean score of Group 1 − Mean score of Group 2

$$\text{Standardized effect size (ES)} = \frac{\text{Mean score of Group 1} - \text{Mean score of Group 2}}{\text{Pooled standard deviation}}$$

$$\text{Pooled standard deviation} = \frac{(N_{exp} - 1)SD^2_{exp} + (N_{control} - 1)SD^2_{control}}{N_{exp} + (N_{control} - 2)}$$

	Outcome Present	Outcome Absent
Intervention Present	Benefit with Intervention (a)	No Benefit with Intervention (b)
Intervention Absent	Benefit without Intervention (c)	No Benefit without Intervention (d)

Absolute Benefit Increase (ABI) = |Experimental group event rate (EER) − Control group event rate (CER)| *or*
ABI = |a/(a + b) − c/(c + d)|

$$\text{Relative benefit increase (RBI)} = \frac{|\text{Experimental group event rate (EER)} - \text{Control group event rate (CER)}|}{\text{Control group event rate (CER)}}$$
or

$$RBI = \frac{|a/(a + b) - c/(c + d)|}{c/(c + d)}$$

	Outcome Present	Outcome Absent
Preventive Intervention Present	Harm with Intervention (a)	No Harm with Intervention (b)
Preventive Intervention Absent	Harm without Intervention (c)	No Harm without Intervention (d)

Absolute Risk Reduction (ARR) = |Control group event rate (CER) − Experimental group event rate (EER)| *or*

ARR = $|c/(c + d) − a/(a + b)|$

Relative Risk Reduction (RRR) = $\dfrac{|\text{Control group event rate (CER) − Experimental group event rate (EER)}|}{\text{Control group event rate (CER)}}$ *or*

RRR = $\dfrac{|c/(c + d) − a/(a + b)|}{c/(c + d)}$

Number needed to treat (NNT) = 1/ABI

Number needed to harm (NNH) = 1/ARR

INDEX

Note: Page numbers followed by *f*, or *t* indicate material in figures, or tables, respectively.